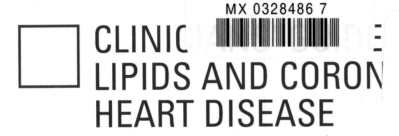

CLINICAL GUIDE LIPIDS AND CORONARY HEART DISEASE

Second edition

D. J. Betteridge
Professor of Endocrinology and Metabolism,
Royal Free and University College Medical School,
University College, London, UK

and

J. M. Morrell
Beaconsfield Road Surgery, Hastings, East Sussex, UK

ARNOLD

A member of the Hodder Headline Group
LONDON

First published in Great Britain in 2003 by
Arnold, a member of the Hodder Headline Group,
338 Euston Road, London NW1 3BH

http://www.arnoldpublishers.com

Distributed in the United States of America by
Oxford University Press Inc.,
198 Madison Avenue, New York, NY10016
Oxford is a registered trademark of Oxford University Press

Whilst the advice and information in this book are believed to be true and accurate at the date of going to press,
neither the authors nor the publisher can accept any legal responsibility or liability for any errors or omissions that
may be made. In particular (but without limiting the generality of the preceding disclaimer) every effort has been made
to check drug dosages; however, it is still possible that errors have been missed. Furthermore, dosage schedules are
constantly being revised and new side-effects recognized. For these reasons the reader is strongly urged to consult the
drug companies' printed instructions before administering any of the drugs recommended in this book.

British Library Cataloguing in Publication Data
A catalogue record for this book is available from the British Library

Library of Congress Cataloging-in-Publication Data
A catalog record for this book is available from the Library of Congress

ISBN 0 340 76408 2

1 2 3 4 5 6 7 8 9 10

Commissioning Editor: Joanna Koster
Development Editor: Sarah Burrows
Production Editor: Wendy Rooke
Production Controller: Deborah Smith
Cover Designer: Terry Griffiths

Typeset in 11/13.5 pt Adobe Jenson by Charon Tec Pvt. Ltd, Chennai, India
Printed and bound in Italy

What do you think about this book? Or any other Arnold title?
Please send your comments to feedback.arnold@hodder.co.uk

My efforts in writing this second edition are dedicated to my partner, Jacqui Lynas, for her love, support and boundless inspiration.

Jonathan Morrell

CONTENTS

Foreword   vii

Preface   ix

Abbreviations   xi

Part One: Background   **1**

1. Lipid and lipoprotein metabolism – the basics   3

2. Epidemiology   23

Part Two: Screening and assessment   **61**

3. Diagnosis   63

4. Screening   92

5. Risk factors and their assessment   101

Part Three: Intervention   **157**

6. Non-lipid risk factor modification   159

7. Diet   172

8. Lipid-lowering drugs   208

9. Lipid-lowering trials   236

Part Four: Practical considerations and special areas   **287**

10. Meeting the challenge   289

11. Special areas   308

12. Economic aspects   338

13. Case studies   345

Index   362

FOREWORD

Clinician's Guide to Lipids and Coronary Heart Disease by Betteridge and Morrell is a remarkably comprehensive text to educate the practising physician about the relationship of lipids to coronary heart disease and to assist in patient management. Because of the astonishing results of recent clinical trials of lipid-lowering therapies, the proper selection of patients for lipid management has become a critical issue for clinical care. This is a rapidly moving field and continuous updating of the evidence base has become of paramount importance for appropriate patient care. It is imperative that clinicians keep abreast of new developments and concepts. The current guide represents an important step in this direction.

Clinicians frequently request simplicity of guidelines for management of patients with lipid disorders; however, the lipid and lipoprotein systems are complex, as are the relationships of these systems to coronary heart disease. The challenge for experts in the field is to simplify concepts as much as possible without oversimplification to the point that proper management is impaired. Clinicians routinely learn to deal effectively with complex issues, such as work-up of anaemia, reading of electrocardiograms and X-rays, and treatment of chronic renal failure. These activities are such an integral part of medical practice that they become routine in spite of their complexity. The need for lipid management, although relatively new for many clinicians, is rapidly emerging as another major area of clinical practice that must be incorporated into routine practice. Going beyond over simplification of lipid management, therefore, will require increased attention to many of the details. This clinicians' guide strikes the correct balance between being too simple and being overly complicated. The guide certainly is up-to-date and incorporates the essentials that are needed for an informed practice.

Appropriate clinical judgment cannot be made without a basic understanding of the metabolism of lipids and lipoproteins, which is provided in this book. Moreover, lipid management no longer stands alone as an isolated discipline. Since lipid disorders are risk factors for coronary heart disease, they must be placed in juxtaposition with other risk factors – cigarette smoking, hypertension, age, family history and diabetes. The integration of all risk factors into a global risk assessment is required for proper selection of therapy. Increasingly, prevention strategies are directed towards 'treatment of risk' rather than treatment of individual risk factors. On the other hand, risk is 'treated' by modifying the individual risk factors. Thus prevention must go beyond 'risk management' to the details of risk factor management. This guide strikes the proper balance between these two approaches. It further provides a valuable discussion of the modalities of lipid management including lipid-lowering diets and lipid-lowering drugs.

Increasingly risk factor management must be placed into the context of medical care in general. Advances in medical research are making it possible to modify the course of diseases in many ways. For this reason, choices must be made on investment of health-care resources into different forms of clinical management. Limited resources require national policy decisions about expenditures on clinical practice. First, policy must consider the strength of the evidence of efficacy of therapies. Fortunately, several large clinical trials confirm the efficacy of lipid-lowering therapies for reducing risk for coronary heart disease. And second, the costs of therapies, particularly lipid-lowering therapies, must be integrated into policy. This guide provides a useful discussion of the economic aspects of lipid management.

A particularly valuable section of the guide is found under case studies. These studies provide practical insights into how to implement lipid management in practice. A wide range of potential cases is considered.

In summary, this text offers both a practical guide to lipid management and a resource document on the rationale for decision-making in clinical practice. It should be a useful document for physicians in several areas of primary care, internal medicine and medical specialty.

Scott Grundy
Director, Center for Human Nutrition,
University of Texas, Southwestern Medical Center,
Dallas, Texas, USA
January 2003

PREFACE

In the preface to the first edition of this book in 1998 we wrote of its timeliness given the wealth of new information on lipids and heart disease in the preceding few years. Astonishingly the momentum in this area continues apace with exciting new and important information more than justifying this second edition which has been extensively re-written.

We are confident that this book will provide a comprehensive background for colleagues and students from a wide range of backgrounds interested in this increasingly important area of medicine. Divided into four main parts – Background, Screening and assessment, Intervention and Practical considerations – the book reflects our complementary expertise and experience across a wide range of important aspects of lipid metabolism, lipid disorders, non-pharmacological and pharmacological therapy and healthcare delivery. Illustrative case studies are included which hopefully will distil for the reader important management issues.

Lipid management has become an important aspect of clinical practice over a wide range of medical and surgical specialties in both hospital and primary care. It is no longer solely the province of the lipid specialist or cardiologist; general physicians, diabetologists, gerontologists, neurologists, nephrologists and vascular surgeons, amongst others, will need to consider lipid-lowering in their everyday practice. However, a large burden of responsibility in terms of effective health care delivery falls on primary care physicians and specialist nurses. We hope that our book will be of interest and practical help to all these colleagues.

We are grateful for the support, encouragement and forbearance of our publishers, Arnold, in the production of this second edition. It will succeed principally if it stimulates and aids physicians across many specialties to provide appropriate evidence-based lipid-lowering management to the benefit of their patients at risk of vascular disease.

D. J. Betteridge
J. M. Morrell
January 2003

ABBREVIATIONS

4D	Die Deutsche Diabetes Dialyse (study)
4S	Scandinavian Simvastatin Survival Study
A to Z	Aggrastat to Zocor (study)
ABC	ATP binding cassette
ACAT	acyl-CoA:cholesterol acyltransferase
ACE	angiotensin-converting enzyme
ADA	American Diabetes Association
ADP	adenosine diphosphate
ADS	average diameter of segments
AF	atrial fibrillation
AFCAPS/TexCAPS	Air Force/Texas Coronary Atherosclerosis Prevention Study
AHA	American Heart Association
ALLHAT	Antihypertensive and Lipid Lowering Treatment to prevent Heart Attack Trial
AMORIS	Apolipoprotein-related Mortality Risk
Apo	apoprotein
ASAP	Atorvastatin vs Simvastatin on Atherosclerosis Progression (study)
ASBT	apical sodium-dependent bile acid transporter
ASCOT	Anglo-Scandinavian Cardiac Outcomes Trial
ASPEN	Atorvastatin as Prevention of Coronary Heart Disease in Patients with type 2 Diabetes (trial)
ASPIRE	Action on Secondary Prevention through Intervention to Reduce Events (study)
ATBC	Alpha Tocopherol, Beta Carotene Cancer Prevention study group
ATP	adenosine triphosphate
AVERT	Atorvastatin versus Revascularization Treatment
BECAIT	Bezafibrate Coronary Atherosclerosis Intervention Trial
BFHS	British Family Heart Study
BIP	Bezafibrate Infarction Prevention
BMI	body mass index
BP	blood pressure
BRHS	British Regional Heart Survey
BUPA	British United Provident Association

CABG	coronary artery bypass graft
CAD	coronary artery disease
CAM	circulating adhesion molecule
CAPPP	Captopril Primary Prevention Project
CARDS	Collaborative Atorvastatin Diabetes Study
CARE	Cholesterol and Recurrent Events (trial)
CARET	Beta Carotene and Retinol Efficacy Trial
CCAIT	Canadian Coronary Atherosclerosis Intervention Trial
CCF	congestive cardiac failure
CDP	Coronary Drug Project
CERP	cholesterol efflux regulatory protein
CETP	cholesterol ester transfer protein
CHAOS	Cambridge Heart Antioxidant Study
CHD	coronary heart disease
CHF	congestive heart failure
CI	confidence interval
CLAS	Cholesterol Lowering Atherosclerosis Study
COC	combined oral contraceptive
COURAGE	Clinical Outcomes Utilizing Revascularization and Aggressive Evaluation (study)
CPK	creatinine phosphokinase
CPR	cardiopulmonary resuscitation
CRP	C-reactive protein
CVA	cerebrovascular accident
CVD	cerebrovascular disease
DAIS	Diabetes Atherosclerosis Intervention Study
DART	Diet and Reinfarction Trial
DBP	diastolic blood pressure
DHA	docosahexaenoic acid
EAS	European Atherosclerosis Society
ECG	electrocardiograph
EDRF	endothelial-derived relaxing factor
eNOS	endothelial nitric oxide synthase
EPA	eicosapentaenoic acid
EPIC	European Prospective Investigation into Cancer and Nutrition
ERA	Effects of Oestrogen Replacement on the Progression of Coronary Artery Atherosclerosis (study)
ESC	European Society of Cardiology
ESH	European Society of Hypertension
ESR	erythrocyte sedimentation rate
EWPHE	European Working Party on Hypertension in the Elderly
FATS	Familial Atherosclerosis Treatment Study

FCH	familial combined hyperlipidaemia
FDB	familial ligand defective apoprotein B
FED	fish eye disease
FH	familial hypercholesterolaemia
FIELD	Fenofibrate Intervention and Event Lowering in Diabetes (trial)
GGPP	geranylgeranylpyrophosphate
GP	glycoprotein
HAART	highly active antiretroviral therapy
HARP	Heart and Renal Protection (study)
HATS	HDL Atherosclerosis Treatment Study
HDL	high density lipoprotein
HELP	Heparin Extracorporeal LDL Precipitation (system)
HERS	Heart and Estrogen/Progestin Replacement Study
HHS	Helsinki Heart Study
HIV	human immunodeficiency virus
HMG-CoA	hydroxymethylglutaryl coenzyme A
HOPE	Heart Outcomes Prevention Evaluation (study)
HPS	Heart Protection Study
HRT	hormone replacement therapy
HSPG	heparin sulphate proteoglycan
ICAM-1	intercellular circulating adhesion molecule 1
IDDM	insulin-dependent diabetes mellitus
IDEAL	Incremental Decrease in Endpoints Through Aggressive Lipid Lowering (trial)
IDL	intermediate density lipoprotein
IFN	interferon
IGT	impaired glucose tolerance
IL	interleukin
IMT	intima-media thickness
ISH	International Society of Hypertension
LCAT	lecithin cholesterol acyltransferase
LDL	low density lipoprotein
LHT	Lifestyle Heart Trial
LIPID	Long Term Intervention with Pravastatin in Ischaemic Disease (study)
LIT	Leiden Intervention Trial
Lp	lipoprotein
LPL	lipoprotein lipase
LRC	Lipid Research Clinics
LRCCPPT	Lipid Research Clinics Coronary Primary Prevention Trial
LRP	LDL-related protein

LTAP	Lipid Treatment Assessment Project
LVH	left ventricular hypertrophy
MAAS	Multicentre Anti-Atheroma Study
MARS	Monitored Atherosclerosis Regression Study
MI	myocardial infarction
MIRACL	Myocardial Ischaemia Reduction with Aggressive Cholesterol Lowering (study)
MLD	mean lumen diameter; minimal luminal diameter
MONICA	Monitoring Cardiovascular Disease
MRC	Medical Research Council
MRFIT	Multiple Risk Factor Intervention Trial
MRI	magnetic resonance imaging
MTP	microsomal triglyceride transfer protein
MUFA	monounsaturated fatty acids
NCEP	National Cholesterol Education Project
NF-κB	nuclear factor-kappa B
NHANES	National Health and Nutrition Examination Survey
NHLBI	National Heart, Lung and Blood Institute
NIDDM	non-insulin-dependent diabetes mellitus
NNT	number needed to treat
NRT	nicotine replacement therapy
NRTI	nucleoside reverse transcriptase inhibitors
NSP	non-starch polysaccharide
OGTT	oral glucose tolerance test
OPCS	Office of Population Censuses and Surveys
OR	odds ratio
OXCHECK	Oxford Prevention of Heart Attack and Stroke project
P/S	polyunsaturated/saturated fat ratio
PAD	peripheral arterial disease
PAI-1	plasminogen activator inhibitor 1
PLAC	Pravastatin Limitation of Atherosclerosis in Coronary Arteries (trial)
PLTP	phospholipid transfer protein
PON 1	paraoxonase 1
POSCH	Programme on the Surgical Control of Hyperlipidaemias
PPAR	peroxisome proliferator-activated receptor
PPP	Primary Prevention Project
PROCAM	Prospective Cardiovascular Münster (study)
PROSPER	Prospective Study of Pravastatin in the Elderly at Risk
PROVE-IT	Pravastatin or Atorvastatin Evaluation and Infection Therapy (trial)
PTCA	percutaneous transluminal coronary angioplasty
PUFA	polyunsaturated fatty acids

PVD	peripheral vascular disease
RDB	regression dilution bias
REGRESS	Regression Growth Evaluation Statin Study
ROS	reactive oxygen species
RR	relative risk
RUTH	Raloxifene Use for the Heart (study)
RXR	retinoid X receptor
SBP	systolic blood pressure
SCAP	SREBP-cleavage activating protein
SCOR	Specialized Center of Research
SD	standard deviation
SDE	surrogate dilution effect
SE	standard error
SEARCH	Study of the Effectiveness of Additional Reductions of Cholesterol and Homocysteine
SERM	selective oestrogen receptor modulator
SFA	saturated fatty acid
SHEP	Systolic Hypertension in the Elderly Program
SHIP	Southampton Heart Integrated Care Project
SMC	smooth muscle cell
SMR	standard mortality ratio
SPACE	Secondary prevention with antioxidants of cardiovascular disease in end-stage renal disease (study)
SPARCL	Stroke Prevention by Aggressive Reduction in Cholesterol Levels (study)
SR-B1	scavenger receptor class B type 1
SRE1	sterol-response element 1
SREBP	sterol regulatory element binding protein
STARS	St Thomas Atherosclerosis Regression Study
STOP	Swedish Trial in Old Patients with Hypertension
TC	total cholesterol
TFA	*trans* fatty acid
TG	triglyceride
TIA	transient ischaemic attack
TLC	therapeutic lifestyle changes
TNF	tumour necrosis factor
TNT	Treat to New Targets (trial)
TSH	thyroid stimulating hormone
UA	unstable angina
UKPDS	United Kingdom Prospective Diabetes Study
ULN	upper limit of normal
VA-HIT	Veterans Administration HDL Intervention Trial

VCAM-1	vascular cell adhesion molecule 1
VLDL	very low density lipoprotein
VTE	venous thromboembolism
WHO	World Health Organization
WHR	waist–hip ratio
WOSCOPS	West of Scotland Coronary Prevention Study

PART ONE

BACKGROUND

CHAPTER 1

LIPID AND LIPOPROTEIN METABOLISM – THE BASICS

It is the authors' experience that colleagues not in the field often have difficulties getting to grips with lipid and lipoprotein metabolism. This area of biochemistry and physiology has perhaps not been well covered at medical school and has been the subject of some-times confusing and changing nomenclature. This is a pity, as many fundamental and exciting developments have taken place in the last two decades.

Recent advances have provided considerable insight into the control of lipoprotein metabolism, a rational approach to the development of therapeutic agents and an under-standing of some of the dyslipidaemias at the molecular level. The latter development has made possible the first attempts at gene therapy in homozygous familial hyper-cholesterolaemia.

It is not proposed to provide here a detailed description of lipid and lipoprotein metabolism. Rather, the basics of lipoprotein metabolism will be described to enable an understanding of the primary and secondary dyslipidaemias, the action of lifestyle and drugs in modulating plasma lipid levels and the role of lipoproteins in atherosclerosis and arterial function.

LIPIDS AND LIPOPROTEINS

The two major lipids in plasma – cholesterol and triglyceride – have essential functions in the overall structure and fuel economy of the body.

Cholesterol

In its free, unesterified form (Figure 1.1), cholesterol is a major component (together with phospholipid) of cell membranes. Its presence helps to stabilize membrane fluidity and therefore the barrier between cell and environment. Cholesterol is also important as a

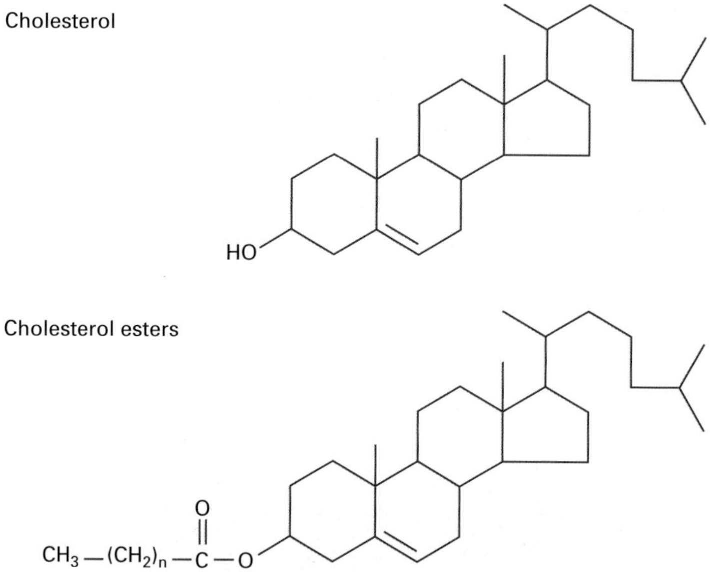

Cholesterol

Cholesterol esters

$$CH_3 - (CH_2)_n - \overset{\overset{\displaystyle O}{\|}}{C} - O$$

FIGURE 1.1 • Structure of free and esterified cholesterol.

precursor of steroid hormones and of bile acids. Cholesterol present in the plasma and extracellular fluid is largely in the esterified form (Figure 1.1).

Triglycerides

Triglycerides are produced by the esterification of glycerol with three fatty acid molecules (Figure 1.2). They are the body's major energy store, particularly in adipose tissue. Fatty acids are released through the action of hormone-sensitive lipase, an enzyme that becomes active during fasting when insulin levels are low. They can be utilized directly as fuel by muscle or, following partial oxidation to ketone bodies in the liver, by other tissues, including brain.

Triglyceride and cholesterol ester are insoluble in the aqueous environment of the plasma and are solubilized by their incorporation into lipoproteins.

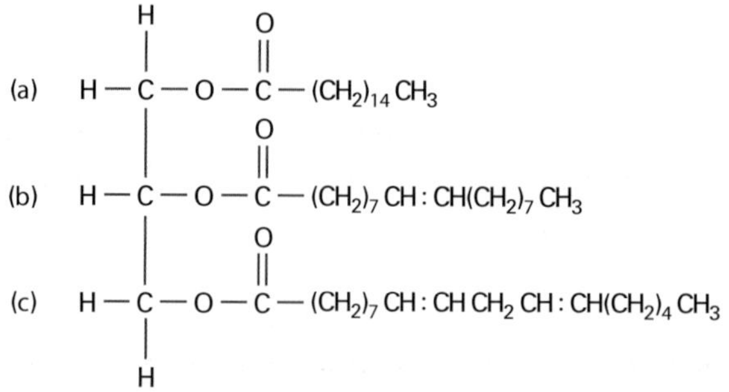

(a) $\quad H - \overset{\overset{\displaystyle H}{|}}{C} - O - \overset{\overset{\displaystyle O}{\|}}{C} - (CH_2)_{14} CH_3$

(b) $\quad H - \overset{|}{C} - O - \overset{\overset{\displaystyle O}{\|}}{C} - (CH_2)_7 CH : CH(CH_2)_7 CH_3$

(c) $\quad H - \overset{|}{C} - O - \overset{\overset{\displaystyle O}{\|}}{C} - (CH_2)_7 CH : CH CH_2 CH : CH(CH_2)_4 CH_3$

$\quad\quad\quad\quad \overset{|}{H}$

FIGURE 1.2 • Structure of triglyceride (triacylglycerol) with, for illustration, (a) a saturated fatty acid, (b) a mono-unsaturated fatty acid and (c) a polyunsaturated fatty acid.

LIPOPROTEIN STRUCTURE

There are several different lipoprotein species found in plasma but their basic structures are similar (Figure 1.3). The insoluble lipid (cholesterol ester and triglyceride) forms a central core in the form of a lipid droplet. This is surrounded by an outer monolayer of molecules such as free cholesterol, phospholipids and proteins termed apoproteins which give the complexes their name. These molecules are able to sit at the water/fat interface because they are partly water-soluble and partly lipid-soluble.

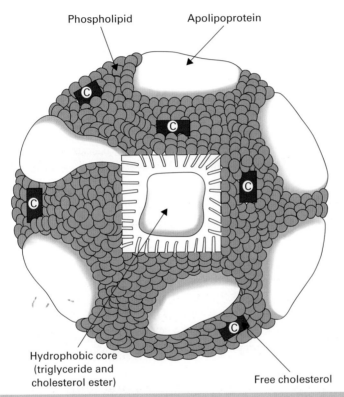

FIGURE 1.3 • Structure of lipoprotein.

Apoproteins

Apoproteins not only have important roles in the secretion and stabilization of lipoproteins, but also have other important regulatory functions in lipoprotein metabolism. There are two translational products of apoprotein (Apo) B. Apo B_{100}, the largest of apoproteins (4536 amino acid residues) and the major apoprotein of the very low density lipoprotein (VLDL) cascade, is important in lipoprotein secretion, structural integrity and is a major ligand for the low density lipoprotein (LDL) receptor. Apo B_{48} (2152 amino acid residues) represents the NH_2-terminal 48 per cent of apo B_{100} and does not possess the binding domain for the LDL receptor. It is synthesized in the intestine and is a structural component of chylomicrons and chylomicron remnants. Apo A-I and A-II are the major proteins of high density lipoproteins (HDL) but, in addition, have other important functions. A-I interacts with the ABCAI [a member of the large protein family known as adenosine 5′-triphosphate (ATP)-binding cassette (ABC) transporters] in the active removal of cholesterol from cells in the initial stage of reverse cholesterol transport. Apo A-I also activates lecithin cholesterol acyltransferase (LCAT), which converts free cholesterol to cholesterol ester. Apoproteins C-I and C-III, constituents of triglyceride-rich lipoproteins and HDL, slow the clearance of triglyceride-rich lipoproteins by a variety of mechanisms.

Apo C-III is an inhibitor of lipolysis through inhibition of the enzyme lipoprotein lipase and also interferes with lipoprotein binding to glycosaminoglycan matrix at cell surfaces where lipoprotein receptors and enzymes are situated. Apo C-I is a major inhibitor of cholesterol ester transfer protein and inhibits lipoprotein binding to the LDL receptor, LDL receptor-related protein and VLDL receptor. Apo C-II, on the other hand, is an important activator of the lipolytic enzyme lipoprotein lipase.

Apo E is a constituent of several lipoproteins, particularly the partially catabolized remnants of triglyceride-rich lipoprotein chylomicrons and VLDL, which carry dietary and endogenously synthesized cholesterol, but also a subclass of HDL. Apo E is an essential ligand for the hepatic uptake of lipoprotein remnants, facilitates (with Apo A-I) cellular cholesterol efflux and can modify immune responses important in atherosclerosis. Through these mechanisms it can be seen that Apo E is protective against atherogenesis.

LIPOPROTEIN CLASSIFICATION

Lipoproteins are classified predominantly according to their separation in the ultracentrifuge. This separation depends on the hydrated density of the different lipoproteins, which is inversely related to their size and reflects their relative contents of core lipid (low density) and surface apoproteins (high density) (Figure 1.4).

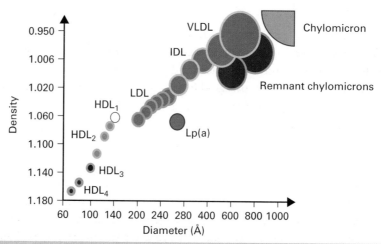

FIGURE 1.4 • Plasma lipoprotein species and subspecies.

LIPOPROTEIN METABOLISM

Lipoproteins serve to transport absorbed dietary fat and endogenously synthesized cholesterol and triglyceride. The pathways of lipoprotein metabolism are complex and there is much interaction between individual lipoprotein species (Figure 1.5). Nevertheless, it is possible to provide a relatively simple overview covering three main interdependent and interconnected areas: the exogenous and endogenous pathways and reverse cholesterol transport. In these various pathways the liver has a pivotal role.

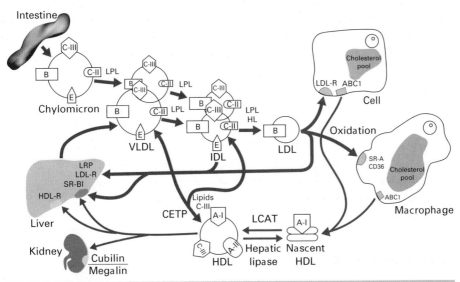

FIGURE **1.5** • Overview of lipoprotein metabolism [Santamarina *et al.* (2001) in *The Metabolic and Molecular Bases of Inherited Disease* (eds C.R. Scriver, J.B. Stanbury, J.B. Wyngaarden and D.G. Fredrickson), 7th edn, McGraw-Hill, New York]. Reproduced with permission of The McGraw-Hill Companies.

EXOGENOUS PATHWAY

In the typical Western diet, approximately 80–140 g triglyceride and 0.5–1.5 g cholesterol are eaten daily. Under normal circumstances, most dietary triglyceride but only about half of the cholesterol is absorbed. Following digestion, absorption and re-esterification, triglyceride and cholesterol are packaged in the jejunal enterocyte with Apo B_{48} in concert with microsomal triglyceride transfer protein (MTP) to form chylomicrons. These are the largest of the lipoprotein species.

Chylomicrons

Chylomicrons as nascent lipoproteins are transported from the endoplasmic reticulum to the Golgi apparatus where they are packaged into secretory vesicles and leave the enterocytes by exocytosis. They enter the circulation via intestinal lymphatics and finally the thoracic duct. Here they acquire additional apoproteins, principally the C group and Apo E, which transfer from HDL. They are rapidly metabolized in two discrete phases

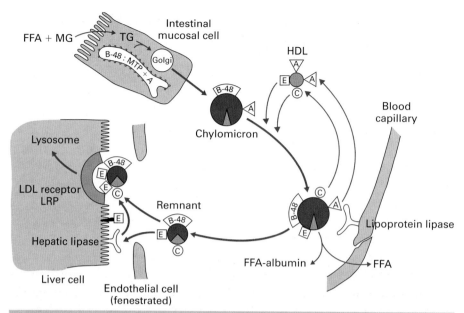

FIGURE **1.6** • Exogenous lipoprotein pathway [Kane, J.P. and Havel, R.J. (2001). Disorders of the biogenesis and secretion of lipoproteins containing the B apolipoproteins, in *The Metabolic and Molecular Bases of Inherited Disease* (eds. C.R. Scriver, J.B. Stanbury, J.B. Wyngaarden and D.G. Fredrickson), 7th edn, McGraw-Hill, New York, pp. 169–81]. Reproduced with permission of The McGraw-Hill Companies.

(Figure 1.6). They bind to the enzyme lipoprotein lipase on the surface of capillary endothelial cells where the large triglyceride component is hydrolysed to fatty acids and glycerol. Apo C-II is an important activator of the enzyme.

The hydrolysis of chylomicron triglyceride by lipoprotein lipase enables the targeted delivery of fatty acids either for oxidation as fuel in muscle or for re-esterification to triglyceride and storage in adipose tissue. As chylomicron triglyceride is progressively removed, some of the surface components of the particle (principally A apoproteins and phospholipid) become redundant and transfer to HDL. Along with this the particles lose their affinity for C apoproteins, which also transfer to HDL.

Chylomicron remnant

The chylomicron following rapid hydrolysis of the bulk of triglyceride and transfer of apoproteins to HDL is released from the enzyme and becomes a chylomicron remnant particle. The remnant particles are rapidly removed by the liver through complex receptor-mediated mechanisms dependent on Apo E (Figure 1.6). The current concept for the hepatic removal of chylomicron remnants involves at least three processes. First, remnants are sequestered to the space of Disse, a lymphatic area containing abundant heparin sulphate proteoglycans (HSPGs) and microvilli projections of hepatocytes. Here Apo E secreted by hepatocytes enriches the remnants and further hydrolytic processing by the enzyme hepatic lipase occurs. Hepatic lipase can also act as a ligand to facilitate remnant uptake independent of its enzymatic activity. Hepatic remnant uptake is receptor-mediated. Remnants can bind to the LDL (Apo B/E) receptor through Apo E as Apo B_{48} does not possess the ligand-binding domain of Apo B_{100}. However, an important role in remnant uptake involves a unique chylomicron remnant receptor, the LDL-related protein (LRP). LRP shows marked structural homology to the LDL receptor; it contains 31 cysteine-rich repeats homologous to the ligand-binding domain of the LDL receptor, which contains seven. Unlike the LDL receptor for which both Apo B_{100} and Apo E are ligands, the major apoprotein ligand for LRP is Apo E. Although LRP is responsible for internalization of Apo E remnants by endocytosis, initial binding also requires HSPG together with hepatic lipase which direct the remnants to LRP. Abnormalities in this process can lead to an important disease, type III (remnant particle disease) dyslipidaemia, as described in Chapter 3.

In relation to overall cholesterol homeostasis it is important to recognize that the cholesterol component of chylomicrons remains with the particle so that dietary cholesterol is delivered to the liver almost quantitatively. The liver is the sole organ that can dispose of cholesterol in significant amounts. Following internalization, remnant lipoproteins are hydrolysed in hepatic lysosomes. Remnant-derived cholesterol can be metabolized in several ways; it can be secreted directly into bile, converted to bile acids stored following esterification or incorporated into nascent lipoproteins.

ENDOGENOUS PATHWAY

Very low density lipoproteins

Triglyceride and cholesterol synthesized in the liver are secreted in VLDL particles which serve to transport the lipids to the periphery. VLDL forms a spectrum of particles that differ in size and metabolic fate.

Regulation of VLDL production in the rough endoplasmic reticulum of hepatocytes is poorly understood. However, it appears that the major VLDL apoprotein, Apo B_{100} is made continuously by liver cells (Figure 1.7). It is degraded in the absence of lipid, which is necessary for lipoprotein assembly to begin. MTP is important in this process as it can transfer triglyceride and cholesteryl esters to Apo B.

The nature of the lipid(s) essential for VLDL assembly remains controversial but cholesterol ester appears to be critical, together with intrahepatic triglyceride lipolysis to fatty acids and their subsequent re-esterification just prior to the incorporation of triglyceride into the particle. VLDL enters the bloodstream via the fenestrae of hepatic sinusoidal endothelium. Each VLDL particle contains one molecule of Apo B_{100} and small amounts of Apo E and Apo C. In a similar way to chylomicrons VLDL receive additional apoproteins C and E by transfer from HDL. VLDL triglyceride is hydrolysed by lipoprotein lipase – the rate of hydrolysis being slower than that of chylomicron triglyceride probably related to the smaller size of the VLDL particle. The residence time in blood of chylomicron triglyceride is 5–10 minutes compared with 15–60 minutes for VLDL triglyceride. Some VLDL remnants are removed by the liver via LDL receptors which recognize Apo B_{100} and Apo E. It is only when apoproteins C transfer from the VLDL particle to HDL as the triglyceride core is hydrolysed that the

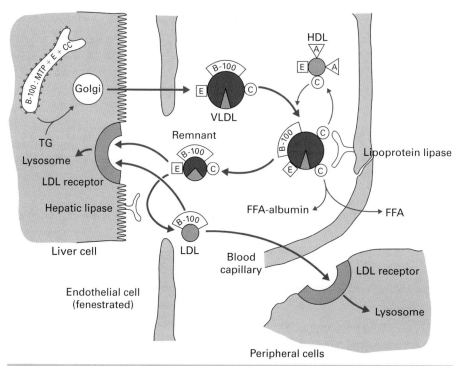

FIGURE 1.7 • Endogenous lipoprotein pathway [Kane, J.P. and Havel, R.J. (2001). Disorders of the biogenesis and secretion of lipoproteins containing the B apolipoproteins, in *The Metabolic and Molecular Bases of Inherited Disease* (eds. C.R. Scriver, J.B. Stanbury, J.B. Wyngaarden and D.G. Fredrickson), 7th edn, McGraw-Hill, New York, pp. 169–81]. Reproduced with permission of The McGraw-Hill Companies.

receptor-binding domains of Apo B and Apo E are exposed. Other VLDL remnants (~50 per cent) are further processed by hydrolysis after binding to hepatic lipase to form LDL.

Hepatic cholesterol synthesis

This is a highly complex process beginning with acetyl-CoA formed from fatty acid oxidation or from carbohydrate breakdown. The rate-determining reaction, which is the conversion of hydroxymethylglutaryl (HMG)-CoA to mevalonate, is catalysed by the enzyme HMG-CoA reductase (Figure 1.8). It is the activity of this enzyme that largely determines the rate of cholesterol synthesis.

Hepatic triglyceride synthesis

Fatty acid flux to the liver from adipose tissue appears to be an important determinant of hepatic triglyceride synthesis and VLDL secretion. Hepatic lipogenesis from carbohydrate substrates is also important. In addition, chylomicron remnant uptake makes a significant contribution to the hepatic lipid pool, providing an important interaction between the exogenous and endogenous pathways.

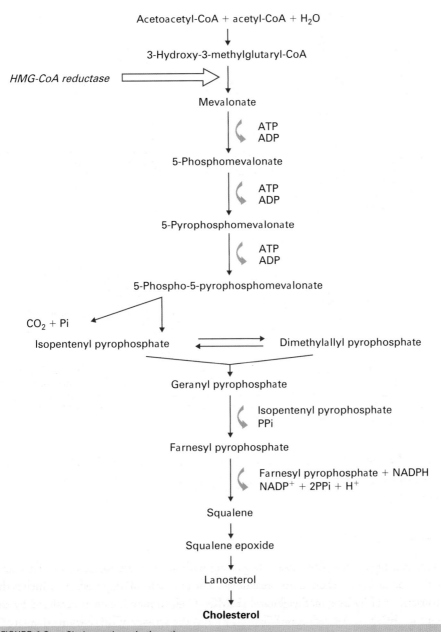

FIGURE **1.8** • Cholesterol synthetic pathway.

Intermediate density lipoproteins

As with chylomicrons, the triglyceride component of VLDL is hydrolysed by lipoprotein lipase. Resulting VLDL remnants, which, like chylomicron remnants, share intermediate density lipoprotein (IDL) on ultracentrifugation, are either removed directly by the liver or further metabolized to LDL through the action of hepatic lipase.

Low density lipoprotein

LDL is the major cholesterol-rich lipoprotein carrying approximately 70 per cent of plasma cholesterol. It serves to transport cholesterol to peripheral cells. Much is now understood about how LDL interacts with the cell membrane and its subsequent internalization and regulation of cellular cholesterol homeostasis (Figure 1.9).

The Nobel laureates Brown and Goldstein identified the LDL receptor that recognizes Apo B_{100} of LDL particles (Brown and Goldstein, 1986). The receptors are large glycoproteins situated on the surface of cells in specialized areas termed coated pits. Coated pits are organelles necessary for the internalization of macromolecules.

The LDL receptor gene has been cloned and localized to the short arm of chromosome 19. The structure (Figure 1.10) and function of the receptor are well understood. The region responsible for binding LDL Apo B_{100} is a negatively charged region at the amino-terminal end of the molecule which consists of seven repeating units of a 40 amino acid sequence rich in cysteine residues. At the carboxyl-terminal end is a 50 amino acid domain, which is responsible for localization of the receptor in the coated-pit regions of cell membranes.

The clinical relevance of this structural detail of the receptor will be appreciated when the inborn error of cholesterol metabolism, called familial hypercholesterolaemia (FH), is discussed. In this condition there are defects in the gene coding for the receptor.

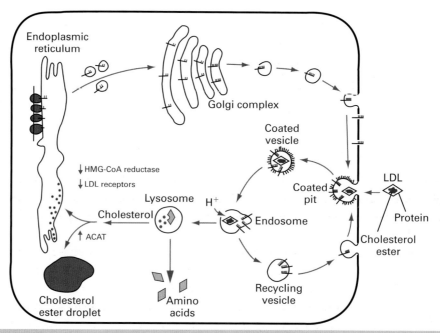

FIGURE **1.9** • LDL receptor pathway. Increasing cellular cholesterol derived from internalization of LDL decreases HMG-CoA reductase activity, activates ACAT and decreases LDL receptor activity. The LDL receptor is formed in the endoplasmic reticulum and travels to the coated pit region of the cell membrane. Source: Brown and Goldstein (1986).

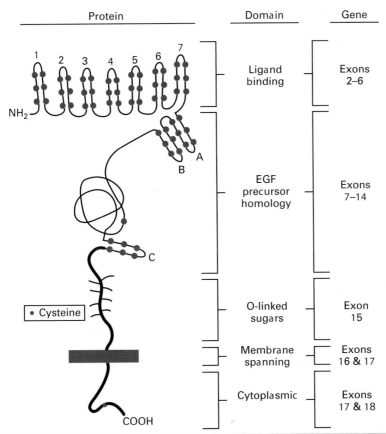

| Protein | Domain | Gene |

FIGURE **1.10** • LDL receptor structure. The LDL receptor consists of 839 amino acids. The various receptor domains are shown together with the exons that code for them. Source: Hobbs, H.H., Russell, D.W., Brown, M.S. and Goldstein, J.L. (1990) *Annu Rev Genet* **24**, 133–70. With permission, from *Annual Review of Genetics*, Volume 24 © 1990 by Annual Reviews www.annualreviews.org.

LDL receptor pathway

Following binding, the receptor/LDL complex is internalized by absorptive endocytosis. The endocytotic vesicle fuses with cellular lysosomes where LDL cholesterol ester is hydrolysed to free cholesterol and protein to amino acids. The LDL receptor recycles to the cell surface.

The increasing cellular free cholesterol generated by this process regulates the activities of two enzymes that are of crucial importance in cholesterol homeostasis (Figure 1.9). HMG-CoA reductase (the major rate-determining enzyme in the cholesterol synthetic pathway) is inhibited, reducing cholesterol synthesis. Acyl-CoA : cholesterol acyltransferase (ACAT) is activated, thus facilitating the re-esterification of cholesterol to cholesterol ester. In addition, the expression of LDL receptors is reduced as cellular cholesterol increases.

These processes are now understood in some detail. A family of transcription factors called sterol regulatory element binding proteins (SREBPs) has been identified. SREBPs are membrane-bound molecules and their activity is controlled by cellular sterol concentrations. To become active and enter the cell nucleus, SREBPs are cleaved by protease enzymes (S1P and S2P) to release the N-terminal domain which is the active transcription factor. The activity of the protease enzyme is in turn regulated by a regulatory protein, the SREBP-cleavage activating protein (SCAP). When cellular sterol content is increased, S1P activity is abolished. Conversely, when cells are depleted of sterol, S1P is active. Within the cell nucleus SREBPs increase transcription of the LDL receptor gene and also genes for important enzymes in cholesterol synthesis including HMG-CoA synthase and HMG-CoA reductase. It is SREBP-2 that is more specific for cholesterol metabolism. These effects are determined by the binding of SREBP to the promoter regions of target genes, one of which is the sterol-response element 1 (SRE1). In experimental animals treated with a combination of statin and bile acid-binding resin, SREBP-2 concentration in hepatic cell nuclei is markedly increased and this is associated with increased LDL receptor messenger RNA. It is likely that the statins lower LDL primarily through activating proteolytic cleavage and hence activation of SREBP-2 (Goldstein *et al.*, 2001).

Thus the LDL receptor pathway is a closely integrated system by which cells acquire cholesterol and cellular cholesterol homeostasis is maintained. The therapeutic potential of interrupting this pathway will become apparent when the statin drugs, which are inhibitors of HMG-CoA reductase, are discussed as it is likely that these drugs lower LDL by activating proteolytic cleavage of hepatic SREBP-2.

It is the activity of LDL receptors in the liver that largely controls plasma LDL levels. Approximately 70 per cent of LDL is removed by this pathway. The importance of the receptor pathway is clear from consideration of the disease familial hypercholesterolaemia (FH) (see Chapter 3). LDL receptor activity is substantially reduced in patients heterozygous for FH and virtually absent in homozygotes. As a result, the plasma half-life of LDL is extended from approximately 2.5 days in normal individuals to 4.5 days in FH heterozygotes and 6 days in homozygotes. Non-receptor-mediated removal of plasma LDL is not well understood.

High density lipoproteins

High density lipoproteins (HDL) are the smallest of the lipoprotein species and transport approximately 20–30 per cent of plasma cholesterol. They are a heterogeneous class of lipoproteins sharing a high density (>1.063 g/mL). Many of their components are subject to rapid exchange with other lipoproteins and to modification by enzyme activity.

Nascent HDL in the form of bilayer discs containing Apo A and phospholipid are secreted by the liver and intestine. These transient particles rapidly become spherical as they take up free cholesterol from cell membranes and other lipoproteins and esterify it to cholesterol ester (which forms a lipid core in the centre of the particle) through the action of lecithin cholesterol acyltransferase (LCAT) enzyme. This enzyme circulates with HDL, and Apo A-I (the major HDL apoprotein) is important in its activation. HDL is also modified by lipid exchange with lipoproteins of lower density through its content of a cholesterol ester transfer protein (CETP) and a phospholipid transfer protein (PLTP).

Mature HDL consists of two principal subclasses on ultracentrifugation; HDL_2 ($d = 1.063-1.125\,g/mL$) and HDL_3 ($d = 1.125-1.21\,g/mL$) and their respective concentrations are in part determined by the metabolism of triglyceride-rich lipoproteins. It is likely that the more dense HDL_3 is converted to HDL_2 by the acquisition of phospholipid and free cholesterol shed from VLDL and chylomicrons during their lipolysis. On the other hand the triglyceride-enriched HDL_2 may be converted back to HDL_3 through the action of hepatic lipase.

More recently, HDL particles have been subclassified by serial use of anti-Apo A-I and Apo A-II immunoaffinity chromatography according to whether they contain one or both of the principal HDL apoproteins, A-I and A-II. Whereas virtually all HDL particles contain A-I, not all contain A-II so that on the basis of Apo A composition particles are designated lipoprotein A-I (Lp A-I) or lipoprotein A-I/A-II (Lp A-I/A-II). The metabolism of these particles is likely to be different and further work is needed to delineate the pathways in detail. However, there is increasing evidence that Lp A-I containing particles, which predominate in HDL_2, are of particular importance in protecting against coronary heart disease (CHD).

Reverse cholesterol transport

HDL is central to reverse cholesterol transport. In this process, first proposed by Glomset (Glomset, 1968), cholesterol surplus to cellular requirements is returned from the periphery to the liver for excretion (Figure 1.5). HDL can act as an acceptor for free cholesterol from tissues. The free cholesterol is esterified by the enzyme LCAT and enters the hydrophobic lipid core of the particle. There is accumulating evidence that a tiny fraction (accounting for approximately 5 per cent of Apo A-I) of HDL, termed pre-beta HDL, is the most efficient HDL subclass for inducing cellular cholesterol efflux.

The cholesterol ester on HDL can return to the liver directly with subsequent recirculation of the particle. However, this process is quantitatively less important than the indirect transfer of HDL cholesterol ester to the liver. Cholesterol ester transfers from HDL to lipoproteins of lower density such as VLDL and LDL via CETP. Thus the major part of cholesterol ester formed within HDL returns to the liver in other lipoproteins. A more detailed understanding of reverse cholesterol synthesis at a molecular level has become possible recently through the identification of important new receptor-mediated processes. The first step in reverse cholesterol transport involves the efflux of cholesterol from cells. This may involve a passive diffusion of free cholesterol from cell membranes to HDL Apo A-I and a receptor-mediated efflux. By the study of an extremely rare condition, Tangier disease (see page 87), which is characterized by marked deficiency of HDL and accumulation of cellular cholesterol ester, it has become clear that the product of the *ABCA1* gene, cholesterol efflux regulatory protein (CERP), is important in the early stage of reverse cholesterol transport. *ABCA1* is a member of the ATP-binding cassette (ABC) gene family, which produce transmembrane proteins that utilize the energy produced by hydrolysis of ATP to transport a variety of substances across cell membranes. Mutations of *ABCA1* have been identified in Tangier disease and also in familial HDL deficiency, providing additional evidence of the importance of this gene in HDL metabolism and reverse cholesterol transport. CERP facilitates the translocation of cholesterol from intracellular compartments to the cell membrane where it can be taken up by pre-beta HDL.

The relationship between cellular cholesterol efflux and HDL concentrations, together with an assessment of arterial wall changes in patients with impaired *ABCA1* function has recently been reported (van Dam *et al.*, 2002). Individuals ($n = 30$) with mutations in *ABCA1* had lower plasma HDL cholesterol concentrations (0.8 ± 0.3 SD versus 1.40 ± 0.4) and increased carotid intima-media thickness (IMT) as assessed by B-mode ultrasound compared to controls. Cellular cholesterol efflux was measured in cultured fibroblasts from a subset of patients and controls. A strong correlation was observed between plasma HDL concentrations and cholesterol efflux ($r = 0.9$, $P = 0.001$). Furthermore, in the patients with *ABCA1* mutations, negative correlations were observed between efflux and IMT. These important results emphasize the importance of *ABCA1* to HDL cholesterol and the relationship to early atherosclerosis.

Important advances have also been made in the understanding of reverse cholesterol transport at the target organ for the delivery of cholesterol, the liver. The selective uptake of HDL cholesterol by the liver is mediated by the scavenger receptor class B type 1 (SR-B1). Knockout mice (SR-B1$-/-$) have shown a twofold increase in total cholesterol due to increased HDL cholesterol whereas animals over-expressing SR-B1 showed reduction in HDL cholesterol. Recently SR-B1 gene polymorphisms have been shown to correlate with plasma lipid levels in a human population.

LIPIDS, LIPOPROTEINS AND ATHEROGENESIS

LDL cholesterol explains the link between plasma cholesterol, atherosclerosis and CHD. Perhaps the most dramatic confirmation of the atherogenicity of LDL comes from familial hypercholesterolaemia. In this condition, characterized by elevations of LDL cholesterol due to LDL receptor defects, homozygotes develop extensive atherosclerosis in childhood. In recent years much has been learned about the interaction of this lipoprotein with cells important in atherogenesis. Essential insights have come from studies of non-human primates. These experiments have pointed to the important role of the monocyte/macrophage in the formation of foam cells which comprise the fatty streak – the initial lesion of atherosclerosis.

When experimental animals (including primates) are fed a high-fat, high-cholesterol diet, the first identifiable lesion is the adhesion of monocytes to arterial endothelium. At a later stage, monocytes penetrate the endothelium, accumulate in the subendothelial space and acquire the characteristics of macrophages, which engulf lipid and become lipid-laden foam cells.

This process appears to be toxic to the overlying endothelium, which is disrupted. This allows platelet adhesion and aggregation with release of potent growth factors that stimulate smooth muscle proliferation and connective tissue accumulation, with consequent development of the mature atherosclerotic plaque.

MODIFIED LDL

When the importance of the monocyte/macrophage in foam cell formation was established, important experiments to study their interaction with LDL were performed. When incubated with native LDL, monocyte/macrophages did not accumulate lipid to any great extent and foam cells were not formed. This result was perhaps to be expected as the LDL receptor is protective in the sense that it is the major pathway by which LDL is cleared from the circulation by the liver. Furthermore, patients with familial hypercholesterolaemia who lack functioning LDL receptors develop premature and extensive atherosclerosis.

In landmark experiments, Goldstein and Brown and colleagues showed that if LDL was chemically modified it was taken up avidly by monocyte/macrophages with foam cell formation (Brown and Goldstein, 1983). This process appeared to be receptor-mediated and the receptor was termed the scavenger receptor. A crucial difference between this receptor and the classical LDL receptor is its lack of down-regulation with increasing cellular cholesterol accumulation. Therefore by this process massive cholesterol accumulation can occur, resulting in lipid-laden foam cells.

Steinberg and colleagues showed that a likely *in vivo* modification of LDL resulting in uptake by monocyte/macrophages is peroxidation (Steinberg *et al.*, 1989). Indeed, oxidatively modified LDL may contribute to atherogenesis in other ways, including direct cytotoxicity to arterial endothelium and the stimulation of monocyte adhesion and monocyte chemotaxis (Figure 1.11). Modified LDL may also interact with the coagulation system through increased expression of tissue factor (thromboplastin) and increased expression of plasminogen activator inhibitor I. These effects enhance the likelihood of activation of the coagulation cascade. Oxidized LDL may also have important effects on arterial tone through inhibition of endothelium-derived relaxing factor and enhanced expression of endothelin, which is a potent vasoconstrictor.

Support for the concept of the atherogenicity of oxidatively modified LDL has come from studies in experimental atherosclerotic animals. In these experiments, antioxidants have been shown to inhibit LDL modification, reduce LDL uptake into the arterial wall

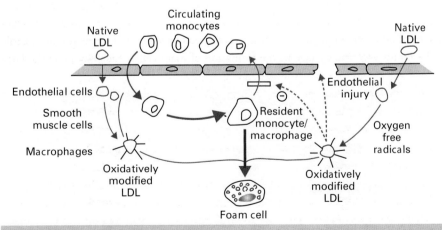

FIGURE **1.11** • Oxidized LDL and atherosclerosis.

and protect against atherosclerosis. So far, the impact of individual antioxidants and antioxidant cocktails have not shown benefit in large CHD prevention trials. Clearly, however, this does not disprove the LDL oxidation hypothesis.

LDL SUBFRACTIONS

LDL is heterogeneous (Krauss and Burke, 1982) and can be separated on density gradient ultracentrifugation into subclasses that vary in size, density and lipid content (Figure 1.12). In healthy subjects the most abundant LDL subclass is LDL-II. Women have proportionately more of the larger, less dense LDL-I particles than men. Conversely, men have proportionately more of the smaller, denser LDL-III particles. LDL heterogeneity can also be assessed on gels where smaller, denser particles give rise to pattern B and larger, less dense particles to pattern A.

It is clear from the work of Austin and Krauss and others that LDL pattern B is strongly related to CHD risk (Austin *et al.*, 1988). This relationship remains to be fully explained but possible explanations include the slower fractional catabolic rate of dense LDL and its increased susceptibility to oxidation.

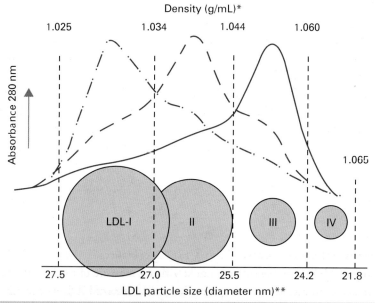

FIGURE **1.12** • LDL subfractions: distribution of human plasma LDL subclass density and particle size. *LDL subclass density profiles obtained by density gradient ultracentrifugation and representative of a typical normal, healthy female (·—· ·—·), male (— — —) and coronary artery disease (CAD) patient (——). **LDL particle size as determined by 2–16 gradient gel electrophoresis. Reproduced from Griffin, B.A. (1995) in *Dyslipidaemia* (ed. D.J. Betteridge) *Clin Endocrinol Metab* **9**, 687–703.

HDL AND PROTECTION FROM CHD

HDL cholesterol is inversely related to CHD risk, as discussed in detail in Part Two. The mechanisms by which increasing HDL concentrations are protective and low levels increase risk remain to be determined fully. The involvement of HDL in reverse cholesterol transport is an attractive explanation for its protective role. This has been given added credibility with the identification of important genetic abnormalities at key regulatory sites such as *ABCAI* in conditions such as Tangier disease, which is associated with markedly low HDL cholesterol and atherosclerosis. Furthermore, there is an impressive consistency from experimental animal models of atherosclerosis showing that over-expression of Apo A-I is associated with protection from atherosclerosis.

An alternative hypothesis does not attach a specific protective role to HDL but suggests that the plasma HDL concentration reflects the efficiency or otherwise of the metabolism of triglyceride-rich lipoproteins, this process being directly related to atherogenesis. Other potential ways by which HDL may protect against atherogenesis and CHD include inhibition of the oxidative modification of LDL lipid and protein. The enzyme paraoxonase circulates bound to HDL. Paraoxonase promotes the breakdown of oxidized lipid. Effects of HDL on thrombotic tendency through inhibition of platelet aggregation and stimulation of the production of the potent platelet inhibitor and vasodilator, prostacyclin, from arterial endothelium may also be important.

Insight into the relation between HDL and aterosclerosis has come from the identification of genetic disturbance in humans. Low HDL cholesterol concentrations associated with Apo A-I gene mutations appear in many cases to be related to premature CHD. However, some structural variations in Apo A-I with alterations in HDL show no apparent increase in CHD risk. An interesting missense mutation, A-I Milano (173 Arg to Cys) for instance is associated with low HDL cholesterol concentration but no increase in CHD and possible longevity. Furthermore, mutations in genes for proteins important in lipoprotein processing, such as CETP and LCAT, are associated with altered HDL cholesterol concentrations but the expected effects on CHD risk are not always observed. Much remains to be learned about HDL metabolism and its relationship to CHD. This will be particularly important as pharmaceutical compounds that profoundly affect HDL cholesterol become available. Clearly, increasing HDL cholesterol is associated with protection against CHD in the overall population. However, in individuals such as the family from Limone sul Garda in Italy with A-I Milano, low HDL cholesterol was not associated with CHD risk (Franceschini *et al.*, 1980). Given the complexity of HDL metabolism, it is unlikely that a measure of total HDL cholesterol will, in all cases, indicate whether the protective mechanisms of HDL are operative or not.

TRIGLYCERIDES AND ATHEROGENESIS

Triglyceride accumulation is not a feature of the atherosclerotic plaque but triglyceride-rich lipoproteins also contain cholesterol esters and it is likely that some of these are directly atherogenic. There is little doubt that remnant particles fall into this category. It was Zilversmit who originally proposed that triglyceride-rich lipoproteins might be atherogenic and that the degree of postprandial lipoprotein metabolism may be central to atherogenesis (Zilversmit, 1979).

In the rare but important disease, type III or dysbetalipoproteinaemia (discussed in detail in Chapter 3), there is marked accumulation of remnant particles and this is associated with premature extensive atherosclerosis not only in coronary but also in peripheral arteries. Laboratory studies have demonstrated that these lipoproteins can interact directly with monocyte/macrophages to produce foam cells.

Hypertriglyceridaemia is associated with alterations in the metabolism of other lipoproteins, which may explain its relationship to CHD risk. It is often inversely related to HDL such that as triglycerides increase, HDL cholesterol concentrations decrease.

Triglycerides are also related to alterations in the distribution of LDL subclasses. In hypertriglyceridaemic individuals there is a preponderance of small, dense LDL particles. As discussed earlier, there is evidence that these particles are highly atherogenic. It has been calculated that the plasma triglyceride concentration accounts for much of the variability in LDL subfraction distribution. This relationship can be explained by the lipid exchange promoted by hypertriglyceridaemia together with the action of hepatic lipase. Triglyceride exchanges for cholesterol ester via CETP to LDL, and triglyceride-rich LDL is a substrate for hepatic lipase resulting in the formation of lipid-poor, protein-rich LDL particles.

A further explanation for the link between plasma triglyceride and CHD risk relates to the association between hypertriglyceridaemia and coagulation factors. Factor VII is an important component of the extrinsic coagulation system and in prospective studies has been shown to be an independent predictor of CHD. Increasing plasma triglycerides are positively correlated with the activity of factor VII and some of the day-to-day variation in factor VII coagulation activity is related to dietary fat intake.

Plasma triglyceride concentration is also positively correlated with activity of plasminogen activator inhibitor 1 (PAI-1). PAI-1 is an inhibitor of plasminogen activation and has been shown to be increased in young myocardial infarction patients.

LIPOPROTEIN(a)

Lipoprotein(a) [Lp(a)] consists of LDL with an additional apoprotein – Apo(a) – attached to it via a disulphide bond (Figure 1.13). Apo(a) has striking structural homology with plasminogen, a zymogen of the coagulation and fibrinolytic system. It has a high degree of internal repeat structure due to a variable number of repeats of kringle 4 plasminogen. Lp(a) concentrations vary widely within and between populations. African populations have several-fold higher Lp(a) concentrations than Caucasians or Asians.

In Europeans most individuals have low levels but there is a pronounced positive skew to the distribution with very high levels in some people, in fact concentrations can vary over 1000-fold. This variation appears to be largely determined by the Apo(a) gene locus. Plasma concentrations correlate inversely with the molecular mass of Apo(a), which exists in many different size polymorphisms.

The physiology of Lp(a) remains poorly understood but its rate of production appears to be a major determinant of its plasma concentration. It is likely that Apo(a) is directly secreted by the liver and then associates with LDL in plasma or at the hepatocyte cell

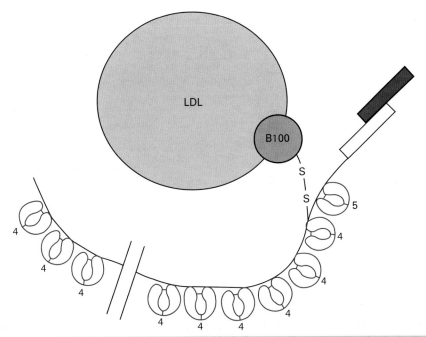

FIGURE **1.13** • Lipoprotein(a). Lipoprotein(a) consists of LDL joined by a single disulphide bridge to apoprotein(a), which consists of the protease domain, kringle 5 and a variable number of kringle 4 repeats of plasminogen. Source: Scanu, A.M. (1990) Lipoprotein(a), in *Baillière's Clinical Endocrinology and Metabolism: Lipid and Lipoprotein Disorders* (ed. D.J. Betteridge), vol. 4, no. 4.

membrane. The site of catabolism of Lp(a) is not known. The LDL receptor plays little, if any, role. However, the kidney may be involved in catabolism. End-stage renal disease is associated with increased Lp(a) concentrations.

The importance of Lp(a) relates to its association with CHD risk. High Lp(a) concentrations are a primary genetic risk factor for CHD, for stroke and peripheral vascular disease. The mechanism of the relationship between Lp(a) and vascular risk remains to be fully determined. It may involve modulation of the balance between thrombosis and fibrinolysis at the endothelial surface. Fibrin thrombosis has the capacity to bind Lp(a). High homocysteine concentrations enhance fibrin binding of Lp(a). Lp(a) induces cellular responses in endothelial and smooth muscle cells which are atherogenic.

Lipid-lowering drugs have no effect on Lp(a), apart from nicotinic acid which may interfere with Lp(a) assembly. Tamoxifen (antioestrogen) and tibolone (synthetic steroid) decrease Lp(a) by a third.

REFERENCES

Austin, M.A., Breslow, J.L., Hennekens, C.H. *et al.* (1988) Low density lipoprotein subclass patterns and risk of myocardial infarction. *J Am Med Assoc* **260**, 1917–21.

Brown, M.S. and Goldstein, J.L. (1983) Lipoprotein metabolism in the macrophage. *Annu Rev Biochem* **52**, 223–61.

Brown, M.S. and Goldstein, J.L. (1986) Receptor-mediated control of cholesterol metabolism. *Science* **191**, 150–54.

Franceschini, G., Sirtori, C.R., Capurso, A., Weisgraber, K.H. and Mahley, R.W. (1980) A-1 Milano apoprotein. Decreased high-density lipoprotein cholesterol levels with significant lipoprotein modifications and without clinical atherosclerosis in an Italian family. *J Clin Invest* **66**, 892–7.

Glomset, J.A. (1968) The plasma lecithin:cholesterol acyltransferase reaction. *J Lipid Res* **9**, 155–67.

Goldstein, J.L, Hobbs, H.H. and Brown, M.S. (2001) Familial hypercholesterolaemia. In *The Metabolic and Molecular Bases of Inherited Disease* (eds C.R. Scrivener, A.L. Beaudet, W.S. Sly and D. Valle), 8th edn, McGraw-Hill, New York, 2863–913.

Krauss, R.M. and Burke, D.J. (1982) Identification of multiple subclasses of plasma low density lipoproteins in normal humans. *J Lipid Res* **23**, 97–104.

Steinberg, D., Parthasarathy, S., Carew, T.E. *et al.* (1989) Beyond cholesterol: modifications of low density lipoprotein that increase its atherogenicity. *N Engl J Med* **320**, 915–24.

Van Dam, M.-J, de Groot, E., Clee, S.M. *et al.* (2002) Association between increased arterial-wall thickness and impairment in ABCAI-driven cholesterol efflux: an observational study. *Lancet* **359**, 37–42.

Zilversmit, D.B. (1979) Atherogenesis: a postprandial phenomenon. *Circulation* **60**, 473–85.

EPIDEMIOLOGY

CHAPTER 2

HISTORICAL PERSPECTIVE

The roots of pathological inquiry extend back to the early eighteenth century. In 1727, Brunner, conducting his father-in-law's autopsy, described the atherosclerotic aorta as 'ruptured, lacerated and rotten, like fruit'. In 1755, Albrecht von Haller passed comment on another post-mortem specimen. Opening into the aortic plaques, he found a yellow mush between the muscular fibres and the intima, which was soft and pultaceous. Since Greek times, the word atheroma had been used to describe any closed sac filled with a porridge-like material (*athere* means mush or gruel) and he likened the plaques to 'atheromata'. He also noted that the same aorta had harder and drier plaques (more fibrotic) and inferred that a gradual process of hardening took place, eventually culminating in a hard, bone-like structure. John Hunter's own post-mortem examination in 1793 at St George's Hospital revealed vascular tissue covered with an 'exudation of coagulating lymph' and the coronary arteries were said to 'ramify through the substance of the heart in the state of bony tubes'.

Even in the eighteenth century human atherosclerosis was not a new disease. Modern palaeopathological studies on Egyptian mummies, dating from the time of the Pharoahs, have revealed the presence of atherosclerotic plaques. Hippocrates observed that 'persons who are naturally of a full habit die suddenly, more frequently than those who are slender' and was presumably describing sudden coronary death. There are clear descriptions of angina from the eighteenth century but syphilis and valvular disease may have been more significant aetiologically than atherosclerosis.

Cholesterol was also first described in the eighteenth century, having been crystallized from alcoholic extracts of gallstones. In 1816 it was named from the Greek *chole* (bile) and *steros* (solid). Its presence in blood was demonstrated in 1838 and in 1843 Vogel showed that it was present in atherosclerotic plaques. As so often in the early epidemiology of heart disease, the finding received little attention.

The advent of systematic cell microscopy in the second half of the nineteenth century elucidated the morphological characteristics of the atheromatous plaque, confirming the deposition of free and esterified cholesterol as the hallmark lesion. By the early twentieth century, study of several diseases – hypothyroidism, nephrotic syndrome and what became later identified as familial hypercholesterolaemia – showed that premature severe atherosclerosis was linked to the level of cholesterol.

Following the first description of acute myocardial infarction in 1911, it soon became known that people recovering from myocardial infarction had higher mean serum cholesterol levels than controls. Nutritional changes in the Western world and the increasing popularity of cigarette smoking led to an increase in coronary atherosclerosis and thrombosis until, by the 1930s, it was evident that the modern pandemic of coronary heart disease was under way, a scourge that few industrialized countries have been able to escape.

Once it was realized, in the early twentieth century, that geographical differences in the frequency of coronary heart disease existed, 'geographical pathology' became a respectable research interest. Initially, differences between populations were identified largely by European investigators working in the colonies and many studies linked low dietary fat intake with a low level of atherosclerosis. Conversely, in 1925 Kuczynski studied Asian Kirghiz plainsmen and correlated their diet rich in meat and milk to their excessive prevalence of obesity, arcus senilis and premature atherosclerosis.

In 1916, De Langen, a physician from Utrecht, showed that Indonesian nationals had lower levels of blood cholesterol than their Dutch counterparts and he related this to the increased incidence of atherosclerosis in the Netherlands. His significant observation was that Indonesian stewards on Dutch passenger ships eating Dutch food had levels similar to those found in the Netherlands. Unfortunately, this forerunner of later important migration studies was published in a Dutch language journal and passed unnoticed.

After the great depression and World War II, there was an explosion of interest in 'geographical pathology' when it was discovered that in countries such as the USA, Finland and much of northern Europe, atherosclerotic disease accounted for more than half the total mortality.

America was further shocked in 1953 when Major William Enos examined the coronary arteries of 300 soldiers (mean age 22.1 years) killed in action in the Korean War. Only 25 per cent were free of visible atherosclerotic lesions, in complete contrast to their Korean counterparts. This should have been no surprise as in 1915 Monckeberg had drawn similar conclusions from German troops killed in World War I – another piece of research that failed to surface. By contrast, some countries such as Japan, those bordering the Mediterranean and most of the underdeveloped world were enjoying much lower rates of coronary mortality and the search was on to identify individual risk factors to explain these differences.

Ancel Keys, a nutritional physiologist from Minnesota, became the dominant figure through the 1950s and 1960s as his high-quality research began to establish the cholesterol hypothesis. With the development of the risk factor concept in 1961 there evolved a predictive capacity for identifying coronary heart disease unparalleled in almost any other condition. Many studies began to tell the same story with the major risk factors of hypercholesterolaemia, high blood pressure and smoking coming to the fore and with

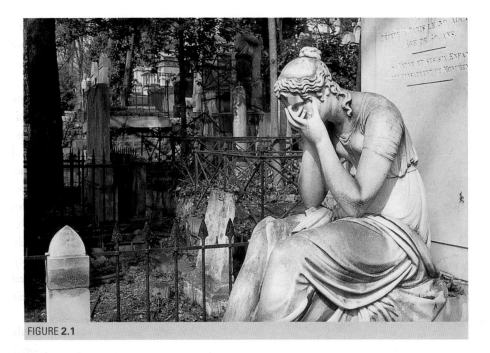

FIGURE **2.1**

hypercholesterolaemia assuming a pivotal central role. Quantitative estimates of how much coronary disease can be accounted for by each risk factor became possible and with them the beginnings of opportunities for effective prevention.

CARDIOVASCULAR DEATH

THE WORLDWIDE POSITION

In 1997, Murray and Lopez estimated that there had been 50.5 million deaths world wide in 1990. Medically certified information was available for less than 30 per cent of deaths but by incorporating other sources and correcting for miscoding they were able to estimate causes of death across a range of age–sex groups around the world. The 30 leading causes of death worldwide are shown in Table 2.1.

Leading causes of death 1990 – the Global Burden of Disease Study

Five of the ten leading killers are communicable, perinatal and nutritional disorders largely affecting children. Four of the ten, CHD, cerebrovascular disease, chronic obstructive pulmonary disease and lung cancer, may be partly prevented by discouraging smoking, correcting pollution and unhealthy diets and by encouraging physical activity.

About a quarter of all deaths world wide are caused by cardiovascular diseases (mostly CHD and strokes). In developed countries, about 50 per cent of deaths are due to cardiovascular disease, whereas in developing countries the proportion is only about 15 per cent. However, as 80 per cent of the world's deaths occur in developing countries,

Epidemiology

TABLE **2.1** • Thirty leading causes of death world wide in 1990

Rank	Cause of deaths	No. deaths ($\times 10^3$)
	All causes	50 467
1	Ischaemic heart disease	6260
2	Cerebrovascular disease	4381
3	Lower respiratory infections	4299
4	Diarrhoeal diseases	2946
5	Perinatal disorders	2443
6	Chronic obstructive pulmonary disease	2211
7	Tuberculosis (HIV seropositive excluded)	1960
8	Measles	1058
9	Road-traffic accidents	999
10	Trachea, bronchus and lung cancers	945
11	Malaria	856
12	Self-inflicted injuries	786
13	Cirrhosis of the liver	779
14	Stomach cancer	752
15	Congenital anomalies	589
16	Diabetes mellitus	571
17	Violence	563
18	Tetanus	542
19	Nephritis and nephrosis	536
20	Drowning	504
21	War injuries	502
22	Liver cancer	501
23	Inflammatory heart diseases	495
24	Colon and rectum cancers	472
25	Protein–energy malnutrition	372
26	Oesophagus cancer	358
27	Pertussis	347
28	Rheumatic heart disease	340
29	Breast cancer	322
30	HIV	312

Source: Murray and Lopez, 1997.

the total number of cardiovascular deaths is roughly equally divided between developed and developing nations.

Figure 2.2 shows CHD mortality rates for men and women in the industrialized world. There are two main observations:

- In this age range, coronary events in men outnumber those in women three- to fourfold. There is also a high correlation between CHD rates in the two sexes across national populations, i.e. in countries with high rates of CHD for men, the rates for women are also high.
- Second, there are marked contrasts in the rates for northern and eastern European countries and those of the Mediterranean countries and Japan. The differences can be understood in terms of lifestyle (in essence dietary and smoking habits) and

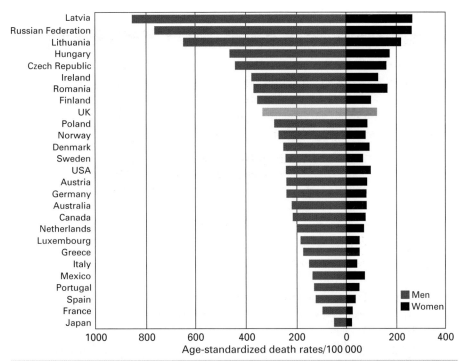

FIGURE **2.2** • Death rates from CHD, men and women aged 35–74, 1994, selected countries.
Source: Reproduced from British Heart Foundation Statistics Database, 1999 with permission.

socioeconomic factors. That they are not due to in-built genetic factors is demonstrated by studies of migrants.

The Ni Hon San Study, 1977

Despite high levels of smoking and hypertension, the natural population of Japan has a low rate of CHD. The Ni Hon San study (Table 2.2) followed migrants from Japan (**Nippon**) to Hawaii (**Honolulu**) and California (**San** Francisco). Although rates of hypertension and smoking fell, mean total serum cholesterol rose and with it the CHD rate.

As a change in gene structure over such a short period of time is untenable, the differences must have been brought about by environmental change, namely the assimilation of an increasingly westernized, atherogenic diet.

TABLE **2.2** • Ni Hon San study (1977) of migrants from Japan to Hawaii and California

Factor	Japan	Honolulu	San Francisco
Acute MI rate/1000	7.3	13.2	31.4
Hypertensive heart disease/1000	9.3	1.4	4.6
Non-smokers (%)	26.0	57.0	64.0
Mean serum total cholesterol (mmol/L)	4.7	5.6	5.9

CHD AND ECONOMIC DEVELOPMENT

International comparisons, like other 'league tables', are not static but dynamic and countries shift their positions as their CHD rates alter (Figure 2.3).

CHD rates are falling in the wealthy countries of Europe and in the USA and Australia. The rates of fall vary, however. For example, between 1970 and 1985 they fell by 48 per cent in the USA, but by only 11 per cent in England over the same period.

CHD rates are rising in many countries of central and eastern Europe and the Russian Federation. In addition, CHD is emerging as a major cause of death in developing countries.

A pattern has emerged of increasing CHD with advancing economic development (industrialization, 'westernization'). Once they have become mature, industrialized countries then show reducing levels. In 1921, the number of CHD and cancer deaths in the UK equalled those from infectious disease. Within 10 years, cardiovascular diseases were pre-eminent as increasing prosperity reduced the incidence of deaths from infection. This is mirrored in Latin America at present where, over the next 25 years, deaths from cardiovascular disease are expected to number five times those from infectious and parasitic disease compared with roughly equal numbers in the two groups in 1985.

Two basic trends explain these changes. The first relates to the contribution of improved food supplies and the control of infectious disease to improvements in the death rate in

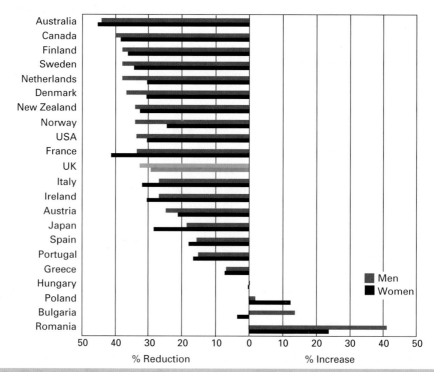

FIGURE **2.3** • Changes in death rates from CHD, men and women aged 35–74, between 1984 and 1994, selected countries. Source: Reproduced from British Heart Foundation Statistics Database, 1999 with permission.

childhood. The net effect of this is to increase the average age of the developing population and over time and with more prolonged exposure to risk factors CHD emerges. The second reason relates to urbanization. The migration from rural to urban areas is largely complete in developed countries but accelerating in undeveloped countries. Urbanization means improved access to food and a change from more vegetarian diets to more carnivorous ones. A 'rich' Western diet is adopted, with its relationships to raised serum cholesterol and hypertension. With a 'rich' diet the secondary role of smoking in the aetiology of atherosclerotic disease becomes manifest on a large scale. A 'rich' diet is high in total fat (especially saturated fat), high in cholesterol, sugar, salt, alcohol and unnecessary calories and low in potassium, fibre and other essential nutrients. With a lower level of energy expenditure resulting from the use of the car, the television and automated labour, the 'couch potato' is born. In essence, the developing world is trading early death and disability from infectious disease for later death and disability from atherosclerosis and its sequelae.

Epidemiologists have described the acquisition of cardiovascular risk, inherent in the transition from a low development culture to a highly developed one, in a series of phases:

- The phase of pestilence and famine – the influence of infectious disease and diets inadequate in quantity and quality mean the incidence of death from cardiovascular disease is only 5–10 per cent. A modern example is tropical Africa.
- The phase of receding pandemics – here a society increasingly geared to agriculture produces adequate food but with a tendency to high dietary sodium. Cardiovascular death begins to increase to 10–35 per cent. North Asian countries typify this scenario at present.
- The phase of degenerative, man-made disease – the supply of food is adequate but there is emphasis on high fat with low fruit and vegetable consumption. Cardiovascular death rises further to 35–55 per cent and this situation is currently seen in East Europe and South Asia.
- The phase of delayed degenerative diseases – again, diet is adequate in amount but reduced saturated fat consumption offsets the cardiovascular death rate, which drops below 50 per cent. Such a situation is seen in western Europe and North America at present.

The high carbohydrate consumption inherent in the last phase has prompted epidemiologists to consider a fifth phase:

- The phase of stabilization/recrudescence – wherein diet high in carbohydrate and calorific content may cause cardiovascular disease rates to soar, as a new pandemic of obesity and type 2 diabetes gets under way.

MONICA is an ongoing World Health Organization (WHO) programme for MONItoring trends and determinants in CArdiovascular disease in 37 populations across 21 countries around the world. MONICA was set up in 1978 when the declining rate of CHD in advanced populations was first noted. The brief was to monitor CHD mortality and to assess whether the noted declines were due to declining event rates or improved survival. The 10-year results were published in 1999 and overall, using MONICA criteria, CHD mortality in the selected populations has fallen by 2.7 per cent in men and 2.1 per cent in women. There is considerable variation between the individual populations, with changes ranging from −6.5 per cent in Finnish men to +2.3 per cent and +2.8 per cent in Chinese and Russian men, respectively. The MONICA analysis attributes about one-third of the improvements to improved survival (reduced case fatality) but two-thirds to improvements in risk factors. A separate American analysis attributed 50 per cent of the decline in mortality to reductions in risk factors, with the impact of medication being 'substantial'. In Scotland, a country with high rates of CHD, 51 per cent of the reduction in CHD between 1975 and 1994 has been attributed to modification of the four risk factors of smoking, cholesterol, blood pressure and social deprivation, thus emphasizing the importance of prevention strategies.

In the USA, CHD rates have approximately halved in the last two decades. Much of this fall results from the improved risk factor status of the population (Figure 2.4). Consumption of total fat, saturated fat, cholesterol, salt and cigarettes have fallen whereas consumption of polyunsaturates, fish and fibre and rates of physical activity have risen. Surprisingly, as in the UK, mean body weight has risen.

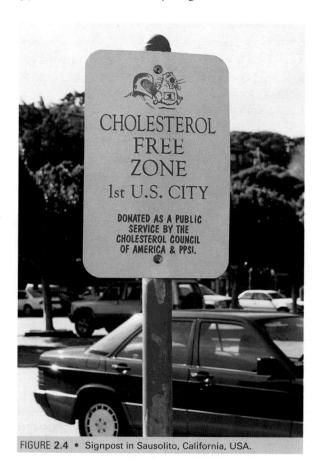

FIGURE **2.4** • Signpost in Sausolito, California, USA.

In the 1980s, a national system for monitoring CHD trends was established and in 1988 the National Cholesterol Education Program recommended the testing of all adults every 5 years and issued guidelines to physicians. The 'Know your Number' campaign was launched and by 1989 two-thirds of the population had been screened and 25 per cent knew their result. The 1980s also saw a fivefold increase in the prescribing of lipid-lowering drugs and a ninefold increase in CHD prevention consultations. Mean cholesterol levels dropped by 3–4 per cent.

In 1987, the life expectancy at birth of Russian men had increased to 64.9 years. Seven years later, life expectancy had declined dramatically to only 57.6 years and this has been attributed to an increasing prevalence of high rates of smoking and drinking, a high intake of saturated fat and a low consumption of fruit and vegetables (Figures 2.5 and 2.6).

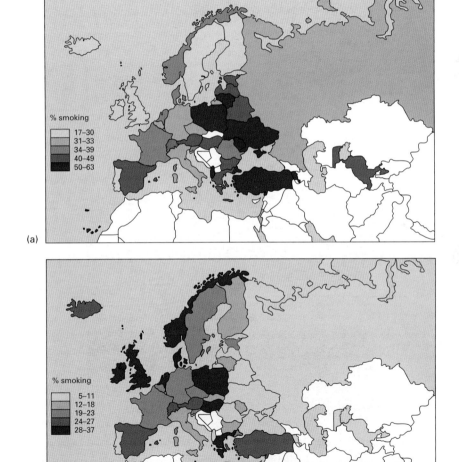

FIGURE 2.5 • (a) Prevalence of smoking, men aged 15 and over, latest available year. (b) Prevalence of smoking, women aged 15 and over, latest available year. Source: Reproduced from European Cardiovascular Disease Statistics, 2000 with permission.

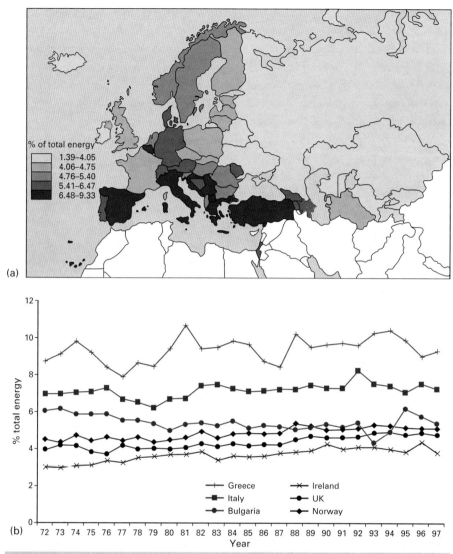

FIGURE **2.6** • (a) Percentage of total energy from fruit and vegetables, 1997. (b) Percentage of total energy from fruit and vegetables, 1972–97, selected countries. Source: Reproduced from European Cardiovascular Disease Statistics, 2000 with permission.

Such trends are seen in other eastern European countries and it is not completely clear what drives populations to adopt lifestyle patterns associated with increasing risk. Certainly, economic factors can influence a population's dietary habits and fascinating data from Hungary illustrate how differential price rises in commodities can favour life-style habits that are responsible for higher levels of CHD (Figure 2.7).

Japan has proved the exception, so far, to the 'industrialization' pattern. Although two-thirds of Japanese men smoke and there are high levels of hypertension, CHD rates have been amongst the lowest in the world. This is attributed to low saturated fat in the diet and low mean serum cholesterol (cf. the Seven Countries Study). Despite an already

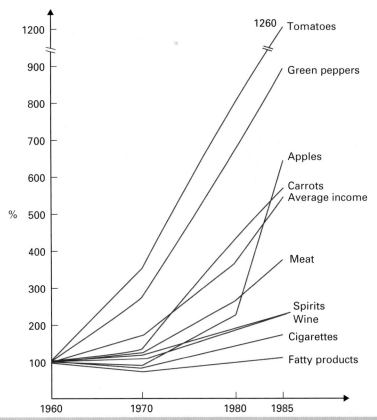

FIGURE **2.7** • Differential price rises in Hungary. Source: Kaposvari and Bales (1988) *Mag yarovszag*, Feb. 26.

low mortality, the rates of further improvement have been amongst the highest in the world. This probably relates to the improved detection and management of hypertension and a reduction of dietary sodium rather than further changes in lipid factors. Indeed, there is some evidence for adverse change in saturated fat consumption and the future may see worsening circumstances.

Deaths from other cardiovascular causes also show international variation. Stroke is a leading cause of death in China, cardiomyopathies and hypertensive heart disease predominate in Africa and in many countries rheumatic heart disease remains common.

Table 2.3 shows the number of CHD deaths for each cerebrovascular death in males (1985–89). This clearly shows that different risk factors or different levels of similar risk factors are at work around the world. In essence, this is reflected by the central importance of dyslipidaemia in the development of CHD and the importance of hypertension in the aetiology of stroke.

Population studies reveal the relative influence of different cardiovascular risk factors and we will now look at studies both between and within individual countries that have characterized the contribution of individual risk factors to the development of CHD.

TABLE **2.3** • Number of CHD deaths for each
cerebrovascular death in males, 1985–89

Country	No. deaths
USA	4.63
New Zealand	4.19
Australia	3.61
England and Wales	3.58
Singapore	2.20
Sri Lanka	1.94
France	1.44
Hong Kong	0.91
Japan	0.46
Korea	0.08

STUDIES BETWEEN POPULATIONS

THE SEVEN COUNTRIES STUDY

In 1980, Ancel Keys published his analysis of CHD in 12 763 middle-aged men divided into 16 cohorts within the seven countries, Japan, Italy, Greece, the Netherlands, Yugoslavia, Finland and the USA. These countries were deliberately chosen because they were known to have differing prevalence rates for CHD death. Initially, 5- and 10-year follow-up data were collected but such was the significance of the study that survivors are still being studied and important reports are still being produced. By 25 years of follow-up, nearly half the subjects had died, 1500 from CHD.

There were four major findings:

1 Within each cohort, the risk of CHD was associated with the level of serum cholesterol. This was evident after 10 years in the cohorts from northern Europe and the USA but only showed at 25 years in the cohorts where absolute death rates were lower. A difference of 0.5 mmol/L was associated with a relative risk of 1.12 (1.17 after correction for regression dilution bias).

2 The mean serum total cholesterol concentration of each cohort was directly related to that cohort's CHD mortality (Figure 2.8). East Finland recorded the highest mean serum total cholesterol at 6.6 mmol/L and had CHD mortality rates more than 15 times those of Ushibaka in Japan where the mean serum total cholesterol was 4.1 mmol/L.

3 The mean serum total cholesterol concentration in a community (and by inference, therefore, the CHD mortality) is directly related to the saturated fat content in the usual diet of that community (Figure 2.9).

4 The mean serum total cholesterol concentration is the key factor in determining a community's risk of CHD. The effect of hypertension, smoking, diabetes and lack of

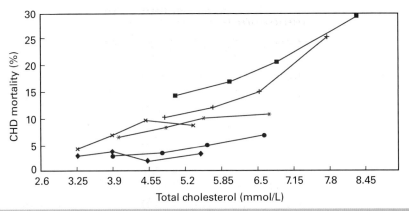

FIGURE 2.8 • 25-year coronary heart disease mortality rates to baseline cholesterol quartile adjusted for age, smoking and blood pressure. ■——■ = Northern Europe; +——+ = USA; ✕——✕ = Serbia; ✳——✳ = Inland Southern Europe; ◆——◆ = Japan; ●——● = Mediterranean Southern Europe. Reprinted from *European Heart Journal* **20**, Kromhout, D., On the waves of the Seven Countries Study: a public health perspective on cholesterol, pp. 796–802, Copyright (1999), with permission from Elsevier Science.

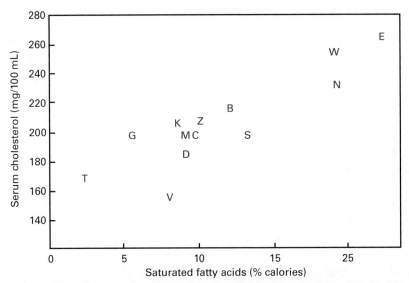

FIGURE 2.9 • Average intake of saturated fat and medium cholesterol levels in the Seven Countries Study around 1960. B = Belgrade, Serbia; C = Crevalcore, Italy; D = Dalmaria, Croatia; E = East Finland; G = Corfu, Greece; K = Crete, Greece; M = Montegiorgio, Italy; N = Zutphen, The Netherlands; S = Slavonia, Croatia; T = Tanushimaru, Japan; V = Velika Krsna, Serbia; W = West Finland; Z = Zrenjanin, Serbia. Source: Keys, A., Aravanis, C., Blackburn, H. *et al.* (1980) *Seven Countries: a Multivariate Analysis of Death and Coronary Heart Disease.* Harvard University Press, Cambridge, MA.

exercise was only additional when the coronary arteries were susceptible because of hypercholesterolaemia. Communities with low mean serum total cholesterol levels had low rates of CHD despite high levels of other risk factors (e.g. Japan).

A number of other international comparative studies have since found similar associations. In 1986, Simons presented data from 19 countries indicating the same relationship for serum cholesterol and CHD death.

STUDIES WITHIN POPULATIONS

Studies within populations establish that the frequency distribution of cholesterol within a cohort, like many biological variables, is almost gaussian with a slight positive skew (Figure 2.10). There are slight differences between men and women, younger women tending to have lower levels of serum cholesterol. The level tends to rise in men until their 40s and then flattens off, whereas in women the rise is maintained (Figure 2.11).

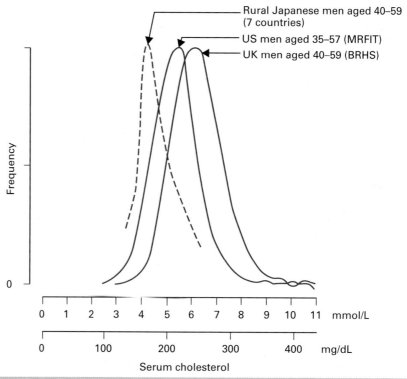

FIGURE **2.10** • Serum cholesterol distribution curves. Source: Durrington (1989) *Hyperlipidaemia – Diagnosis and Management.* Wright, Bristol.

STUDIES IN THE USA

Framingham

Data collection in this small town, 18 miles west of Boston, began with 740 volunteers in 1948. Eventually more than 5000 volunteers were amassed from the town's very stable 28 000 population and research is ongoing. Much of our understanding of the multifactorial aetiology of CHD stems from these data and multivariate statistical analysis has helped to determine the net and joint effects of each risk factor.

The major findings establish a list of CHD risk factors that act in both sexes and at all ages but with different strengths:

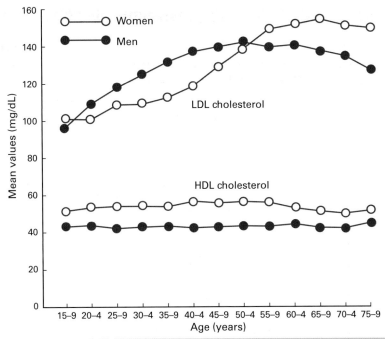

FIGURE **2.11** • Trends in lipoprotein levels in men and women according to age. Source: Kannel, W.B. (1988) *Nutr Rev* **46**, 66–78.

■ Total cholesterol (TC) is positively related to CHD. After only 6 years it was apparent that TC concentrations were powerfully related to the subsequent rate of heart disease.

■ LDL cholesterol is positively related to CHD.

■ HDL cholesterol is negatively related to CHD, the higher values being associated with lower CHD rates.

■ The ratio TC/HDL is established as an efficient lipid risk predictor (Table 2.4). Subjects whose TC/HDL cholesterol ratio exceeds 4.5 are at increased risk. Although pivotal to Framingham data and in widespread use, the concept of ratios is debated. For example, in Japan, where both total cholesterol and HDL cholesterol levels are low, calculated ratios are high but, of course, CHD incidence is low.

TABLE **2.4** • Likelihood ratios for various lipid profiles of CHD, Framingham Study, Examination 11

Lipid profile	Men	Women
TC	1.98 NS	2.26 NS
LDL-C	4.39	4.53
HDL-C	14.03	21.21
Triglyceride	0.51 NS	9.52
TC/HDL-C	17.11	20.41

The table estimates the relative power of a test to predict CHD from asymptomatic subjects. HDL-C, high density lipid cholesterol; LDL-C, low density lipid cholesterol; TC, total cholesterol.

- *Hypertension.* There is a curvilinear relationship between blood pressure and the subsequent development of CHD. Both systolic and diastolic pressures, such as systolic blood pressure (SBP)>160 mmHg or diastolic blood pressure (DBP)>95 mmHg, are equally good predictors. At these levels, CHD is increased two- to threefold, atherothrombotic brain infarction, sevenfold. Left ventricular hypertrophy is an especially dangerous finding.
- *Smoking.* Cigarette smokers in Framingham run about one and a half times the risk of non-smokers.
- *Glucose.* Framingham subjects show an increase in CHD even at modest glucose elevations. Patients with diabetes mellitus show a dramatic increase in risk. Female diabetics completely lose the normal gender advantage.
- *Lack of exercise.*
- *Weight.* The relationship to death appears to be U-shaped, with cancer deaths at lower weights and cardiovascular deaths at higher weights.
- *Stress.* Type A personality, characterized by the need to excel, bossiness, time urgency, eating quickly, impatience and a workaholic nature was associated with a doubling of risk in both sexes.
- *Family history.* Persons whose father died before the age of 60 have double the rate of heart disease. There is a 30 per cent increased risk if a parent died before age 65.

Composite analysis confirmed that combinations of risk factors were not merely additive in terms of effect, but multiplicative. The quantification and interaction of risk associated with combinations of smoking, hypertension and hypercholesterolaemia is shown in Figure 2.12.

Framingham data show that all cardiovascular risk factors contribute to CHD and confirm the central role of dyslipidaemia.

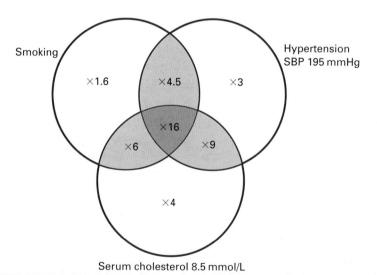

FIGURE **2.12** • Quantification and interaction of risk associated with combinations of smoking, hypertension and hypercholesterolaemia.

The Multiple Risk Factor Intervention Trial – MRFIT

Inspired by the findings of the Seven Countries Study, MRFIT was designed as a flagship trial to see if risk factor modification, especially dietary change and smoking reduction, would reduce CHD events. As a trial, the study was unsuccessful: there were no statistically significant differences between the usual care and intervention groups. In mitigation, the trial was conducted at a time of rising population awareness of CHD risk factors and it proved impossible to curtail the activities of the usual care group, who ceased to remain a genuine control population.

In total, 361 662 men aged 35–37 years from 18 US cities were screened between 1973 and 1975. Data on 356 222 men followed up for 6 years was published in 1986 and 12-year data are now available. The value of the study is in its statistical precision, for at 70 times the size of the Framingham database the conclusions are very powerful (Figure 2.13).

MRFIT revealed that the relationship between CHD and cholesterol was continuous, strong and graded across the range of cholesterol concentrations. There is no threshold level below which CHD events do not occur but the risk increases dramatically from a cholesterol level of about 5.2 mmol/L.

MRFIT also reaffirmed the multiplicative effect of the major risk factors. At any level of a given risk factor, the coincidence of other factors increased the CHD risk. As only 3 per cent of the study population were non-smokers with low SBP (<118 mmHg) and low total cholesterol (<4.7 mmol/L), the findings are relevant to virtually the whole population of American males. The absolute risk of CHD for individuals in the lowest 3 per cent was 3.09 per 10 000 person-years, whereas for the group at highest risk (smokers, SBP >142 mmHg and TC >6.3 mmol/L) it was 62.11 per 10 000 person-years. This 20-fold increase corresponds to 684.6 excess deaths per 10 000 men for 11.6 years of follow-up.

The findings of MRFIT are impressive but it is important to recognize that they represent underestimates as, being based on single initial measurements, they neither

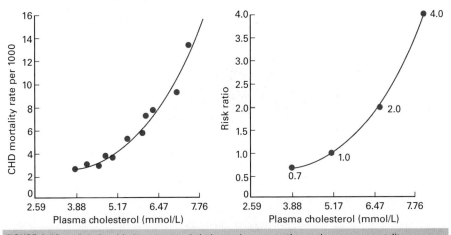

FIGURE 2.13 • Relationship between total cholesterol concentration and coronary mortality in the Multiple Risk Factor Intervention Trial (MRFIT). Source: Reproduced from Grundy, S.M. (1986) *J Am Med Assoc* **256**, 2849–58 with permission.

correct for regression-dilution bias (see page 53) nor control for change in risk factor status over time.

STUDIES IN THE UK

British Regional Heart Study (BRHS)

Regional differences in the UK, with a pronounced north/south divide, have been known for some time (Figure 2.14). The BRHS was designed to determine the personal and environmental risk factors active in the UK and whether they would explain the geographical variation in CHD mortality.

Between 1978 and 1980, 7735 men aged 40–59 years, randomly chosen from general practices in 24 towns in England, Scotland and Wales, were examined. After 4.2 years of follow-up, there had been 202 major CHD events and it is interesting to note that in 197 of them either raised cholesterol, high blood pressure or smoking were present.

There were three main areas of data collection:

Prevalence of CHD

Electrocardiograph (ECG) findings and a questionnaire established that 25 per cent of the study population had evidence of CHD and the prevalence correlated well with local mortality rates. Even in the lowest age group (40–44 years) prevalence was 1 in 6.

Personal risk factors

Each risk factor was divided into quintiles (fifths) with approximately 1500 men in each. The top and bottom quintiles were compared to produce a figure of relative risk (Table 2.5). The predictive capacity of these data led to the development of a primary care scoring system.

Fifteen-year follow-up of 7142 initially healthy men now shows that a non-smoking, low body mass index (BMI), physically active 50-year-old man has an 88 per cent chance of living to 65 years. By contrast, an obese, inactive smoker's chance is reduced to only 30 per cent.

Regional influences

It was found that mean serum total cholesterol levels were fairly constant across the 24 towns (6.0–6.6 mmol/L) and that there was no correlation with regional differences. It is important to note that this mean level is high and therefore the cholesterol factor is active right across the UK. By contrast, smoking and blood pressure (BP) levels did vary, in keeping with geographical and social class differences.

Social class differences in the UK

Social class differences are a manifestation of the socioeconomic forces at work in CHD causation (Figure 2.15). Sixty years ago CHD was more common in social classes I and II, but there has been a complete reversal, with the crossover at some stage in the 1950s.

(a)

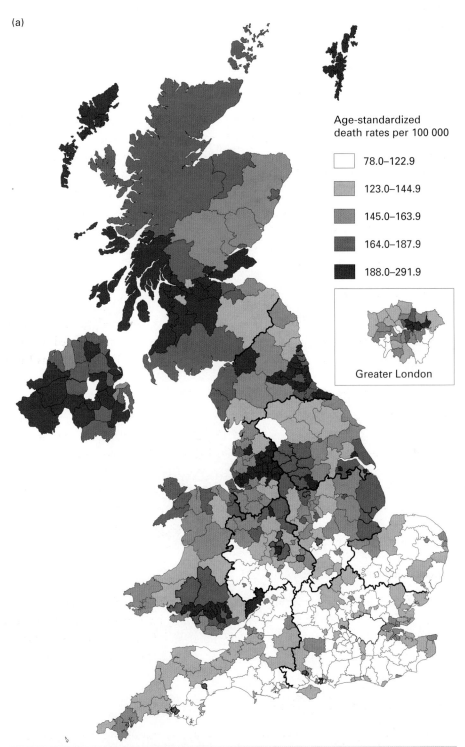

Age-standardized
death rates per 100 000

☐	78.0–122.9
	123.0–144.9
	145.0–163.9
	164.0–187.9
	188.0–291.9

Greater London

FIGURE **2.14** • (a) Age-standardized death rates from CHD for men under 75 by local government district, 1992–96, UK.

(b)

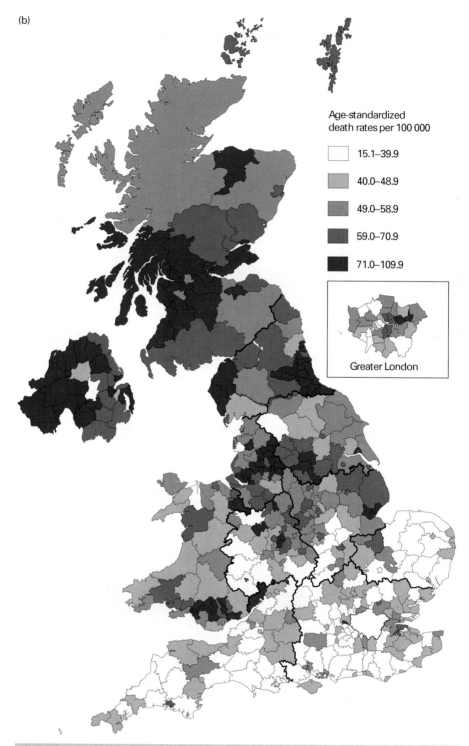

Age-standardized
death rates per 100 000

☐	15.1–39.9
▨	40.0–48.9
▨	49.0–58.9
▨	59.0–70.9
■	71.0–109.9

Greater London

FIGURE 2.14 • (continued) (b) Age-standardized death rates from CHD for women under 75 by local government district, 1992–96, UK. Source: Reproduced from British Heart Foundation Statistics Database, 1999 with permission.

TABLE **2.5** • Coronary risk factors in the British Regional Heart Study

Factor	Relative risk	Comment
Age	4.7	Even the middle quintile, the 'average man' had ×2 risk
Total cholesterol (TC)	3.1	
Low HDL	2.0	
Triglyceride (TG)		Association disappeared when adjusted for TC and HDL
Systolic BP	3.0	
Diastolic BP	3.1	
'Smoking years'	5.1	Smokers:non-smokers 3.0
Body mass index (BMI)	1.8	Association disappeared when adjusted for TC, HDL, TG, BP
Alcohol		No association

The decline in CHD in social classes I and II almost completely accounts for the recent decline in CHD seen in the UK, there being no change in the rates for manual occupations.

Whilst serum cholesterol levels are highest in social class I and lowest in V, levels of blood pressure and smoking, fibrinogen and obesity show the reverse trend (Table 2.6). Unemployment has an increased relative risk of 3.56.

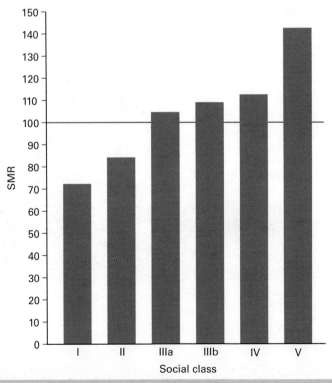

FIGURE **2.15** • CHD: social class differences. SMR, standardized mortality ratio. Source: Reproduced from British Heart Foundation Statistics Database, 1999, with permission.

TABLE **2.6** • Smoking and obesity trends by social class in the UK, 1998

Factor		Social class					
		I	II	IIIN	IIIM	IV	V
Smoking (%)	M	15	21	23	33	38	45
	F	14	20	24	30	33	33
Obesity (%)	M	12	16	16	20	16	18
	F	14	18	18	24	25	28

Social class: I, professional; II, intermediate; IIIN, skilled non-manual; IIIM, skilled manual; IV, partly skilled manual; V, unskilled manual.
Source: Data (used with permission) from British Heart Foundation Statistics Database 2002.

Clearly, important interventions could be targeted at obese social class IV/V women and class IV/V male smokers.

Immigrant populations in the UK

It has become apparent from an increasing number of reports since the 1950s that there are large differences in CHD rates between immigrant populations and UK nationals (Table 2.7). People from ethnic minorities now comprise 5.9 per cent of the UK population and 2.9 per cent come from South Asia. The scale of the problem has become a major public health issue in communities where immigrant residence is high. It is estimated that by 2007, one-third of London's population will be from the ethnic minorities.

For Afro-Caribbeans, the danger of stroke is greater than the risk of CHD and relates to an increased prevalence of hypertension in both sexes and obesity in women.

High rates of CHD are found amongst immigrants from India, Pakistan and Bangladesh and this finding has been duplicated in other countries. Mortality rates are higher for women than men and, in addition, the increased risk also applies to second-generation immigrants. There are very few data from South Asia itself but two studies suggest a low prevalence of CHD in rural India. In two north Indian cities, the prevalence of CHD, judged by ECG changes, showed rates equivalent to those in the UK.

TABLE **2.7** • Mortality rates in immigrant populations aged 20–69 years in UK

1979–83	Country of birth	Standardized mortality ratio (SMR) (England + Wales = 100)	
		Men	Women
CHD mortality	Scotland	111	119
	Ireland	114	120
	South Asia	136	146
	Caribbean	45	76
CVA mortality	Caribbean	176	210

CVA, cerebrovascular accident.

The increased risk of South Asian immigrants is not explained in terms of standard risk factors.

- Hindus from Gujurat in western India are vegetarian and have low levels of cholesterol, whereas Sikhs from the Punjab in north India and Muslims from Pakistan and Bangladesh have average levels.
- Blood pressure is average in Gujuratis, increased in Punjabis and reduced in Muslims.
- Smoking is low in Sikhs and all South Asian women, and average in Hindus and Muslims. Smoking is very high in Bangladeshi Muslims (82 per cent).

Hypotheses for the high rates of CHD in South Asians initially included the use of traditional foods such as ghee and other cooking oils, stress, racism and poverty. Although ghee, which is rich in saturated and *trans* fatty acids, was much cited as a culprit, dietary analyses have shown that South Asians tend to derive less energy from fat in the diet and have lower saturated fat intakes than the UK norm.

The first real clues to the puzzle were found in a 1988 study of Bangladeshi migrants to East London, where a high prevalence of type 2 diabetes was found. This was confirmed in McKeigue's 1991 Southall study, which revealed the findings shown in Table 2.8.

The aggregation of diabetes, low HDL, high triglyceride, hypertension, central distribution of body fat and high levels of insulin is known as the **insulin resistance syndrome** (see page 120), described by Reaven, and it is very likely that some sort of genetic predisposition to develop insulin resistance exists in this group. Unfortunately, when adjusted for all the features of the insulin resistance syndrome, there is still an excess mortality in the South Asian group and other factors must be active.

Similar findings have been described in New Zealand Maoris and Australian Aborigines consuming a western diet. The failure of insulin to suppress non-esterified fatty acids from adipose tissue may increase VLDL triglyceride, which may reduce HDL and produce smaller, more atherogenic LDL. This may have been a mechanism to use triglyceride rather than glucose as fuel at times of deprivation. The presence of this 'thrifty genotype' interacting with the calorie-rich western diet, replete with fat and carbohydrate, to promote weight gain and insulin resistance may be the explanation for the increased susceptibility to CHD. An alternative explanation, using the fetal programming hypothesis (see page 57), is that the increased susceptibility to CHD is

TABLE **2.8** • Southall study, 1991. Risk factors in Europeans and South Asians

Risk factor	European	South Asian
Mean BP	121/78	126/82
BMI	25.9	25.7
Total cholesterol (mmol/L)	6.11	5.98
Diabetes (%)	4.8	19.6
Waist:hip ratio	0.94	0.98
HDL	1.25	1.16
TG	1.48	1.73
Fasting insulin (mU/L)	7.2	9.8

the result of a mismatch of fetal/early life metabolism and that of middle age. Low levels of exercise, particularly amongst South Asian women, compound the situation further.

Strategies to control CHD in South Asians should emphasize all important factors and include social and environmental ones, such as poverty and employment. Health promotion activities should be aware of linguistic and cultural differences (for example, central obesity is regarded as a sign of prosperity) and consider the heterogeneity of different racial subgroups.

STUDIES IN OTHER COUNTRIES

Many other intrapopulation studies confirm the establishment of serum cholesterol as the major risk factor for CHD. The continuous relationship extends across the range of cholesterol values with no evidence of a threshold. Chen *et al.* (1991) studied 9021 men and women in Shanghai, China for 8–13 years. Average serum cholesterol was low by western standards at 4.2 mmol/L but even though there were only 43 CHD deaths (7 per cent of the total recorded) in the time period, there was still a strongly positive, independent association with serum cholesterol concentration. Experimental data on the transfer of cholesterol from the blood into atheromatous plaques indicates a threshold as low as 1 mmol/L.

It has been important to verify the conclusions of the major cohort studies by reproducing their findings across a range of populations. The **Pro**spective **Ca**rdiovascular **M**ünster Study (PROCAM) was initiated in Germany in 1979 to examine the cardiovascular risk factors, mortality and prevalence data of cardiovascular events in working people. Data exist for more than 25 000 men and women based on an intensive initial examination. Severe hypercholesterolaemia (>7.8 mmol/L) was found in 5 per cent of men and 8 per cent of women aged 45–64 years. In the same age range, 4849 men had a second examination and over 8 years of follow-up, 258 major coronary events were recorded (Table 2.9). The greatest difference between the subgroup with major coronary events and the group without, was seen in the LDL cholesterol to HDL cholesterol ratio, where a ratio of more than five was associated with a substantial increase in the incidence of CHD (Table 2.9).

In addition, a quarter of the total CHD events recorded over 8 years in the whole population occurred in the 4.3 per cent where a ratio of more than five existed with hypertriglyceridaemia. This pattern, known as the atherogenic lipoprotein profile, is increased two- to threefold in type 2 diabetes and contributes to the excess cardiovascular risk of these patients.

TABLE **2.9** • LDL cholesterol:HDL cholesterol (LDL-C:HDL-C) ratios and events in PROCAM 8-year follow up

LDL-C:HDL-C ratio	CHD events/1000 men
<3	18
4–4.9	64
5–5.9	171
>7	278

THE FRENCH PARADOX

The low CHD mortality rate in France is the envy of most industrialized countries and because it is not explained by an analysis of standard risk factors, has generated an academic debate that continues to explore a number of elucidatory hypotheses. The debate has been colourful, enriched by international skepticism, the influence of numerous vested interests and the undoubted attraction of elements of the French way of life.

Table 2.10 shows the age-standardized death rates from CHD in men aged 35–74 in five European countries in 1995, together with data regarding the main risk factors from MONICA project sites, collected during the mid-1990s.

TABLE **2.10** • CHD death rates and risk factor data in men from five European countries

Country	Deaths/ 100 000	Smoking (%)	Mean SBP (mmHg)	Mean cholesterol (mmol/L)
France (Lille)	92	33	135	5.8
UK (Glasgow)	314	41	133	6.1
Lithuania (Kaunas)	610	35	137	6.0
Germany (Augsburg)	231	35	137	6.2
Spain (Catalonia)	125	41	121	5.6

Despite broadly similar levels of risk factors, the CHD risk of men living in Lille is less than a sixth of that of men living in Kaunas and less than a third of those living in Glasgow. Clearly, variations in risk factors do not explain the inter-country differences.

Further information can be obtained from WHO data collected during the same period in men aged 35–64 (Table 2.11).

The 'Mediterranean' diet is much promulgated as the reason for the French paradox. The Lyon Diet Heart Study (see page 182) used a diet rich in fruits, vegetables, monounsaturated fat and alpha-linolenic acid and demonstrated a substantial decrease in mortality in a secondary prevention population, albeit with wide confidence intervals. Sadly, supportive evidence concerning onions,

TABLE **2.11** • Aspects of dietary composition in men from five European countries

Country	Fruit and vegetable consumption (g/person/day)	Total energy from fat (%)	Amount of pure alcohol per person/year (L)
France	282	37.7	11.4
UK	253	38.0	7.3
Lithuania	349	45.4	–
Germany	231	38.4	11.1
Spain	455	37.5	9.5

THE FRENCH PARADOX

garlic, folate, nuts, fibre and glycaemic load is lacking and many studies have methodological flaws.

Alcohol consumption, however, is high in France and may provide the clue to unlocking the paradox. Cohort studies consistently show about a 20 per cent CHD risk reduction in those who drink one or more units of alcohol per day. Alcohol increases HDL cholesterol production as well as favourably altering haemostatic factors and influencing platelet aggregation.

Lower rates of CHD are commonly seen in wine-drinking countries and this epidemiological association has encouraged the view that the protective effect of alcohol was specific to wine. A plausible mechanism has emerged for the benefits of red wine in particular and this still generates an enormous amount of enthusiasm amongst health professionals and their patients alike! All grape products contain large quantities of phenolic compounds, some of which may have antioxidant properties. Flavonoids, such as quercetin, are phenolic compounds found in grape skins and are thought to have important antioxidant and anti-atherogenic actions. Such compounds are particularly present in red wine, where grape skins are in contact with the developing wine for longer.

Unfortunately, epidemiological and randomized crossover studies consistently show that it is the alcohol that reduces risk, not any added constituent. Furthermore, the large cohort studies show that drinking more than about one unit per day confers little or no extra protection.

For the French there is a significant downside to their high alcohol consumption.

Alcohol-related deaths in French men aged 55–64 were 348 per 100 000 in 1992 (UK 105/100 000) and this excess mortality is so large as to totally abolish the survival advantage of the low mortality from CHD.

There is no doubt that some of the low CHD rate is explained by under-certification. French doctors have had a tendency to certify late sequelae of coronary disease as poorly specified causes. Estimates for the effect of under-certification would increase the reported rate by up to 20 per cent. To compensate, there is evidence, how-ever, that French doctors introduce preventative treatment more extensively. In 1993, 34 per cent of myocardial infarction (MI) survivors in France took lipid-lowering medication, compared with only 4 per cent in the UK.

Recently, Law and Wald (1999) suggested that the French paradox might indeed be artefactual. It is only in the last 15 years that animal fat consumption and serum cholesterol concentrations in France have approached those of countries where CHD is more prevalent and, due to the 'time lag' between risk factor exposure and the appearance of symptomatic atherosclerotic disease, France may soon see a dramatic rise in CHD death.

The existence of the French paradox is also questioned by commentators from other Mediterranean countries who point out that MONICA data from Barcelona and sites in Italy are of the same order as France and that the paradox is essentially a southern European one, not exclusively French. Whatever the outcome, the debate is sure to run.

WHAT ARE NORMAL CHOLESTEROL LEVELS? ▰▰▰▰▰

We have seen that serum cholesterol is distributed almost normally through a population and that the mean value differs with age and sex. We have also seen that the mean value is raised in countries with high rates of CHD and that this in turn relates to the saturated fat content of the diet. The mean value of serum cholesterol for a population should not, therefore, be regarded as normal. Laboratories tend to express results in terms of standard deviations from the mean, some suggesting a 'normal range' for cholesterol of 5.2–7.8 mmol/L.

Around the world, mean cholesterol levels vary (Table 2.12). Subsistence farming and hunter-gatherer societies have serum cholesterol levels of about 3.5 mmol/L and this probably provides the best definition of 'normal'. It should be remembered that the relationship between serum cholesterol and CHD is continuous and graded and that even at low levels of mean cholesterol, some CHD events still occur.

TABLE **2.12** • Typical cholesterol values in men aged 45–64 years in different populations

Population	Cholesterol (mmol/L)
Hunter-gatherer societies	3–3.5
Rural China	3.5
Rural Japan	4.5
Urban Japan	5.0
Mediterranean countries	5.2–5.6
USA	5.7
Northern Europe	6–6.4
Finland 1980	7.0

Levels from reference population surveys in the UK and USA are shown in Table 2.13. The UK data come from the 1998 Health Survey for England, in which the cholesterol level of 10 569 subjects was measured. Only 237 (2.2 per cent) reported taking lipid-lowering drugs and their results are included. The American data come

TABLE **2.13** • Mean serum cholesterol levels in the UK and USA (mmol/L)

Age (years)	UK men	UK women	Age (years)	US men	US women
16–24	4.4	4.6	0–24	4.0	4.1
25–34	5.1	4.9	25–34	4.8	4.7
35–44	5.5	5.2	35–44	5.3	4.9
45–54	5.8	5.7	45–75	5.6	5.5
55–64	5.8	6.2			
65–74	5.8	6.4			
75+	5.5	6.3	75+	5.3	6.0
All	5.5	5.6			

from the Lipid Research Clinics Program reference values and National Health and Nutrition Examination Survey (NHANES) 3.

The 1998 Health Survey for England also showed that 67.5 per cent of those sampled had serum cholesterol levels over 5.0 mmol/L and 26.5 per cent had a total cholesterol to HDL cholesterol ratio of more than 5. From this it is easy to extrapolate that in a practice of 10 000 patients, with about 3000 patients in the 25–59 age group, approximately 2000 patients would have raised cholesterol levels and at least 750 would be at significant risk. The burden of this work is beyond the resource of secondary care and, like hypertension, cholesterol management must become a primary care discipline.

IS LOW CHOLESTEROL SAFE?

We have seen that lower serum cholesterol concentrations are associated with lower risk of coronary disease and that this relationship is consistent regardless of whether serum cholesterol is high, such as in Western populations, or low, such as in China. Prospective studies, however, report higher non-atherosclerotic death rates in subjects with low cholesterol with the net effect of increased total mortality at these levels (Figure 2.16).

The excess non-atherosclerotic mortality occurring at low cholesterol levels chiefly reflects increased rates of cancer, accidents and suicide. In addition, there is a small increase in the incidence of haemorrhagic stroke (see page 55). When some of the earlier trials of cholesterol lowering not only failed to show improvements in overall mortality (despite reductions in CHD) but also highlighted increased non-atherosclerotic mortality, major doubts began to emerge about the safety of reducing cholesterol to lower levels in at-risk populations.

The statin trials have largely resolved the issue of safety because they show no excess non-atherosclerotic mortality and cholesterol lowering can be viewed as safe, at the very least for 5–6 years and probably for longer when further data are available. The excess mortality is attributable to cancer and depression causing low cholesterol, not the reverse.

The latest prospective study to examine this question has reported from Korea, where 482 472 men aged 30–65 years were followed for 6.4 years, during which there were 7894 deaths. Serum cholesterol levels are low in Korea compared with Western populations, with a mean level reported of 4.9 mmol/L. The risk of death from coronary heart disease was low, as expected, but increased significantly in the top 5 per cent of the cholesterol distribution, where total cholesterol was more than 6.5 mmol/L. The bottom 5 per cent of the cholesterol distribution, where total cholesterol was less than 3.5 mmol/L, was, however, also associated with an increased total mortality.

The U-shaped mortality curve is very similar to that found in populations with higher mean serum cholesterol concentrations. An inverse relationship was observed between cholesterol level and mortality from cancer, violent causes, stroke and other causes. Deaths from any

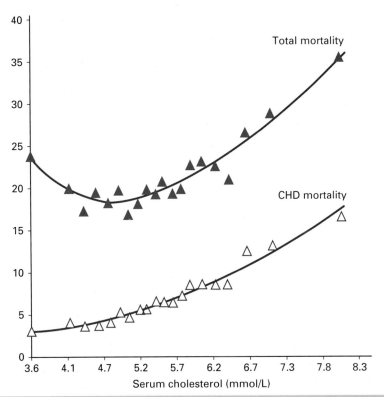

FIGURE **2.16** • Age-adjusted 6-year CHD and total mortality in MRFIT subjects by baseline cholesterol level. Note: Entire cohort of 361 662 men was divided into approximate twentieths, and each point represents the mortality (either CHD or total) and the mean cholesterol level in one of those twentieths. Hand-fitted lines are drawn through the points. Source: Reprinted from Martin, M.J., Hulley, S.B., Browner, W.S., Kuller, L.H. and Wentworth, D. (1986) *Lancet* **2**, 933–6 with permission from Elsevier Science.

cancer were more frequent at low cholesterol levels. Stomach and liver cancers, which accounted for half of all cancer deaths, both remained significantly raised even when deaths in the first 5 years of follow-up were deleted to reduce any confounding pre-morbid effect.

Cholesterol is reduced as part of the acute phase response to injury or disease and may remain depressed for many years, thus complicating the interpretation of these epidemiological findings.

For example, chronic infection with *Helicobacter pylori* and hepatitis B virus, relevant to stomach and liver cancer, may persist over many years. Thus, both chronic inflammatory states and pre-symptomatic cancer may be present for more than the arbitrary 5 year cut-off used in this study.

Depression is accompanied by decreased appetite, inadequate food intake and weight loss, all factors that reduce serum cholesterol. The theory that low cholesterol leads to low serotonin

IS LOW CHOLESTEROL SAFE?

IS LOW CHOLESTEROL SAFE?

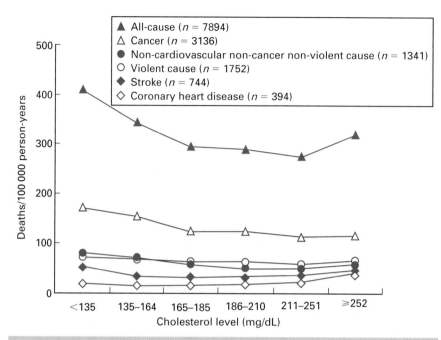

FIGURE 2.17 • Age-adjusted rate of cause-specific mortality among 482 472 men aged 30–65 years by baseline cholesterol level, Korea, 1990–96. Reproduced from *Am J Epidemiol* (2000) **151**, No. 8, p. 742, by permission of Oxford University Press.

levels, which in turn leads to violent behaviour and suicide, is not supported by careful behavioural studies in which cholesterol is found to be unrelated to hostility or risk-taking behaviour. In addition, reducing cholesterol concentrations in animals does not alter brain serotonin concentrations.

Further reassurance of the safety of low cholesterol is provided by the condition of heterozygous familial hypobetalipo-proteinaemia. Here, serum cholesterol levels as low as 2–3 mmol/L are associated with longevity without additional adverse effects.

THE CHOLESTEROL PAPERS

The association between serum cholesterol and CHD was examined in an influential review by Law *et al.* (1994a–c) who published three papers addressing three major questions:

■ the strength of the relationship between serum cholesterol and CHD;
■ the extent and time course of CHD reduction with a given degree of cholesterol reduction;
■ the possible adverse effects of cholesterol lowering (see page 239).

In the first paper, the authors used data from 21 515 men aged 35–64 years attending the British United Provident Association (BUPA) centre in London between 1975 and 1982. In the follow-up to 1991, there were 538 deaths. Two statistical corrections were applied to the results to prevent underestimation of the association between serum cholesterol and CHD:

1 *Regression dilution bias (RDB)*. This factor corrects for the natural variation of serum cholesterol within an individual over time and also for variation in laboratory measurement. Taking a single measurement for a cohort study might place an individual in a false risk quintile and this adds bias.

2 *Surrogate dilution effect (SDE)*. Cohort studies tend to measure total serum cholesterol; 1 mmol/L of total cholesterol is equivalent to 0.67 mmol/L of LDL cholesterol. Intervention studies show that a 1 mmol/L drop in total cholesterol is equivalent to a 1 mmol/L drop in LDL cholesterol because it is largely LDL cholesterol that is lowered by diet and drugs. It follows that extrapolations of the effect of lower cholesterol from cohort trials will underestimate the associated rate of CHD.

The paper analysed the BUPA data to produce a figure for reduction in CHD associated with a reduction of 0.6 mmol/L total cholesterol. This figure was chosen because it was roughly 10 per cent of the UK average and the sort of improvement that could be brought about by lifestyle and dietary change.

For every 0.6 mmol/L reduction in total cholesterol, there were reductions in CHD of 17 per cent, 24 per cent when corrected for RDB and 27 per cent when corrected for SDE. Moreover, all-cause mortality after correction was also reduced by 10 per cent, i.e. a 10 per cent reduction in cholesterol led to a 10 per cent reduction in total mortality.

The second paper, using data from the 10 largest cohort studies (including MRFIT, BRHS, BUPA and Whitehall) and three international studies (including Seven Countries and Ni Hon San), extended the statistical corrections to a cumulative database of nearly half a million men. The percentage decrease in the CHD risk for every 0.6 mmol/L reduction in total cholesterol is shown in Table 2.14. In the international studies, 0.6 mmol/L reduction is associated with a reduction of CHD by 38 per cent at 55–64 years.

Although the reduction of cholesterol is weaker with increasing age, the absolute effects are greater. It is estimated that a 54 per cent reduction in CHD in men aged 40

TABLE **2.14** • Estimated percentage decrease in CHD risk for differing serum cholesterol reductions

Age (years)	0.6 mmol/L (10%)	1.2 mmol/L (20%)	1.8 mmol/L (30%)
40	54	79	90
50	39	63	77
60	27	47	61
70	20	36	49
80	19	34	47

would save 400 deaths per year in the UK whereas a reduction of 19 per cent at 80 would save 20 000.

If a 30 per cent drop in cholesterol (1.8 mmol/L) such as observed in the Scandinavian Simvastatin Survival Study (4S) is used as the baseline cholesterol reduction, the postponement of CHD death is predicted to average 9 years for a 60-year-old man.

The findings regarding the speed of effect and safety of cholesterol lowering are discussed in Chapter 9 (page 237).

CHOLESTEROL AND STROKE

Stroke is the third leading cause of death in the world and the leading cause of disability. It is estimated that 4 million strokes occur each year (600 000 in the USA and 519 000 in Europe) and approximately one-third are fatal. Survivors pose a significant burden to health-care systems and society as:

- 48 per cent suffer hemiparesis;
- 32 per cent are clinically depressed;
- 22 per cent are unable to walk;
- 12–18 per cent are aphasic;
- 24–53 per cent are dependent on carers.

The well-established risk factors for stroke (Table 2.15) include the majority of those for CHD with the remarkable exception of cholesterol. The Prospective Studies Collaboration, published in 1995, found no association between serum cholesterol and stroke rates in an analysis of 13 397 strokes in more than 450 000 individuals from 45 cohorts, studied for 16 years.

Several explanations have been proposed for this finding. Most strokes occur in later life when serum cholesterol is often lower and many individuals whose serum cholesterol was high earlier will already have succumbed to coronary disease. When the data from MRFIT are analysed, there is a clear dose–response

TABLE **2.15** • Established risk factors for stroke

- Age (>80 risk = 2% per annum)
- Male sex
- Family history
- Race
- Geographical location
- Hypertension/systolic BP
- Left ventricular hypertrophy
- Smoking
- Diabetes mellitus/impaired glucose tolerance
- Transient ischaemic attack
- Carotid stenosis
- Cardiac disease (AF, endocarditis, mitral stenosis, recent MI)
- Hyperhomocysteinaemia
- Hypercoagulable states

AF, atrial fibrillation.

relationship between thrombotic stroke and serum cholesterol and it seems that the type of stroke is important. Strokes are either thrombotic or haemorrhagic, about half originating from large vessel atheroma and the other half from small cerebral artery disease, arrhythmias and cortical degeneration.

MRFIT also shows a slight negative association between fatal haemorrhagic stroke and low cholesterol levels.

Epidemiologists debate whether this is a genuine association as there is no plausible explanation for the finding and the number of individuals with low cholesterol included in the studies was low.

The early clinical trials of cholesterol lowering showed no reduction in cerebrovascular events and it was a surprise when the statin trials showed benefits (see Table 2.16).

TABLE **2.16** • Reduction in the risk of stroke in the statin trials

Trial	Statin	No. strokes (treatment v placebo)	Risk reduction (%)
4S	Simva-	70 v 98	29
CARE	Prava-	54 v 78	31
PAIP	Prava-	5 v 13	62NS
LIPID	Prava-	169 v 204	19
WOSCOPS	Prava-	46 v 51	10NS

CARE, Cholesterol and Recurrent Events trial; LIPID, Long Term Intervention with Pravastatin in Ischaemic Disease; PAIP, Pravastatin Atherosclerosis Intervention Project (PLAC 1, PLAC 11, REGRESS, KAPS); 4S, Scandinavian Simvastatin Survival Study; WOSCOPS, West of Scotland Coronary Prevention Study.

Significant reductions in stroke are only seen in patients with existing CHD. The table does, however, include the findings of carotid imaging studies, which support the concept of lipid lowering in large vessel disease to reduce stroke risk.

Retrospective meta-analyses of the statin trials have corroborated the findings of individual trials with risk reductions ranging from 24 to 31 per cent. The confidence intervals, however, are wide and most of the benefit seems to be a reduction of non-fatal stroke with the effect on fatal stroke being unclear. The

recently published Heart Protection Study (HPS) confirms a similar level of stroke and transient ischaemic attack (TIA) reduction in high-risk subjects without an excess of haemorrhagic cerebrovascular events. Major vascular events were also significantly reduced in subjects without CHD but with prior stroke or peripheral arterial disease. Forthcoming studies include Stroke Prevention by Aggressive Reduction in Cholesterol Levels (SPARCL), where atorvastatin will be compared with placebo in patients with minor CVA or TIA.

CHOLESTEROL AND STROKE

CHOLESTEROL AND STROKE

How might statins reduce stroke risk?

The observed reductions in cerebro-vascular disease with statins may relate to their greater LDL cholesterol lowering potency compared to older therapies and, therefore, their capacity to retard atherosclerosis progression. Interestingly, however, cerebrovascular event reduction was also seen in the Veterans Administration HDL Intervention Trial (VA-HIT), where LDL cholesterol concentration was not affected by therapy. Patients taking gemfibrozil had a 25 per cent risk reduction for stroke and a 59 per cent lower risk for TIA. Apart from beneficial effects on HDL cholesterol and triglycerides, fibrates are well known to have favourable effects on coagulation factors and other factors may be operative.

Speculation for the effect of statins has also included plaque stabilization and improved endothelial function. Small blood pressure reductions are also observed over time with continued treatment and this, too, may contribute.

Cerebral magnetic resonance imaging (MRI) examination of 3658 men and women over 65 years of age showed that, whilst only 5 per cent reported a history of cerebrovascular disease, 31 per cent had silent 'infarct-like lesions'. Such 'silent strokes' may result in reduced cognitive function and impaired motor coordination. Whether brain lesions can be prevented and cognitive function preserved will be the subject of the ongoing trial, the Prospective Study of Pravastatin in the Elderly at Risk (PROSPER).

THE FUTURE BURDEN OF CORONARY HEART DISEASE

Although first published in 1798, Malthusian principles continue to explain the exponential rise in world population. More people were added to the world's population in the last 50 years than in the preceding million and by 2050 there will be about nine billion people. Reductions in fertility and increased survival due to public health measures, famine control and medical advances mean that the low birth and death rates of developed countries are now being seen in developing nations. Unfortunately, due to the high fertility of previous generations, the cohorts of future parents in developing countries are already born and inevitably substantial growth in world population will continue. The largest increases will occur in regions such as Africa, where poverty and unemployment are endemic.

Falling birth rates and increasing longevity will lead to ageing populations everywhere. The number of people aged over 60 will increase fourfold by 2050, representing 21 per cent of the world's population. An increasing burden of health and social needs will pose major problems and cardiovascular disease, cancer, psychiatric conditions and injuries will predominate (Table 2.17).

In developed countries the proportionately reduced number of working-age people will find it difficult to support an increasingly dependent population and in developing countries managing the triple burdens of poverty, communicable disease and rising non-communicable disease will bring enormous pressures on resources.

TABLE **2.17** • Ten projected leading causes of disability- adjusted life years in 2020

1. CHD
2. Depression
3. Road-traffic accidents
4. Cerebrovascular disease
5. Chronic obstructive pulmonary disease
6. Lower respiratory infections
7. Tuberculosis
8. War injuries
9. Diarrhoeal disease
10. HIV

Source: Murray, C.J.L. and Lopez, A.D. (1997) Global Burden of Disease Study. *Lancet* **349**, 1498–504.

FROM WOMB TO TOMB

The identification of the causative risk factors responsible for cardiovascular disease is one of the triumphs of modern epidemiology and most individuals appreciate that adult exposure to an unhealthy lifestyle accords well with the development of atherosclerosis and eventually, outcome events. The publication of research that suggests that the origins of cardiovascular disease could be 'pre-programmed' before birth has generated much interest and controversy.

The story begins more than a hundred years ago when the first evidence for biological programming was discovered in birds during observations of the imprinting phenomenon. Since the 1960s, considerable evidence has shown that, in animals, nutrition in early life can have long-term effects on metabolism, growth and future disease processes.

To test these observations in human cohorts, Barker's group from Southampton, UK, identified the birth records of individuals from historic registers constructed as long ago as 1911. In more than 50 papers they have established the associations between low birth weight and cardiovascular parameters for both sexes. Subsequently, other independent epidemiologists have confirmed similar findings in different populations. The associations with low birth weight include:

■ raised serum cholesterol;
■ glucose intolerance and diabetes;
■ hypertension;
■ raised fibrinogen and other clotting factors;
■ increased cardiovascular death.

Barker's hypothesis is that poor fetal nutrition, in middle to late gestation, induces growth retardation and fetal adaptations that programme disease in later life. Lack of nutrients or oxygen produces a pattern of growth retardation resulting in thin, low birth weight babies with disproportion in head size, length

FROM WOMB TO TOMB

FROM WOMB TO TOMB

and weight. Cigarette smoking in pregnancy provides a contemporary illustration. Babies in developing countries, who tend to be small, do not progress to cardiovascular disease because they are proportionate in head size, length and weight.

The problem with the hypothesis is that without randomized intervention studies the evidence is easily misinterpreted. It is difficult to separate off the multiplicity of confounding postnatal influences and chief amongst these are adjustment for adult weight and socioeconomic influences. In particular, poor maternal circumstances in pregnancy predict future deprivation in the lives of her offspring, the uptake of adverse lifestyles and consequently, the development of increased cardiovascular risk.

Some of the original records from which Barker extrapolated his findings do not represent the total birth record of the area and inevitably some individuals have been lost to follow-up. This has allowed detractors to level accusations of incomplete sampling and selection bias.

Gestational age is rarely recorded and there are no measures of the actual nutritional intake of the mothers. Some of the papers are inconsistent in their findings and there is evidence of publication bias, in that the protagonists of the argument do not always cite conflicting studies that do not support the hypothesis. The effects of migration, wherein migrants assume the cardiovascular risk of their new environment, is not explained and it is hard to reconcile the position in some countries, such as Scotland, Norway and Finland, where both birth weights and cardiovascular disease are distributed in the upper range.

Despite the objections, the public health implications of the fetal origins theory demand further inquiry. Prospective methods should be used, measuring fetal growth and placental function. Until that information becomes available, common sense dictates that health professionals should promulgate good nutrition and health practices 'from womb to tomb'.

REFERENCES AND FURTHER READING

American Heart Association (1999) *Heart and Stroke Statistical Update*. American Heart Association, Dallas, TX.

Assman, G. (1991) The Prospective Cardiovascular Munster Study. *Am J Cardiol* 68, 30A–34A.

Barker, D.J.P. (ed.) (1993) *Fetal and Infant Origins of Adult Disease*. BMJ Publishing Group, London.

Beaglehole, R. (2001) Global cardiovascular disease prevention: time to get serious. *Lancet* 358, 661–3.

Chen, Z., Peto, R., Collins, R. *et al.* (1991) Serum cholesterol concentrations and coronary heart disease in population with low cholesterol concentrations. *Br Med J* 303, 276–82.

Coronary Heart Disease Statistics (1999) British Heart Foundation, London.

European Cardiovascular Disease Statistics (1999) British Heart Foundation, London.

Kannel, W.B. (1990) Contribution of the Framingham Heart Study to preventative cardiology. *J Am Coll Cardiol* 15, 206–11.

Keys, A. (1980) *Seven Countries: a Multivariate Analysis of Death and Coronary Heart Disease.* Harvard University Press, Harvard.

Law, M.R., Thompson, S.G. and Wald, N.J. (1994a) Assessing possible hazards of reducing serum cholesterol [see comments]. *Br Med J* **308**, 373–9.

Law, M.R., Wald, N.J. and Thompson, S.G. (1994b) By how much and how quickly does reduction in serum cholesterol concentration lower risk of ischaemic heart disease? [see comments]. *Br Med J* **308**, 367–72.

Law, M.R., Wald, N.J., Wu, T., Hackshaw, A. and Bailey, A. (1994c) Systematic underestimation of association between serum cholesterol concentration and ischaemic heart disease in observational studies: data from the BUPA study [see comments]. *Br Med J* **308**, 363–6.

Law, M.R., Wald, N.J. (1999) Why heart disease mortality is low in France: the time lag explanation. *Br Med J* **318**: 1471–80.

McKeigue, P.M., Shah, B. and Marmot, M.G. (1991) Relation of central obesity and insulin resistance with high diabetes prevalence and cardiovascular risk in South Asians. *Lancet* **337**, 382–6.

Murray, C.J.L. and Lopez, A.D. (1997) Global Burden of Disease Study. *Lancet* **349**, 1269–76, 1347–52 and 1436–42.

Shaper, A.G., Pocock, S.J., Walker, M. *et al.* (1981) British Regional Heart Study. *Br Med J* **283**, 179–86.

Song, Y., Sung, J. and Kim, J. (2000) Which cholesterol is related to the lowest mortality in a population with low mean cholesterol level: a 6.4-year follow up study of 482 472 Korean men. *Am J Epidemiol* **151**, 739–47.

Stamler, J. (1986) Findings of the Multiple Risk Factor Intervention Trial. *J Am Med Assoc* **254**, 2823–8.

Tunstall-Pedoe, H., Kuulasmaa, K., Mahonen, M. *et al.* (1999) Contributions of trends in survival and coronary-event rates to changes in coronary heart disease mortality: 10-year results from 37 WHO MONICA Project populations. *Lancet* **353**, 1547–57.

PART TWO

SCREENING AND ASSESSMENT

DIAGNOSIS

The interpretation of blood lipid concentrations should not be performed in isolation. The results should be applied to the individual in the knowledge of other risk factors and concurrent diseases, the family history and clinical evaluation, as discussed in Chapter 5.

There has been a tendency to see the results of blood lipid investigations as diagnoses in themselves – hypercholesterolaemia, hypertriglyceridaemia, etc. This is unfortunate and probably relates to the first classification of lipid disorders proposed by Fredrickson and colleagues at the National Institutes of Health in the USA and later adopted by the WHO (Beaumont *et al.*, 1970). This classification was based solely on laboratory parameters using a combination of cholesterol and triglyceride measurements and lipoprotein electrophoresis (Table 3.1).

It is likely that many readers will remember struggling to get to grips with the various types of hyperlipidaemia the evening before examinations, instantly forgetting them thereafter. Although now largely abandoned, there is no doubt that this classification enabled much progress to be made in understanding lipoprotein metabolism and the biochemical basis of the hyperlipidaemias.

New ways of classifying hyperlipidaemias have been developed because the WHO classification does not provide insight into the underlying diagnosis or pathophysiological abnormalities. Type II hyperlipidaemia, for example, may be due on the one hand to hypothyroidism (an important secondary cause of hypercholesterolaemia) and on the other to an inborn error of cholesterol metabolism such as familial hypercholesterolaemia (FH). In addition, HDL is not considered in the WHO classification.

The most useful classification of blood lipid disorders is into primary and secondary dyslipidaemias. Dyslipidaemia is preferable to hyperlipidaemia because qualitative as well as quantitative abnormalities occur, and in the case of HDL the abnormality is often low concentrations.

Most laboratories will provide cholesterol and triglyceride concentrations, but unfortunately some laboratories still resist clinicians' requests for HDL cholesterol measurements.

TABLE **3.1** • WHO classification of hyperlipidaemias and hyperlipoproteinaemias

Type	Appearance of serum	Lipids		
		Cholesterol	Triglycerides	Fasting chylomicrons
I	'Cream layer'; clear infranatant	Normal or ↑	Greatly ↑	↑
IIa	Clear	↑	Normal	Absent
IIb	Clear or faintly turbid	↑	↑	Absent
III	Usually turbid, may be also faint 'cream layer'	↑	↑	Present, may be ↑
IV	Usually turbid	Normal or ↑	↑	Absent
V	'Cream layer'; turbid infranatant	Normal or ↑	Greatly ↑	↑

Type	Lipoprotein pattern			Electrophoretic mobility
	LDL	VLDL	HDL	
I	Normal or ↓	Mildly ↑, normal or ↓	↓	Chylomicron at origin
IIa	↑	Normal or ↓	Normal or ↓	β band ↑
IIb	↑	↑	Normal or ↓	β band ↑, pre-β band ↑
III	Density 1.006[a]–1.019 ↑ Density 1.019–1.063 ↓	↑[b]	Normal or ↓	'Broad β' band
IV	Normal or ↓	↑	Normal or ↓	Pre-β band ↑
V	Normal or ↓	↑	Usually ↓	Chylomicrons and pre-β band ↑

[a] Intermediate density lipoproteins. Source: Beaumont, J.L., Carlson, L.A., Cooper, G.R. *et al.* (1970) *Bull WHO* **43**, 891–915.
[b] 'Floating' β-lipoproteins – density <1.006 g/mL with β-electrophoretic mobility.

It is difficult to understand this attitude. In defence, some laboratories claim budgetary problems, but perhaps the real reason is that the measurement of HDL cholesterol is still a manual method and therefore inconvenient for the laboratory. It is hoped that the introduction of direct methods will make HDL cholesterol concentrations easier to obtain.

Without a full lipid profile including HDL, the situation is akin to assessing a patient with a low haemoglobin without access to red cell morphology or measures of haematinics. HDL cholesterol is important in its own right in helping better to determine individual CHD risk. Furthermore, with knowledge of the full profile it is possible to calculate LDL cholesterol – which is the major therapeutic target in most patients. LDL cholesterol is determined using the Friedewald formula (Friedewald *et al.*, 1972) (all concentrations in mmol/L):

LDL cholesterol = total cholesterol − HDL cholesterol − total triglyceride/2.19

The function, total triglyceride/2.19, provides an estimate of VLDL cholesterol based on the usual lipid composition of this lipoprotein. It is reasonably accurate when total triglyceride levels are below 4.5 mmol/L, but the formula is unreliable when triglycerides are high. In this situation, LDL cholesterol can be measured after removal of triglyceride-rich lipoproteins by ultracentrifugation, which is available in specialist centres. It is best to obtain at least two and preferably three lipid profiles before making long-term decisions on management, particularly before deciding on drug therapy in primary prevention.

Most laboratories report biochemical parameters as locally determined reference ranges. These are derived from measurement of the particular analyte in many samples (often obtained from blood donors) with calculation of the mean together with a measure of the distribution of the measurements around the mean. The reference range is often reported as the mean ±1 or 2 standard deviations.

This traditional method of reporting reference ranges is inappropriate for lipid measurements. It is useful, however, to report results in relation to desirable lipid levels in terms of CHD risk. Many laboratories have adopted this approach and emphasize on the report form the importance of assessing overall risk. Taking into account major findings from epidemiological studies relating increasing cholesterol to CHD, several cut-points have evolved somewhat arbitrarily but have received general acceptance by national and international bodies.

Countries where the standard unit is mmol/L are at a disadvantage as the cut-point levels are often not round numbers. This is because the original cut-points were defined as round numbers in mg/dL which, when converted to mmol/L, are no longer round numbers. Thus the desirable level of cholesterol is taken as below 200 mg/dL. This becomes 5.2 when converted to mmol/L. More recently, bodies producing guidelines have sensibly rounded this to 5 mmol/L.

The goals of therapy and guidelines adopted by the National Cholesterol Education Program (NCEP) Adult Treatment Panel III (Anonymous, 2001) and the European Atherosclerosis Society (Wood *et al.*, 1998) are shown in Table 3.2 for comparison. Although there are major similarities between these two major sets of guidelines, there are differences in detail, which are worthy of comment. The NCEP focus is on LDL cholesterol (<100 mg/dL; 2.6 mmol/L is considered optimal) the measurement of which is widely available in the USA. In the European guidelines, total cholesterol is the primary lipid criterion (<5.0 mmol/L; 190 mg/dL is considered optimal); although an LDL cholesterol goal is also given (<3.0 mmol/L; 115 mg/dL is considered optimal). When the decision has been made to treat, whether in primary or secondary prevention, identical treatment goals apply in the European guidelines. In the NCEP, LDL cholesterol goals are determined by the category of CHD risk. The current European guidelines, as with previous ones, emphasize the importance of the calculation of individual CHD risk when considering lipid-lowering drug therapy for primary prevention. Useful

TABLE **3.2(a)** • National Cholesterol Education Program, Adult Treatment Panel III

Categories of risk which modify LDL-C goals

Risk category	LDL goal (mg/dL)
CHD and CHD risk equivalents[a]	<100
Multiple (2+) risk factors[b]	<130
0–1 risk factor	<160

[a] Diabetes is regarded as a CHD risk equivalent.
[b] Major risk factors (exclusive of LDL-C): cigarette smoking; hypertension (blood pressure $\geq$140/90 mmHg); low HDL-C (<40 mg/dL)[c]; family history of premature CHD (CHD in male first-degree relative <55 years; CHD in female first-degree relative <65 years); age (men $\geq$45 years; women $\geq$55 years).
[c] HDL-C $\geq$60 mg/dL counts as a 'negative' risk factor; its presence removes one risk factor from the total count.

LDL cholesterol goals and cut-points for therapeutic lifestyle changes (TLC) and drug therapy in different risk categories

Risk category	LDL goal (mg/dL)	LDL level to initiate TLC	LDL level to consider drug therapy
CHD or CHD risk equivalents (10-year risk >20%)	<100	$\geq$100	$\geq$130 (100–129 drug optional)
2 + risk factors (10-year risk <20%)	<130	$\geq$130	10-year risk 10–20% $\geq$130 10-year risk <10% $\geq$160
0–1 risk factor	<160	$\geq$160	$\geq$190 (160–189 drug optional)

Source: Executive Summary of the Third Report of the National Cholesterol Education Program (NCEP) Expert Panel on Detection, Evaluation and Treatment of High Blood Cholesterol in Adults (Adult Treatment Panel III) (2001). *J Am Med Assoc* **285**, 2486–97.

TABLE **3.2(b)** • European Atherosclerosis guidelines: management of hypercholesterolaemia[a]

Therapeutic group	Conservative measures (weight loss, lipid-lowering diet)	Drugs (based on LDL-C)
Cholesterol 5.2–6.5 mmol/L	Effective in majority	Only in CHD or very high risk and unresponsive to diet
LDL-C 3.5–4.5 mmol/L Cholesterol 6.5–7.8 mmol/L	Need close dietary compliance	CHD or high risk if LDL >3.5 mmol/L and unresponsive to diet
LDL-C 4.5–5.5 mmol/L Cholesterol 7.8 mmol/L	Most respond adequately	Justified even in absence of other risk factors in genetic
LDL-C >5.5 mmol/L	Needs close dietary compliance Three-month trial	forms of hypercholesterolaemia

Factors affecting risk. Modifiable factors: hypertension, cigarette smoking, diabetes mellitus, obesity, low HDL-C, high fibrinogen; other factors: personal history of CHD, family history of premature vascular disease, male sex, postmenopausal women.
[a] Source: International Task Force (1992) Prevention of coronary heart disease: scientific background and new clinical guidelines. Recommendations of the European Atherosclerosis Society. *Nutr Metab Cardiovasc Dis* **2**, 113–56.

TABLE **3.3** • Clinical identification of the metabolic syndrome

Risk factor	Defining level
Abdominal obesity[a] (waist circumference)[b]	
Men	>102 cm (>40 inches)
Women	>88 cm (>35 inches)
Triglycerides	≥150 mg/dL (1.7 mmol/L)
HDL-C	
Men	<40 mg/dL (1.04 mmol/L)
Women	<50 mg/dL (1.3 mmol/L)
Blood pressure	≥130/≥85 mmHg
Fasting glucose	>110 mg/dL (6.1 mmol/L)

[a] The presence of abdominal obesity is more highly correlated with metabolic risk factors than is an elevated body mass index (BMI). A simple measure of waist circumference is recommended to identify the body weight component of the metabolic syndrome.

[b] Some male patients can develop multiple risk factors when the waist circumference is only slightly increased (94–102 cm, 37–40 inches). Such patients may have strong genetic contribution to insulin resistance and they should benefit from changes in lifestyle.

charts are provided for this purpose based on data from the Framingham prospective study. High-risk individuals are defined as those whose 10-year CHD risk exceeds 20 per cent or will exceed 20 per cent if projected to age 60. NCEP for the first time provides a point scoring system based on Framingham alongside their more traditional risk categories. Other new features of NCEP (ATPIII) (Anonymous, 2001) include increased attention to diabetes mellitus and the metabolic syndrome (Table 3.3). Diabetic patients without symptomatic CHD are considered as CHD risk equivalent; in other words diabetic patients, many of whom will have multiple risk factors, should be treated in terms of lipid lowering as if they already had CHD. Patients with the metabolic syndrome (a syndrome closely linked to insulin resistance), which represents a constellation of lipid and non-lipid risk factors of metabolic origin, are identified as candidates for intensified therapeutic lifestyle changes. Diabetes is discussed in detail in Chapter 11.

Beyond LDL cholesterol, NCEP defines low HDL cholesterol (<40 mg/dL; 1.04 mmol/L) as a major risk factor which modifies LDL goals. High HDL cholesterol (>60 mg/dL; 1.55 mmol/L) is regarded as a negative risk factor and its presence removes one risk factor from the total risk factor count. In the European guidelines, the risk factor charts assume an HDL cholesterol of 1.0 mmol/L (39 mg/dL) for men and 1.1 mmol/L (43 mg/dL) for women. It is acknowledged that CHD risk is higher than indicated in the charts for individuals with low HDL. In some national guidelines, for example the New Zealand and the British, it is the total cholesterol/HDL cholesterol ratio that is the lipid parameter entered in the risk factor charts.

NCEP has lowered serum triglyceride cut-points compared with previous reports. Normal serum triglycerides are regarded as <150 mg/dL (1.7 mmol/L). When serum triglycerides are high (200–499 mg/dL; 2.3–5.6 mmol/L), NCEP identifies non-HDL cholesterol (total cholesterol − HDL cholesterol) as a secondary target of therapy. This takes into account cholesterol carried in atherogenic remnant particles. The treatment goal for non-HDL cholesterol is set 30 mg/dL (0.78 mmol/L) higher than LDL cholesterol. In the European guidelines, raised serum triglycerides are defined as >2.0 mmol/L (>180 mg/dL); CHD risk is higher than indicated in the risk charts in this situation.

Some laboratories measure apoprotein levels for the assessment of dyslipidaemic patients. The usefulness of Apo E phenotyping is discussed in the section on remnant particle disease, and the identification of C-II deficiency in the section on familial chylomicronaemia, later in this chapter. These estimations are available in specialist lipid referral centres.

The question arises as to whether routine laboratories should adopt other apoprotein measurements to help determine CHD risk, such as Apo A-I (the major HDL protein) and Apo B (the major LDL protein). These measurements are relatively easy to perform using automated immunochemical methods. However, standardization of these assays between different laboratories and different countries is not fully developed.

Apo B theoretically should allow the assessment of the atherogenic lipoprotein particle burden. One molecule of Apo B is present per LDL particle and in addition is found in VLDL and remnant particles. Measurement of Apo B may be clinically useful in certain situations. In a patient with CHD and an apparently 'normal' cholesterol concentration, Apo B may be raised as discussed in the section on familial combined hyperlipidaemia. The question arises as to whether the additional measurement of Apo B enables better risk categorization over and above the simple lipid profile of cholesterol, triglyceride, HDL cholesterol and LDL cholesterol. A recent analysis of the huge AMORIS (Apolipoprotein-related Mortality Risk) study based in Sweden has provided important additional information (Walldius *et al.*, 2001). AMORIS has data on 175 553 individuals (76 831 women) followed for 66.8 months during which there were 1223 fatal myocardial infarctions. In multivariate analysis adjusted for age, total cholesterol and triglycerides, Apo B and Apo B/A-I ratio were strongly and positively related to increased risk of fatal infarction in both sexes. Increasing Apo A-I concentrations were inversely related to risk. In this study, Apo B was a stronger predictor of risk than LDL cholesterol in both sexes. These findings are supported by data from the Quebec heart study, amongst others. Whether the Apo B/A-I ratio is a better predictor of risk than LDL cholesterol/HDL cholesterol ratio was not tested in AMORIS and other prospective studies are awaited. Ongoing studies are employing reference materials for measurement of apoproteins B and A-I provided by the WHO International Federation of Clinical Chemistry, which hopefully will overcome previous problems associated with disparate methods and reference materials.

The importance of lipoprotein(a) as a risk factor in the presence of hypercholesterolaemia has been discussed elsewhere (page 21). The authors use lipoprotein(a) measurement in certain groups of patients for further assessment of CHD risk. In young adults with heterozygous FH, particularly females, a high lipoprotein(a) measurement would point to more aggressive treatment. Similarly, in primary prevention a high lipoprotein(a) concentration may tip the balance in favour of drug treatment.

The epidemiological studies that link increasing fibrinogen to CHD risk are convincing and, although not a 'lipid factor', the authors certainly include this parameter in their CHD risk assessment. In addition, C-reactive protein and other inflammatory markers may be useful additional measures of vascular risk in the future.

There is no doubt that new biochemical and genetic measurements to identify vascular risk more precisely will be developed in the future together with non-invasive imaging [such as carotid intima-media thickness (IMT), magnetic resonance imaging (MRI), etc.] to identify significant early disease.

SECONDARY DYSLIPIDAEMIAS

Faced with significantly abnormal lipid concentrations the clinician must, first of all, exclude possible secondary causes of dyslipidaemia. The more common secondary causes together with the resulting lipid abnormalities are shown in Table 3.4. Additional biochemical tests may be needed to exclude or confirm these disorders. Common secondary causes presenting to the primary care physician are hypothyroidism, obesity, non-insulin-dependent diabetes, high alcohol intake and some drug therapies.

Although hypothyroidism is most commonly linked to hypercholesterolaemia due to increased LDL cholesterol concentrations, any dyslipidaemia can occur in this condition. The clinician should have a low threshold for requesting a thyroid stimulating hormone (TSH) estimation. Several secondary and tertiary referrals to the Lipid Clinic have required extremely tactful letters to referring physicians. One lady's diet-resistant

TABLE **3.4** • Secondary causes of dyslipidaemia

Cause	Effects		
	Cholesterol	Triglyceride	HDL
Diabetes mellitus			
NIDDM		↑	↓
IDDM: poor control		↑	↓
IDDM: good control		↓	↑
Hypothyroidism	↑		
Obesity	↑	↑	
Alcohol abuse		↑	
Chronic renal failure	↑	↑	
Nephrotic syndrome	↑ ±	↑	
Cholestasis	↑		
Acute hepatocellular disease	↑	↑	↓
Gout		↑	
Anorexia nervosa	↑		
Bulimia		↑	
Pregnancy		↑	
Immunoglobin excess	↑	↑	

hypercholesterolaemia was attributed to the fact that she worked in a fish and chip shop, but it responded to thyroxine therapy following the diagnosis of hypothyroidism. A referral from a consultant colleague posed a potentially difficult clinical problem: a man with CHD and hypercholesterolaemia was intolerant of statin drugs because of aches and pains. He was hypothyroid clinically as well as biochemically.

Dyslipidaemia often occurs in association with other risk factors that require drug therapy, such as hypertension. Some commonly used antihypertensives may adversely affect blood lipid levels. In patients requiring multiple drug therapy, care should be taken in the choice of antihypertensive agent for the dyslipidaemic patient.

Other drugs may have adverse effects on blood lipid concentrations – particularly the corticosteroids, which can increase both cholesterol and triglyceride (Table 3.5). A drug-induced dyslipidaemia seen more frequently follows the increasing use of isotretinoin compounds for severe acne. These drugs may produce a mixed dyslipidaemia, often accompanied by a reduction in HDL cholesterol. The effects of these drugs (as with most other drugs that adversely affect lipids) are more pronounced in those patients with underlying lipid disorders and other secondary causes such as obesity, excess alcohol and diabetes. The dose of isotretinoin may have to be reduced if the dyslipidaemia fails to respond to dietary measures.

Relatively new causes of dyslipidaemia (often severe) are the antiretroviral drugs often used in combination (highly active antiretroviral therapy; HAART) for human immuno-deficiency virus (HIV) infection. Patients receiving HAART are an increasingly common reason for referral to the Lipid Clinic. This is discussed in Chapter 11 (page 331).

Abnormal liver function tests with modest abnormalities in transaminases and alkaline phosphatase in patients with mixed dyslipidaemia are more likely to be secondary to the dyslipidaemia than a cause of it. Mixed dyslipidaemia, particularly when there is associated glucose intolerance or frank diabetes, is often associated with fatty liver, which is readily seen on ultrasound. These changes resolve when the dyslipidaemia is

TABLE **3.5** • Effects of drugs on lipids, lipoproteins and apoproteins

Drug	Cholesterol	Triglyceride	LDL-C	HDL-C	Apo A-1	Apo B
Retinoids	↑ 25%	↑ 100%	↑ 35%	↓ 30%	→	↑ 35%
Cyclosporin	↑ 40%	↑ 160%	↑ 60%	↓ 15%	↓ 15%	↑ 80%
Phenytoin	→ ↑	→	↓ 20%	↑ 30%	↑ 10%	↑ 15%
Phenobarbitone	↑ 10%	→	↑ 20%	↑ 40%	↑ 10%	↑ 15%
Carbamazepine	↑ 0–15%	↑ 15%	↑ 15%	↑ 15%	↑ 10%	→ ↑
Valproate	↓ 10%	→	↓ 15%	→	→	→
Heparin		↓ 35%				
β-Agonists	→	→	→	↑ 10%		
Oestrogens	*	↑	↓	↑	↑	↓
Progestogens	*	→ ↑	→ ↑	↓	↓	
Corticosteroids	↑	↑	↑	↑		

* Effects depend on type of oestrogen and progestogen and route of administration.

treated. Liver abnormalities resulting in secondary hypercholesterolaemia are usually associated with cholestasis such as primary biliary cirrhosis and sclerosing cholangitis.

PRIMARY DYSLIPIDAEMIAS

Having excluded secondary dyslipidaemias on clinical grounds and, where necessary, with further laboratory analyses, it is important to make a diagnosis of the primary disorder where possible (Table 3.6). The clinical relevance of this process will become apparent following discussion of the various conditions. Diagnosis of the different dyslipidaemias carries different implications for CHD risk, family screening and genetic counselling, and clinical management.

The underlying biochemical and genetic mechanisms are well understood in some of the primary disorders such as FH and dysbetalipoproteinaemia (remnant particle disease, type III dyslipidaemia). In others, such as familial combined hyperlipidaemia, much still needs to be learned.

FAMILIAL HYPERCHOLESTEROLAEMIA (FH)

FH is the best understood of the primary dyslipidaemias. Studies of FH patients have demonstrated the importance of raised cholesterol as a critical CHD risk factor but have also enabled major advances to be made in the understanding of cholesterol metabolism. Experiments on cultured skin fibroblasts from homozygous FH patients helped in the discovery of the LDL receptor by the Nobel laureates Michael Brown and Joseph Goldstein in Dallas (Brown and Goldstein, 1986).

Inheritance

FH is an autosomal dominant condition which in the heterozygous state affects approximately 1:500 in European populations. In some populations, such as the Lebanese and South Africans of Dutch descent, it is more common – approximately 1:100.

A typical family tree is shown in Figure 3.1. Homozygotes or compound heterozygotes are fortunately extremely rare, at approximately one in a million. The vertical transmission through three generations is readily apparent, with roughly equal numbers of offspring affected and an equal sex distribution.

Pathophysiology

The genetic abnormality lies in the LDL receptor gene resulting in either absent or defective LDL receptor activity. Over 400 different mutations in the LDL receptor gene resulting in the FH phenotype have so far been described, and undoubtedly many more remain to be discovered. Halving of normal receptor function in the heterozygote results in LDL cholesterol levels that are increased two- to threefold. The plasma half-life of LDL is also prolonged. In FH homozygotes, LDL cholesterol levels may be elevated sixfold.

TABLE 3.6 • Primary dyslipidaemias[a]

Disease	WHO phenotype	Typical lipid levels (mmol/L)	Lipoproteins	CHD risk	Pancreatic risk	Possible clinical signs
Polygenic hypercholesterolaemia	IIa	Chol 6.5–9, trig <2.3	LDL ↑	+	–	Xanthelasma, corneal arcus
Familial hypercholesterolaemia	IIa	Chol 7.5–16, trig <2.3	LDL ↑	+ + +	–	Tendon xanthoma, arcus, xanthelasma
Familial defective apoprotein B$_{100}$	IIa	Chol 7.5–16, trig <2.3	LDL ↑	+ + +	–	Tendon xanthoma, arcus, xanthelasma
Familial combined hyperlipidaemia	IIa, IIb, IV or V	Chol 6.5–10, trig 2.3–12	LDL ↑, VLDL ↑, HDL ↓	+ +	–	Arcus, xanthelasma
Remnant particle disease	III	Chol 9–14, trig 9–14	IDL ↑	+ + +	±	Palmar striae, tuberoeruptive xanthomata
Familial hypertriglyceridaemia	IV, V	Chol 6.5–12, trig 10–30	VLDL ↑, chylomicrons ↑	?	+ +	Eruptive xanthomata, lipaemia retinalis, hepatosplenomegaly
Lipoprotein lipase deficiency	I	Chol <6.5, trig 10–30	Chylomicrons ↑	–	+ + +	Eruptive xanthomata, lipaemia retinalis, hepatosplenomegaly
High HDL	–	HDL chol >2.0	HDL ↑	–	–	–

Chol, cholesterol; trig, triglycerides.
[a] Source: International Task Force for Prevention of Coronary Heart Disease (1992) Prevention of coronary heart disease: scientific background and new clinical guidelines. Recommendation of the European Atherosclerosis Society. *Nutr Metab Cardiovasc Dis* **2**, 113–56.

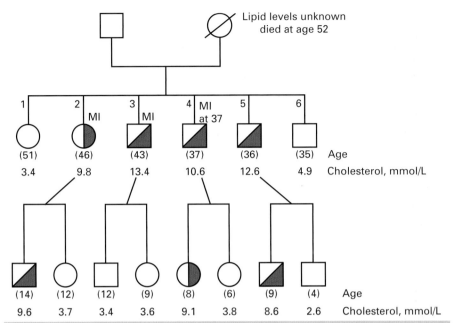

FIGURE **3.1** • Typical family tree demonstrating inheritance of familial hypercholesterolaemia. MI, myocardial infarction. Source: Mann, J.L. (1989) *Lipid Rev* **3**, 33.

Clinical features

The clinical stigmata of FH are often striking and sometimes spectacular. Corneal arcus (Figure 3.2) and xanthelasma (Figure 3.3) can occur in young adults but the clinical hallmark is the presence of tendon xanthomata (Figure 3.4). These cholesterol deposits are seen commonly in the Achilles tendon and in extensor tendons over the back of the hands. Subperiosteal xanthomata also occur at the tibial tuberosity.

The development of xanthomata is a function of age, LDL cholesterol concentrations, local trauma and possibly genetic factors; in some series 70 per cent of patients

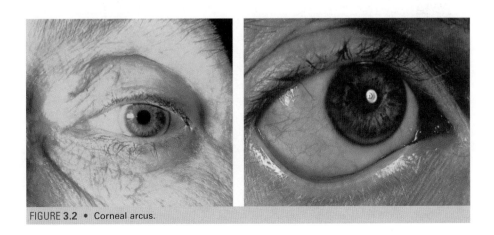

FIGURE **3.2** • Corneal arcus.

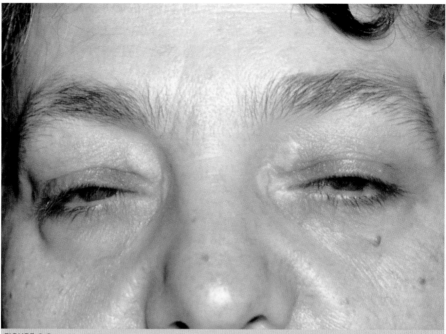

FIGURE **3.3** • Xanthelasmata.

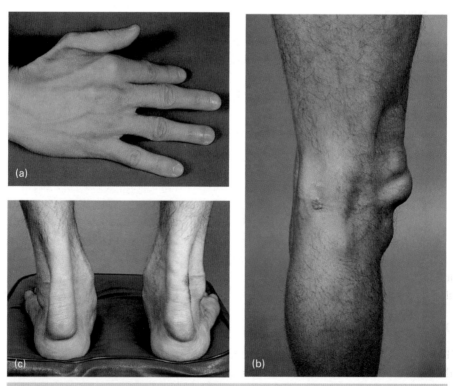

FIGURE **3.4** • Tendon xanthomata in (a) extensor tendons of hand, (b) patellar tendon and subperiosteal xanthomata and (c) Achilles tendon.

have xanthomata by the age of 30 years and 90 per cent by the age of 40 years. Xanthomata are usually asymptomatic but occasionally tenosynovitis occurs, particularly in the ankles. The most important feature of xanthomata (and the reason for their multiple illustration in this book) is their lack of recognition by physicians and surgeons. Our favourite explanation given to one patient was that the xanthomata on the back of the hand were as a result of rugby playing injuries! In FH homozygotes, quite bizarre xanthomata may be present with orange-yellow deposits in the skin (planar xanthomata) over the buttocks, knees and hands and in the interdigital web between the first and second fingers.

Other causes of tendon xanthomata are exceedingly rare but include cerebrotendinous xanthomatosis, phytosterolaemia, familial ligand defective Apo B, an autosomal recessive form of hypercholesterolaemia, and occasionally patients with type III dyslipidaemia.

The most important clinical feature of FH is the development of premature and extensive atherosclerosis. Although the contribution to overall CHD within the population is small, the effect can be devastating in individual families. In the early observational studies the average age of onset of CHD in male heterozygotes was 43 years and in females 53 years. In homozygotes symptomatic CHD can occur in childhood and very few survive past the age of 30 years. In a prospective study of FH heterozygotes in the UK (Table 3.7) a 100-fold increased risk of death was observed in young adults aged 20–39 years (Scientific Steering Committee, 1991).

TABLE 3.7 • Standardized mortality ratios (SMR) for coronary heart disease and all causes in prospective follow-up study of patients with familial hypercholesterolaemia

Age (years)	Coronary heart disease		All causes	
	SMR	95% Confidence intervals	SMR	95% Confidence intervals
20–39	9686[a]	(3670–21 800)	902[a]	(329–1950)
40–59	519[a]	(224–1020)	253[a]	(134–432)
60–74	44[b]	(1–244)	69	(22–160)
20–74	386[a]	(210–639)	183[b]	(117–273)

Source: Scientific Steering Committee, Simon Broome FH Register (1991) *Br Med J* **303**, 893.
[a] $P < 0.001$; [b] $P < 0.01$.

The estimated percentage risk of CHD symptoms, and death from myocardial infarction (MI) in FH heterozygotes based on several reports from different countries is shown in Table 3.8. The earlier onset of symptomatic disease in males is clearly evident.

Diagnosis

The diagnosis of FH is an important one to make. The high risk of premature CHD in the absence of other risk factors warrants aggressive lipid-lowering therapy, often with a combination of drugs. It is the authors' practice to undertake regular non-invasive testing for silent ischaemia in FH heterozygotes, with stress ECGs or thalliums every 1–2 years.

TABLE **3.8** • Estimated percentage risk of CHD symptoms and CHD death in FH heterozygotes

Age	Females		Males	
	CHD symptoms	CHD death	CHD symptoms	CHD death
40	3	0	20	–
50	20	2	45	25
60	45	15	75	50
70	75	30	–	80

Adapted from Goldstein, J.L., Hobbs, H.H. and Brown, M.S. (2001) In *The Metabolic and Molecular Bases of Inherited Disease* (eds C.R. Scriver, J.B. Stanbury, J.B. Wyngaarden and D.G. Fredrickson), 7th edn, McGraw-Hill, New York, pp. 2863–931.

This is particularly important if the age of onset of CHD is early in a particular family. Family screening is mandatory in FH. The majority of heterozygotes remain unidentified and untreated. Screening the families of affected individuals provides a pick-up rate of approximately 50 per cent, given the autosomal dominant transmission. Screening of 200 relatives based on cholesterol concentration revealed 121 new cases in one study in the UK. It was estimated that to identify a similar number of FH heterozygotes, 60 000 people from the general population would be required (Bhatnagar *et al.*, 2000). In Holland where there is a large screening project for FH based on DNA testing in families based on identified LDL receptor mutations, 2000 new cases have been identified in 5 years (Umans-Eckenhausen *et al.*, 2001). The condition exhibits complete phenotypic expression in children and it is our practice to advise testing of children around the age of 10 years.

The diagnosis is straightforward when there is a strong family history of premature CHD together with high cholesterol and xanthomata in the index case (Table 3.9). However, not all individuals have xanthomata and family history may be non-contributory. Here the primary care physician is in an excellent position to help in the diagnosis by family screening. As other hyperlipidaemias do not tend to be expressed in childhood, the finding of high cholesterol in children and adolescents strongly points to the diagnosis of FH. A simple lipid profile with calculation of LDL cholesterol is usually all that is required. Although specialist laboratories can now undertake LDL receptor gene analysis, this is not yet standard practice as there are such a large number of mutations (Figure 3.5) and many remain to be identified. In a family with a known mutation, DNA testing for the receptor gene defect is quick and effective and can be performed on saliva as well as blood samples. The practical and ethical issues concerning genetic testing for familial hypercholesterolaemia have been well discussed (Humphries *et al.*, 1997).

FAMILIAL LIGAND DEFECTIVE APOPROTEIN B (FDB)

FDB was first described in 1986 by Vega and Grundy (reviewed by Kane and Havel, 2001). In lipoprotein kinetic studies it was observed that LDL from some donors was cleared more slowly from the circulation in individuals with normal LDL receptor function.

TABLE **3.9** • Diagnosis of heterozygous familial hypercholesterolaemia

Definite FH	Possible FH
(a) Child under 16: total cholesterol above 6.7 mmol/L or LDL cholesterol above 4.0 mmol/L; adult: total cholesterol above 7.5 mmol/L or LDL-C above 4.9 mmol/L	
Plus	Plus
(b) Tendon xanthomata in patient or relative (parent, child, grandparent, sibling, aunt, uncle)	(b) Family history of myocardial infarction below age 50 in second-degree relative or below 60 in first-degree relative
Or	Or
(c) DNA-based evidence of an LDL receptor mutation	(c) Family history of raised cholesterol in first-degree relative or a history of cholesterol above 7.5 mmol/L in second-degree relative

Based on the Simon Broome FH register diagnostic criteria (1991) *Br Med J* **303**, 893–6.

This LDL did not bind normally to cultured human fibroblasts with consequent decreased endocytosis of accumulation of cellular cholesterol ester. Further *in vitro* studies suggested that there was a defect in LDL Apo B in the region involved in binding to the LDL receptor. Subsequently genomic DNA analysis (Soria *et al.*, 1989) revealed a point mutation in Apo B: a CGG-to-CAG mutation at the codon for amino acid 3500 resulting in an arginine to glutamine substitution. This substitution, surprisingly for a single

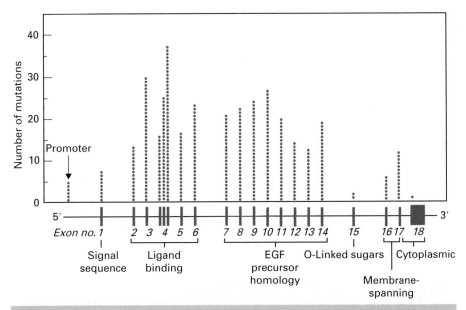

FIGURE **3.5** • Mutations in various exons of the LDL receptor gene in patients with familial hypercholesterolaemia. Source: Goldstein, J.L., Hobbs, H.H. and Brown, M.S. (2001) In *The Metabolic and Molecular Bases of Inherited Disease* (eds C.R. Scriver, J.B. Stanbury, J.B. Wyngaarden and D.G. Fredrickson), 7th edn, McGraw-Hill, New York, pp. 2863–931.

substitution, has quite marked effects on the disposition of Apo B charged amino acid residues in the ligand-binding domain. A further mutation at the same 3500 amino acid involving an arginine-to-tryptophan substitution has also been described. Homozygotes for FDB have been described.

In terms of effects on lipoprotein metabolism, a defect in the ligand-binding domain of Apo B would be expected to cause selective LDL accumulation. Unlike the situation in FH, increased fractional conversion of IDL to LDL would not be expected as Apo B is not a significant ligand for remnant removal. Diminished hepatic LDL uptake leads to up-regulation of LDL receptors and kinetic studies have shown increased fractional catabolic rate for IDL and decreased LDL production rate. Therefore less severe hypercholesterolaemia than in FH is observed in FDB. On average, LDL cholesterol concentrations are 7.3 mmol/L (281 mg/dL) but with significant variation. Triglyceride and HDL cholesterol concentrations are unaffected. In patients with FDB it is likely that plasma LDL cholesterol concentrations are affected by the presence of other genetic factors, e.g. polymorphism of the LDL receptor.

FDB may mimic the FH phenotype with high levels of LDL cholesterol and clinical stigma of early corneal arcus and tendon xanthomata. As a whole, FDB is associated with lower CHD risk than heterozygous FH. However, when FDB and FH are matched for LDL cholesterol, the risk is similar. In individuals of European descent the frequency of FDB has been calculated at between 1:500 to 1:600. It is rare in other populations.

More recently, a further functional significant mutation in the ligand-binding domain of Apo B has been described involving an arginine to cystine substitution at amino acid 3531.

Patients with FDB do respond to statin drug therapy, probably reflecting increased removal of Apo E-containing remnant particles through up-regulated hepatic LDL receptors.

FAMILIAL COMBINED HYPERLIPIDAEMIA (FCH)

FCH is a well-recognized clinical entity. It is more common than FH, with a frequency of approximately 1–2 per cent, but as yet the genetics of the disorder and their interaction with environmental factors remain to be resolved. It is likely that the clinical syndrome represents a heterogeneous group of genetic abnormalities interacting with different environmental and other genetic factors.

Inheritance

FCH was first described in 1973, following a study of 500 MI survivors and their families in Seattle, USA (Goldstein et al., 1973). Of these patients (MI < 55 years), 11 per cent were identified as coming from families in which multiple lipoprotein abnormalities were found. Roughly a third of the affected family members had isolated hypercholesterolaemia, a third had mixed lipaemia and a third had isolated hypertriglyceridaemia.

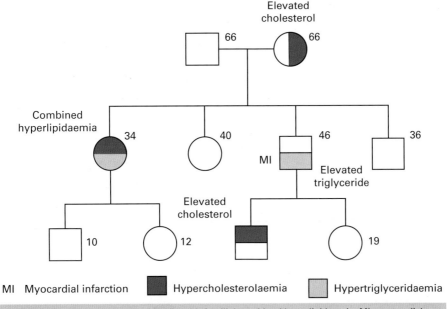

FIGURE 3.6 • Typical pedigree of family with familial combined hyperlipidaemia. MI, myocardial infarction; solid black, hypercholesterolaemia; shaded, hypertriglyceridaemia. Source: Bierman, E.L. (1989) *Lipid Rev* **3**, 81.

It has been estimated that FCH accounts for about 10–15 per cent of myocardial infarction in North America and Europe.

The original interpretation of the family studies was that the condition was inherited as an autosomal dominant. This has been questioned and others have suggested a polygenic inheritance. Until the genetic defects are determined, the exact inheritance will remain an open question. A typical FCH pedigree is shown in Figure 3.6.

Pathophysiology

A consistent finding in FCH is overproduction of Apo B-containing lipoproteins by the liver. The resulting lipid phenotype depends on the efficacy or otherwise of the catabolic pathways. It is interesting that individuals heterozygous for familial lipoprotein lipase deficiency develop a similar lipoprotein profile to FCH.

Obesity and insulin resistance appear to be commoner in FCH and undoubtedly this will contribute to the variable phenotypic expression with hypertriglyceridaemia, low HDL cholesterol, remnant particles and the presence of small, dense LDL. Apo B concentrations are increased in FCH with often a decrease in LDL cholesterol/Apo B ratio, indicating an increased number of lipoprotein particles.

An association has been described between the presence of coronary atherosclerosis and what was termed hyperapobetalipoproteinaemia, i.e. increased Apo B but normal cholesterol levels in LDL. Frequently these individuals were also hypertriglyceridaemic. The question arises as to whether these individuals should be considered as FCH.

Clinical features

There are no typical clinical stigmata to help in the diagnosis of FCH. Tendon xanthomata do not occur. Although affected individuals may have corneal arcus and xanthelasma, these signs are not specific.

The diagnosis is often presumptive in a patient with mixed lipaemia and CHD or a strong family history of CHD. A low HDL cholesterol and increased Apo B concentration (if available) are usually present. The primary care physician or Lipid Clinic specialist is well placed to perform family screening. This forms the crux of the diagnosis: the identification of family members with multiple lipoprotein phenotypes. FCH is seen in childhood but expression is limited until the third decade.

The main reason for making the effort at diagnosis is the high CHD risk of affected individuals, including those where the main abnormality is hypertriglyceridaemia. The high risk warrants effective therapy for primary as well as secondary CHD prevention. Dietary measures are generally insufficient and drug therapy is often required, sometimes with combination therapy. A particularly severe dyslipidaemia is seen in the individual heterozygous for FH and FCH with marked xanthomatosis (tendon and tuberous) and premature CHD.

Interestingly, the lipid phenotype may change with therapy. For instance, an obese individual with mixed lipaemia (type IIb) who responds well to diet may revert to type IIa phenotype. Conversely, an individual treated with a resin drug (which may exacerbate hypertriglyceridaemia) may change from a type IIa to a IIb phenotype. The first-line therapy for most FCH patients is a statin, but in some cases combination with a fibrate or nicotinic acid is necessary.

COMMON POLYGENIC HYPERCHOLESTEROLAEMIA

This diagnosis fits the majority of patients with hypercholesterolaemia. It is really a diagnosis made after exclusion of secondary causes and the monogenic primary disorders. Polygenic hypercholesterolaemia reflects the interaction of multiple genes with environmental factors such as diet. It represents a heterogeneous group of disorders and classification will depend on the fruits of further research to pinpoint the major genetic susceptibility genes. The frequency of this disorder will vary between countries, principally as a result of different dietary intakes of saturated fat and cholesterol. It contributes significantly to differing mean cholesterol concentrations and CHD prevalence observed between countries.

Several common polymorphisms in different gene loci have been shown to determine differences in plasma cholesterol between individuals – the most studied being Apo E, Apo B and the LDL receptor gene (Humphries et al., 1999). For instance, individuals carrying the Apo E_2 allele will on average have lower plasma cholesterol concentrations (roughly 10 per cent) than individuals with other E alleles. Individuals with one or more E_4 alleles will on average have cholesterol concentrations 10 per cent higher.

A particular polymorphism of the Apo B gene (identified by the presence of a cutting site with the enzyme *Xba*I) has been shown to be associated with increased plasma cholesterol. This effect is only modest (3–8 per cent), but it is clear that the effect may be marked if this genetic polymorphism is present in an individual with other known or as yet undescribed polymorphisms at important candidate genes.

In the myocardial infarction survivor study of Goldstein *et al.* (1973), a group of patients with hypercholesterolaemia was identified whose families showed increased cholesterol levels. The prevalence of common polygenic hypercholesterolaemia will vary depending on what cut-point is taken for cholesterol. A cut-point of 7.4 mmol/L was taken in the myocardial infarction survivors study which gave a figure of 14 per cent for the frequency of the disorder.

Patients with polygenic hypercholesterolaemia do not develop any specific physical signs although corneal arcus and xanthelasmata may be present. The degree of therapy will depend mainly on assessment of overall CHD risk. Nutritional and lifestyle measures are the first-line therapy for those considered to be at low to moderate risk, whilst hypolipidaemic drug therapy is reserved for those at highest risk.

PRIMARY ISOLATED HYPERTRIGLYCERIDAEMIA

The large majority of patients with hypertriglyceridaemia have a demonstrable secondary cause, perhaps the most common being the metabolic syndrome, obesity and high alcohol intake. In some cases the disease appears to be familial and with dominant inheritance. The metabolic abnormality appears to be an increased hepatic output of large VLDL with an increased triglyceride/Apo B ratio. The genetic abnormality is not yet determined. LDL and HDL cholesterol concentrations tend to be low.

The degree of hypertriglyceridaemia will depend on whether there are additional acquired or genetic factors present to accentuate overproduction or impair the catabolism of the lipoproteins. Lipoprotein lipase activity is in the normal range but often towards the lower end of normal.

The diagnosis of familial hypertriglyceridaemia is made in an individual with isolated hypertriglyceridaemia together with demonstration of a similar lipid profile in other family members. This will differentiate it from FCH where multiple lipoprotein phenotypes would be expected. Unlike lipoprotein lipase deficiency, reduction of dietary fat will not lead to rapid amelioration of the hypertriglyceridaemia.

Individuals with familial hypertriglyceridaemia have either the type IV or the type V WHO phenotype. Those with the type V phenotype may develop the clinical signs described for the chylomicronaemia syndrome and are at risk of pancreatitis. To what extent CHD risk is increased in familial hypertriglyceridaemia is uncertain. As with other hypertriglyceridaemias (apart from lipoprotein lipase deficiency), glucose intolerance is a common accompaniment and the question arises as to whether it is insulin resistance that causes the hypertriglyceridaemia or vice versa.

Treatment of familial hypertriglyceridaemia is with nutrition and lifestyle measures together with hypolipidaemia drugs. The justification for treatment is to reduce the risk of pancreatitis, particularly in those with the type V phenotype.

The drugs of choice are fibrates, nicotinic acid and fish oils. With treatment, LDL concentrations paradoxically rise, but from low levels towards the normal range. There is evidence that non-receptor-mediated LDL catabolism is increased in hypertriglyceridaemic states and this is reduced when the triglycerides are reduced. LDL from hypertriglyceridaemic patients binds less well to the LDL receptor, which may explain this phenomenon. The use of drugs for moderate hypertriglyceridaemia remains controversial.

REMNANT PARTICLE DISEASE

Although rare, type III hyperlipidaemia (remnant particle disease, broad-beta disease, dysbetalipoproteinaemia) is particularly interesting as it represents an interaction between established genetic and other secondary factors (either genetic or acquired). It has provided evidence of the atherogenicity of remnant particles that is of relevance to other dyslipidaemias, such as those that accompany non-insulin-dependent diabetes mellitus, the metabolic syndrome and renal disease. Furthermore, it has become clear that Apo E isoforms not only form the basis of remnant particle disease but also make an impact on plasma cholesterol levels in the general population (see section above on polygenic hypercholesterolaemia, page 80).

Laboratory findings

Patients with remnant particle disease have roughly equivalent elevations in plasma cholesterol and triglyceride. In addition, there are classical findings on electrophoresis and ultracentrifugation which reflect the accumulation of the remnants of chylomicron and VLDL metabolism, namely β-VLDL. Lipoprotein electrophoresis shows the characteristic broad-beta band, and following separation of VLDL by ultracentrifugation the VLDL cholesterol to total triglyceride molar ratio is increased (>0.6). These investigations can be performed in specialist centres but they are not necessary for effective therapy as long as the clinical syndrome is recognized, together with its importance as a cause of premature atherosclerosis. Of interest is the premature peripheral vascular disease in patients with type III disease.

Pathophysiology

More than 90 per cent of individuals with remnant particle disease are homozygous for the Apo E_2 isoform. There are three common genetically determined isoforms of Apo E, as shown in Figure 3.7. Approximately two-thirds of individuals are homozygous for E_3 (the normal allele) whilst E_2 homozygosity is found in approximately 1 per cent of the population. In Apo E_2, cysteine substitutes for arginine at position 158. As a result, the ability of the apoprotein to bind to the LDL receptor (Apo B, E) is dramatically reduced.

Apo E_2 homozygosity is relatively common (1:100) but remnant particle disease is rare, affecting between 1:5000 and 1:10 000 adults. It is clear, therefore, that further abnormalities are necessary to 'stress' the system so that dyslipidaemia develops. The other factors may be genetic, such as FCH, familial hypertriglyceridaemia and FH, or environmental, such as obesity, diabetes mellitus or hypothyroidism. Type III

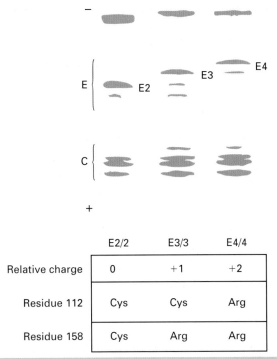

	E2/2	E3/3	E4/4
Relative charge	0	+1	+2
Residue 112	Cys	Cys	Arg
Residue 158	Cys	Arg	Arg

FIGURE 3.7 • Isoforms of Apo E. Source: Mahley and Rall (1999).

hyperlipidaemia is more prevalent in men than women. Affected women are usually postmenopausal, which possibly implicates oestrogen deficiency acting through a reduction in LDL (Apo B/E) receptors. There have been reports of amelioration of the dyslipidaemia with oestrogen replacement therapy. With the increasing availability of isoelectric focusing or PCR techniques, the identification of E_2 homozygosity has become the confirmatory test. As an aside, it is important to remember that possession of the Apo E_4 isoform has been shown to be a risk factor for the development of Alzheimer's disease. Therefore, when requesting Apo E isoforms the request should be: is the Apo E isoform compatible with remnant disease? The laboratory should report along similar lines, i.e. compatible or not compatible with remnant disease, rather than reporting the actual E isoforms.

Rarely, type III hyperlipidaemia results from dominant inheritance of a rare variant of Apo E involving substitution of acidic or neutral amino acid residues for basic ones in the receptor-binding region of Apo E. The presence of these single variants (e.g. arginine 142 – cysteine; lysine 146 – glutamic acid) is sufficient for development of the type III phenotype although it can be exacerbated by other genetic and environmental factors as in E2/2 homozygosity. It is likely that these dominant mutations directly affect receptor binding of Apo E-containing remnants to the receptor. Apoprotein E Leiden, which is characterized by a tandem duplication of amino acid residues 121–127 of Apo E, probably leads to conformation change in the receptor-binding region (Mahley and Rall, 1999).

Clinical features

Remnant disease is associated with striking clinical stigmata (Figure 3.8). Yellow/
orange streaking of the palmar creases together with soft tissue xanthomata either side
of the crease are called palmar xanthoma and are pathognomonic of the disease. In addition, tuberous xanthomata resembling cauliflower florets are often present at the elbows
and knees. Sometimes tuberous xanthomata are surrounded by satellite lesions resembling eruptive xanthomata; these are known as tubero-eruptive xanthomata. With
coexistent FH, tendon xanthomata may be present.

Premature and extensive atherosclerosis is the most important clinical feature of
remnant disease. In one series, about 30 per cent had premature CHD and a similar
proportion had peripheral vascular disease. Occasionally, if the triglycerides are grossly
elevated with hyperchylomicronaemia, pancreatitis may occur.

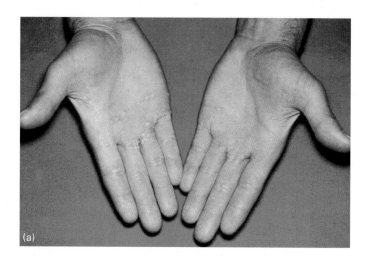

(a)

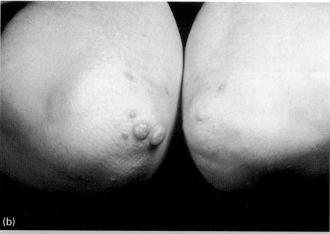

(b)

FIGURE **3.8** • Clinical stigmata of type III dyslipoproteinaemia: (a) palmar
xanthomata; (b) tubero-eruptive xanthomata.

Remnant disease is generally expressed in adult life and the diagnosis is easy when the classical stigmata are present. The contributing secondary factors need to be identified and treated appropriately if present. Treatment is with diet and hypolipidaemic drugs. The response to diet can be encouraging, particularly in the obese. If drugs are required, then excellent responses are observed with either the fibrates or the HMG-CoA reductase inhibitors.

LIPOPROTEIN LIPASE DEFICIENCY (FAMILIAL CHYLOMICRONAEMIA SYNDROME)

This very rare condition is informative in that it emphasizes the importance of the enzyme, lipoprotein lipase, in lipid metabolism and the role of Apo C-II as the essential activator of the enzyme. It can produce severe symptoms, which may go undiagnosed (Bhatnagar, 1999; Brunzell and Deeb, 2001).

Inheritance

Absence (or virtual absence) of lipoprotein lipase activity is inherited as a recessive disorder affecting approximately one in 10^6 of the population. It presents in childhood or early adult life. In some individuals no enzyme protein is detectable; in others the enzyme protein is defective and its catalytic activity markedly reduced. In many patients the genetic defect can be identified at the molecular level. Other individuals possess normal lipoprotein lipase activity but lack Apo C-II, which is necessary for activation of the enzyme. Many structural defects ($>$60) have been described in the lipoprotein lipase (LPL) gene, including deletions, missense mutations with markedly reduced or absent LPL activity. C-II deficiency is inherited as an autosomal recessive and is less common than LPL deficiency. Approximately 14 kindreds have been described with single-base substitutions leading to stop codons, splice-site mutations and frame shift mutations associated with reduced or absent Apo C-II.

Pathophysiology

Loss of LPL activity results in massive accumulation of chylomicrons so that plasma triglyceride concentrations may be as high as 50–100 mmol/L. VLDL concentrations are normal and LDL and HDL concentrations decreased. Absence of lipoprotein lipase or C-II deficiency can be demonstrated in specialist centres. The diagnosis can be predicted from the massive hypertriglyceridaemia, the presence of chylomicrons in fasting plasma and the absence of secondary causes such as uncontrolled diabetes mellitus or type I glycogen storage disease, which can produce high triglyceride concentrations in children. If fasting plasma is refrigerated overnight, the characteristic cream layer is observed (Figure 3.9).

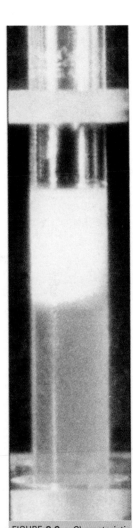

FIGURE 3.9 • Characteristic cream layer of type I hyperlipidaemia plasma. The sample was placed in the refrigerator overnight.

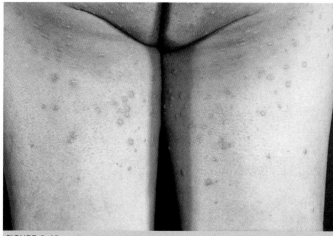

FIGURE **3.10** • Eruptive xanthomata.

Clinical features

Clinically the condition presents with recurrent attacks of abdominal pain and sometimes frank pancreatitis. In addition, eruptive xanthomata (Figure 3.10) may appear over elbows, knees and buttocks. Hepatosplenomegaly can occur, due to the accumulation of lipid-laden macrophages, and lipaemia retinalis may be observed. In one series of patients with LPL deficiency, approximately a third were detected in the first year of life with the majority of the remainder diagnosed in the first decade. Patients with Apo C-II deficiency tend to present later in life – possibly related to the somewhat less severe dyslipidaemia.

Rarely, other symptoms are reported by patients with severe chylomicronaemia including dyspnoea, disturbances of memory and concentration, depression and tinnitus.

An important practical point that has led to management difficulties in our experience is that massive hypertriglyceridaemia can lead to interference with amylase assays, producing falsely low levels. As a result, the diagnosis of pancreatitis may be missed. Other laboratory measurements may be interfered with by chylomicronaemia including haemoglobin and bilirubin and liver transaminases, and, by decreasing water volume in plasma, artificially low sodium (approximately 2–4 mmol/L per 10 mmol/L triglyceride).

Drug therapy is ineffective in this condition and diet is the cornerstone of therapy to prevent recurrent attacks of abdominal pain. A low total fat diet is required with triglyceride intake of less than 20 g/day. This will reduce chylomicron formation and maintain plasma triglyceride levels at a level (<11 mmol/L) unlikely to precipitate pancreatitis. No more than 20 g of fat should be eaten at any one meal. The diet may be supplemented with medium-chain triglycerides, which are absorbed directly into the portal system, but these may not be well tolerated. Other secondary causes of hypertriglyceridaemia should be avoided – including alcohol and drugs, which can increase VLDL. In adults with increased VLDL (shown by an increase in plasma cholesterol), fibrates may reduce triglycerides modestly in association with the low total fat diet. Patients need very careful monitoring during pregnancy. In one case report, dietary fat was reduced to 2 g in the second and third trimester of pregnancy – the infant was normal. In the future, LPL and C-II deficiency are likely to be candidates for therapeutic gene transfer.

VERY RARE DISORDERS

Many rare abnormalities have been described in lipid and lipoprotein metabolism which have thrown considerable light on the understanding of overall metabolism. Genetic studies of well-characterized clinical phenotypes increasingly expand our knowledge and are likely to lead to improved therapy as new targets for therapeutic modulation are identified. The reader is referred to other texts as sources of reference (Betteridge et al., 1999; Scriver et al., 2001).

TANGIER DISEASE

Tangier disease (Tangier island, Virginia, USA, home of first patients described) is a very rare recessive disorder characterized by accumulation of cholesterol ester-rich foam cells leading to hyperplastic orange tonsils and hepato/splenomegaly and corneal opacification. Peripheral neuropathy is a further common feature with lipid deposition in Schwann cells. HDL cholesterol is profoundly decreased together with the major HDL apoproteins, A-I and A-II. Triglycerides are moderately increased and total and LDL cholesterol reduced. Recently it has been shown that Tangier disease is caused by homozygous mutations in the ABCA1 gene located on the long arm of chromosome 9 which encodes the cholesterol efflux regulatory protein, a rate-limiting factor in reverse cholesterol transport. Patients have a moderately increased risk of atherosclerosis. No specific treatment is available for Tangier patients – HDL levels are resistant to usual lifestyle measures and drugs. Attention to CHD risk factors is important. Hyper-triglyceridaemia can be treated with lifestyle and fibrates.

FAMILIAL LCAT DEFICIENCY AND FISH EYE DISEASE

Familial LCAT deficiency is characterized biochemically by markedly reduced HDL cholesterol levels and Apo A-I and Apo A-II, and hypertriglyceridaemia, and clinically by corneal opacities, haemolytic anaemia (possibly associated with abnormal erythrocyte membrane lipids), proteinuria and renal disease with progression to renal failure. The cornea is dull and pale with increasing opacity approaching the limbus. The cloudy appearance of the cornea is due to granular deposits consisting of free cholesterol and phospholipids. Renal biopsies show increased free cholesterol and phospholipids. Abnormal LDL enriched in triglyceride, oxidized phospholipid and little cholesterol ester (similar to lipoprotein X seen in obstructive liver disease) may play a role in the pathogenesis of renal disease. LCAT is the major enzyme for the esterification of free cholesterol in plasma lipoproteins, the preferred substrate being HDL, as discussed in Chapter 1. In LCAT deficiency the decreased HDL cholesterol results from increased catabolism of nascent HDL rich in free cholesterol which cannot be converted to cholesterol ester. Approximately 30 mutations in the *LCAT* gene (located on the long arm of chromosome 16) have been described mostly involving point mutations throughout the six exons. Deletions and insertions resulting in frame shift and premature termination have also been described. From these findings it is likely that all regions of the gene are important for enzyme activity.

Fish eye disease (FED) is characterized by markedly decreased HDL concentrations and cloudy corneas. These patients do not develop anaemia or renal disease. In FED there appears to be a selective deficiency of LCAT activity on HDL. Mutations of the *LCAT* gene associated with FED are thought to affect the hydrophilic surface of the enzyme associated with binding of HDL and cholesterol. Premature CHD is not a feature of either fish eye disease or familial LCAT deficiency.

ABETALIPOPROTEINAEMIA

This rare recessive disorder is characterized clinically by severe neuromuscular disorders (spinocerebellar ataxia) developing in childhood and adolescents, degenerative pigmentary retinopathy and ceroid myopathy. Fat malabsorption is a central manifestation usually starting early in life associated with increased lipid content of intestinal mucosa. Anaemia with abnormal erythrocytes known as acanthocytes are characteristic. Hepatic steatosis and fibrosis have been described. Biochemically, abetalipoproteinaemia is associated with absence of all Apo B-containing lipoproteins from plasma and as a consequence plasma concentrations of cholesterol and triglyceride are very low indeed. The metabolic defect in abetalipoproteinaemia resides in MTP, which is an obligate requirement for synthesis of Apo B-containing lipoproteins. This protein is absent from intestinal and hepatic microsomes of affected individuals; truncations of the C terminus as a result of nonsense mutations, point substitutions and splice mutants have been described in the *MTP* gene.

Treatment is with a low total-fat diet ($\approx 15\,\mathrm{g/day}$) which reduces gastrointestinal symptoms. Supplementation with tocopherol inhibits progression of neurological manifestations as well as the retinal and muscle problems. Supplementation with other fat-soluble vitamins is required.

FAMILIAL HYPOBETALIPOPROTEINAEMIA

Distinct from abetalipoproteinaemia, familial hypobetalipoproteinaemia is an autosomal dominant disorder characterized by low plasma cholesterol and Apo B concentrations. In homozygotes the biochemical features resemble those of abetalipoproteinaemia. Heterozygotes have mean cholesterol concentrations of approximately 4–5 mmol/L and LDL cholesterol of about half that of unaffected siblings. Triglycerides are normal or low.

Hypobetalipoproteinaemia is associated with genetic abnormalities in the Apo B gene. Substitutions or deletions causing frame shifts lead to premature stop codons and varying truncation of the protein. Truncated forms of Apo B are poorly lipidized and secreted at reduced rates.

SITOSTEROLAEMIA

This rare autosomal recessive disorder, also known as phytosterolaemia, is characterized clinically by the development of extensive tendon and subcutaneous xanthomas during childhood with normal cholesterol levels. Biochemically, there are high plasma levels of the plant sterols sitosterol, campesterol and stigmasterol comprising 11–16 per cent of total plasma sterols which accumulate in tissues. Physiologically, there is over-absorption of plant sterols. The metabolic defect is unknown but it has been postulated that sitosterolaemia results from a loss of discrimination between various sterols for esterification – sitosterol is normally a poor substrate for acylcholesterol acyltransferase. Patients are at high risk of premature CHD; why this should be the case is not fully understood. Other clinical features include haemolytic anaemia, platelet abnormalities, splenomegaly and arthritis.

Treatment is dietary with a diet as low as possible in plant sterols which involves elimination of all plant foods with high contents of fat and all sources of vegetable fats. The anion-exchange resin cholestyramine will reduce plasma plant sterol levels by half. Colestipol has similar effects. Sitostanol, which is not absorbed, also lowers plant sterols.

HDL ABNORMALITIES

Twin studies indicate that approximately half the variance in HDL cholesterol in the general population is genetically determined. Variants of several genes coding for proteins involved in HDL metabolism including CETP, LPL and LCAT genes, have an impact on HDL. Common genetic variations in the hepatic lipase gene and the Apo A-I/Apo C-III/Apo A-IV gene loci also account for variability in HDL cholesterol in normotriglyceridaemic Caucasians.

HYPOALPHALIPOPROTEINAEMIA

Genetic determinants of low HDL cholesterol concentration have been described. Mutations occur in the gene for Apo A-I, the major HDL apoprotein, due to nonsense mutations, frame shifts and missense mutations. Some of these abnormalities are associated with barely detectable HDL cholesterol and Apo A-I levels. Some of the patients suffered premature CHD. Tangier disease and LCAT deficiency, which lead to low HDL cholesterol, are described above. Lipoprotein lipase deficiency is associated with low HDL. Heterozygotes for LPL deficiency have been described with mild hypertriglyceridaemia and low HDL.

HYPERALPHALIPOPROTEINAEMIA

Markedly raised HDL has been described in a family due to overproduction of Apo A-I; the nature of the abnormality was not elucidated.

High HDL concentrations are a feature of mutations in CETP. An intron 14 splicing defect in the *CETP* gene was described in a Japanese family. Homozygotes with this defect have no detectable CETP and HDL cholesterol levels two to six times higher than normal. HDL is enriched in cholesteryl esters. Heterozygotes with the intron 14 defect have about a 30 per cent reduction in CETP with a mild increase in HDL cholesterol. The relationship of *CETP* mutations and resulting HDL cholesterol changes to CHD remain unclear.

CEREBROTENDINOUS XANTHOMATOSIS

This rare familial sterol storage disease is characterized clinically by tuberous and tendon xanthomata, early atherosclerosis, dementia, spinal cord paresis, cataracts and cerebellar ataxia. Biochemically, there is accumulation of cholestanol and cholesterol in tissues. The genetic defect resides in the gene for sterol 27-hydroxylase and more than 20 different mutations have been described. Defects in 27-hydroxylase lead to a block in the bile acid synthetic pathway with accumulation of 5β-cholestane 3α,7α,12α-triol and 7α-hydroxy-4-cholestene-3-one. Treatment is with the bile acid chenodeoxycholic acid which reduces 7α-hydroxylase, the first committed step in bile acid synthesis. Improvements in dementia have been described with this treatment.

REFERENCES

Anonymous (2001) Executive Summary of the Third Report of the National Cholesterol Education Program (NCEP) Expert Panel on Dectection, Evaluation and Treatment of High Blood Cholesterol in Adults (Adult Treatment Panel III). *J Am Med Assoc* **285**, 2486–97.

Beaumont, J.L., Carlson, L.A., Cooper, G.R. *et al.* (1970) Classification of hyperlipidaemia and hyperlipoproteinaemias. *Bull WHO* **43**, 891–915.

Betteridge, D.J., Illingworth, D.R. and Shepherd, J. (eds) (1999) *Lipoproteins in Health and Disease*, Arnold, London.

Bhatnagar, D. (1999) Hypertriglyceridaemia. In *Lipoproteins in Health and Disease* (eds D.J. Betteridge, D.R. Illingworth and J. Shepherd), Arnold, London, pp. 737–51.

Bhatnagar, D., Morgan, J., Siddiq, S., Mackness, M.I., Miller, J.P. and Durrington, P.N. (2000) Outcome of case finding among relatives of patients with known heterozygous familial hypercholesterolaemia. *Br Med J* **321**, 1497–500.

Brown, M.S. and Goldstein, J.L. (1986) Receptor-mediated control of cholesterol metabolism. *Science* **191**, 150–4.

Friedewald, W.T., Levy, R. and Frederickson, D.S. (1972) Estimation of the concentration of low density lipoprotein cholesterol in plasma without use of the preparative ultracentrifuge. *Clin Chem* **18**, 499–502.

Goldstein, J.L., Hazzard, W.R., Schrott, H.G. *et al.* (1973) Hyperlipidaemia in coronary heart disease II. Genetic analysis of lipid levels in 176 families and delineation of a new inherited disorder: combined hyperlipidaemia. *J Clin Invest* **54**, 1544–68.

Humphries, S.E., Galton, D. and Nicholls, P. (1997) Genetic testing for familial hypercholesterolaemia: practical and ethical issues. *Q J Med* **90**, 169–81.

Humphries, S.E., Peacock, R. and Gudnason, V. (1999) Genetic determinants of hyperlipidaemia. In *Lipoproteins in Health and Disease* (eds D.J. Betteridge, D.R. Illingworth and J. Shepherd), Arnold, London, pp. 127–62.

Kane, J.P. and Havel, R.J. (2001) Disorders of the biogenesis and secretion of lipoproteins containing the B apolipoproteins. In *The Metabolic and Molecular Bases of Inherited Disease* (eds C.R. Scriver, J.B. Stanbury, J.B. Wyngaarden and D.G. Fredrickson), 7th edn, McGraw-Hill, New York, pp. 169–81.

Mahley, R.W. and Rall, S.C. (1999) Type III hyperlipoproteinaemia (dysbetalipoproteinaemia remnant particle disease). In *Lipoproteins in Health and Disease* (eds. D.J. Betteridge, D.R. Illingworth and J. Shepherd), Arnold, London, pp. 719–36.

Scientific Steering Committee, on behalf of the Simon Broome Register Group (1991) Risk of fatal coronary heart disease in familial hypercholesterolaemia. *Br Med J* **303**, 893–6.

Scriver, C.R., Stanbury, J.B., Wyngaarden, J.B. and Fredrickson, D.G. (eds) (2001) *The Metabolic and Molecular Bases of Inherited Disease*, 7th edn, McGraw-Hill, New York.

Umans-Eckenhausen, M.A.W., Defesche, J.C., Sijbrands, E.J.G., Scheerder, R.L.J.M. and Kastelein, J.J.P. (2001) Review of the first 5 years of screening for familial hypercholesterolaemia in the Netherlands. *Lancet* **357**, 165–8.

Vega, G.L. and Grundy, S.M. (1986) In vivo evidence for reduced binding of low density lipoproteins to receptors as a cause of primary moderate hypercholesterolaemia. *J Clin Invest* **78**, 1410–14.

Walldius, G., Jungner, I., Holme, I., Aastvert, A.H., Kolar, W. and Steiner, E. (2001) High apolipoprotein B, low apolipoprotein A-1, and improvement in the prediction of fatal myocardial infarction (AMORIS study): a prospective study. *Lancet* **358**, 2026–33.

Wood, D.A., De Backer, G., Faergeman, O. *et al.* (1998) Prevention of coronary heart disease in clinical practice. Recommendations of the Second Joint Task Force of the European Society of Cardiology, European Atherosclerosis Society and European Society of Hypertension. *Eur Heart J* **19**, 1434–503.

SCREENING

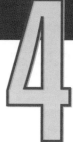

In 1982, the World Health Organization Expert Committee on Prevention of Coronary Heart Disease considered that a comprehensive plan for CHD prevention in the general population should include:

■ a population strategy;
■ a high-risk strategy;
■ secondary prevention.

A population strategy means altering, for the whole population, those lifestyle, environmental, social and economic factors that are the determinants of CHD. In terms of Figure 4.1, this means shifting the risk curve for the whole population in the direction of lower risk by attention to factors such as, nutrition, smoking and exercise.

The high-risk, or individual strategy aims to identify and treat those individuals at the higher end of a risk factor distribution in order to reduce the risk of CHD for that

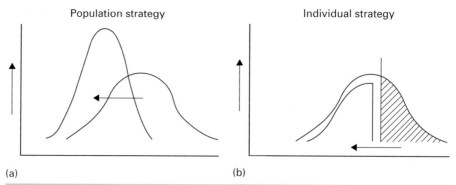

FIGURE **4.1** • (a) The population strategy aims to shift the whole population in the direction of lower risk. (b) The high-risk individual strategy aims to identify and treat individuals in the upper part of the distribution.

individual. The scientific evidence for unifactorial interventions such as lowering cholesterol or blood pressure or stopping smoking is compelling, but in a multifactorial disease, global assessment and intervention are more appropriate. The high-risk approach implies the need for some sort of screening process to identify high-risk individuals. The process is time- and resource-intensive but is highly appropriate for CHD prevention as the first presentation of disease might be fatal or permanently disabling.

Secondary prevention means preventing recurrent events in patients with clinically established CHD. Of course, some high-risk individuals will already have asymptomatic disease but they are hard to identify and targeting secondary prevention patients for intervention produces an immediate impact on overall CHD rates and is endorsed by all consensus authorities.

There is no conflict between the strategies, which can and should run together for maximum preventive effect. They are interactive and mutually supportive.

POPULATION STRATEGY

Since Ancel Keys demonstrated the population differences in the Seven Countries Study, population effects have been seen in several countries – most notably the USA and Australia. Populations tend to behave coherently around the societal norm; so if that norm moves in the direction of health benefit, whole distribution shifts are seen and the large potential of the population strategy is realized. By influencing risk factors in advance, the strategy is seen as radical, rather than the palliative or rescue attempt of the individual approach where risk factors are already established. This has its parallel in famine relief where relief supplies mirror the individual approach while educational and agricultural projects reflect the population approach.

The potential of the population strategy for benefit is large, but the benefit for the individual is small and those at highest risk may be excluded from benefit at all. In terms of serum cholesterol, improved nutritional and other lifestyle habits for everyone would result in the mean cholesterol level of the population falling and the risk of CHD being substantially reduced. Those with genetic hyperlipidaemias, which are less responsive to dietary change, would benefit more from being identified and treated individually using the high-risk approach. However, this would have a relatively small impact on the total number of CHD events occurring in a population, as large numbers exposed to slightly raised cholesterol and the influence of other risk factors produce more cases of CHD than small numbers, exposed to a high level of cholesterol alone.

INDIVIDUAL APPROACH

Most health professionals feel comfortable with the individual approach, as the focus is directly on the patient. Patients, too, are better motivated by a traditional, personal approach but there are drawbacks. First, the identification of patients at high risk requires a feasible screening process which fulfils the criteria shown in Table 4.1.

TABLE **4.1** • Criteria for a successful screening test for CHD risk assessment

The test for CHD risk assessment is valid, precise, easy, acceptable and cost-effective.
The relationship between CHD risk and symptomatic disease is quantified.
There is a defined screening strategy and an intervention and follow-up policy.
Trained staff and facilities for screening and intervention are available.
Screening results in a reduction of coronary mortality and morbidity.
Screening itself has no adverse effects.
The cost of screening and intervention is justified in relation to outcome.

TABLE **4.2** • National Cholesterol Education Program (NCEP) lipid screening in adults

Age	⩾20 years
Appropriate screening	Universal, opportunistic
Non-fasting TC and HDL in:	Healthy individuals
	Fasting lipid profile if high TC, low HDL or borderline high
	TC + ⩾2 other risk factors
Full fasting profile where:	Atherosclerosis present
	Diabetes present
	High multiple risk
	Physician chooses

Second, by its nature, the individual strategy acts later in the disease process and has more limited potential. It may be more difficult to change the behaviour patterns of people after many years, especially against the societal norm, and there is a risk of labelling people as patients and creating a 'worried well' population.

High-risk individuals are identified in two ways: by **selective** or **non-selective** (mass) screening.

SELECTIVE VERSUS NON-SELECTIVE SCREENING

In the USA, the National Cholesterol Education Project (NCEP) recommends cholesterol screening for all adults aged over 20 every 5 years (Table 4.2). Countries that advocate mass screening argue that knowledge of serum cholesterol for an individual provides an incentive for change, but this has not been proved and may even be a disincentive if the level is low. Furthermore, serum cholesterol by itself is not a good screening test and this is shown in the BRHS data (Figure 4.2). There is considerable overlap between the curves in Figure 4.2, showing that knowledge of serum cholesterol alone does not distinguish between the two populations. Of course, this is due to the interaction of other risk factors and thus, the multifactorial approach to screening is favoured.

Cholesterol screening can therefore be offered to those selected patients who would have most to gain, by virtue of their existing risk profile, from the additional knowledge of their lipid parameters. A counter to this argument is the data from the MRFIT (see page 39), where men with high cholesterol as their only risk factor nevertheless were still at greater

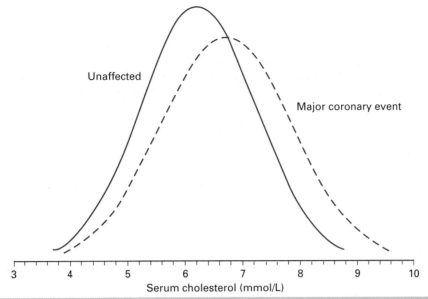

FIGURE **4.2** • Serum cholesterol distribution in 438 men who had a major coronary event and 7252 unaffected men. Source: Pocock, S.J., Shaper, A.G. and Phillips, A.N. (1989) *Br Med J* **298**, 998–1002.

risk. The attraction of selective screening is in its cost-effectiveness. The cost of preventing a CHD event in a low-risk 40-year-old female is 100 times the cost for a 60-year-old male.

If a selective screening policy is adopted, a list of people to be screened can be drawn up. In a practice of 10 000 patients, there might be about 45 patients suffering from genetic hyperlipidaemia and significant numbers of these and other patients with very high cholesterol levels will be missed by even extensive lists of risk criteria, including family history, the presence of lipid stigmata, obesity, hypertension and diabetes. A recent study by Neil *et al.* (2000) showed that in Oxfordshire UK, only a quarter of the potential cases of familial hypercholesterolaemia (frequency 1 in 500) were diagnosed, the majority not until middle age. Clearly there is potential here for screening of all children or sophisticated family tracking of known probands.

HOW MIGHT SCREENING BE ACHIEVED?

Until the time comes when regular checks from cord blood to the grave are standard, there are several available methods.

- Commercial: the advent of portable dry chemistry devices has enabled supermarket and pharmacy testing to be available to the public and this has proved popular. One retail pharmacy chain saw 17 000 patients in 4 weeks in the UK when it offered this service. Private health insurance agencies also undertake health screening.
- Occupational: it is in industry's interest to maintain its workforce and occupational screening is increasingly common.
- In primary care.

Screening in primary care

The development of the primary care team, with its multidisciplinary, patient-centred approach to multifactorial assessment, makes primary care the ideal setting for risk factor screening. Only primary care can cope with the enormity of the task.

Where there is enthusiasm, significant numbers of patients will respond to the invitation to a screening consultation. Up to 90 per cent will accept if that invitation is made opportunistically while the patient is already at the surgery, even though the consultation will mean a return visit. Systematic screening by postal invitation is much less successful.

Opportunistic screening can take place at any primary care contact and the fact that 70 per cent of patients visit their primary care physician annually and 90–95 per cent over a 5-year period means that most of the practice can be screened. As those in social classes IV and V attend more regularly, there is opportunity to address the groups most at need. Spreading the task over years does allow the possibility of tackling the large numbers involved – just screening adults aged 25–60 years means 50 per cent of the practice population. More formal opportunities for screening exist at new patient interviews, well-person checks or designated coronary prevention clinics.

Studies of the effectiveness of risk factor intervention ('health checks') in primary care have been disappointing and this is discussed in Chapter 10.

WHOM TO TEST?

If opportunistic, selective screening is undertaken, cholesterol screening may be offered to patients with:

- a personal history of CHD, peripheral arterial disease (PAD) or CVA (for secondary prevention);
- a family history of CHD or PAD (especially before age 55 years) or hyperlipidaemia;
- hypertension;
- diabetes mellitus;
- physical stigmata of hyperlipidaemia;
- obesity (BMI > 30);
- chronic renal disease;
- smoking habits (reflecting the importance of smoking as a major risk factor).

AGE CONSIDERATIONS

There is no consensus regarding the age at which cholesterol screening can be offered to the population. Even children with heterozygous familial hypercholesterolaemia have abnormal endothelial function and the usual lower limit for screening of 25 years would therefore be inappropriate for cases of genetic hyperlipidaemia.

Subgroup analysis of the older subjects in the major outcome trials (who were up to 75 years old at randomization) strongly supports their treatment. The recent publication of the Heart Protection Study (HPS), which included subjects up to the age of 80, supports this view with huge benefit shown in the over-75s. Although Law's meta-analysis (see page 53) suggested reduced benefit from cholesterol lowering in the elderly, the increased absolute risk that comes with age means that they are more likely to benefit from risk factor modification, particularly cholesterol and systolic blood pressure. There is however, considerable co-morbidity in this group and clinical judgement is required. Evidence for risk factor reduction in the very elderly is not available and clinical judgement is again required on what action, if any, to take.

FREQUENCY OF TESTING

A reasonable frequency for cholesterol testing for primary prevention risk assessment is every 5 years from age 20–25 years to 60–70 years, according to overall risk. Borderline cases can vary from 1 to 5 years. Patients on treatment with diet should be tested initially every 3 months, then every 6–12 months; patients on medication should be tested initially every 6–8 weeks until at target, then every 6–12 months.

WHAT TO TEST?

Fasting has little effect on serum cholesterol levels. In general population screening, where triglyceride estimation is unnecessary, non-fasting specimens are adequate and this makes the test more acceptable to patients. Unlike total serum cholesterol and HDL cholesterol levels, the level of triglyceride is affected by meals (chylomicrons from the gut) and in healthy subjects it takes 6–8 hours to produce a steady triglyceride level.

In the high-risk patient, such as one with pre-existing atherosclerosis or diabetes, where the clinician requires as much information as possible on the levels of risk factor responsible, it is reasonable to estimate the full fasting profile immediately.

NORMAL VARIATION

We have already seen (Figure 2.11) that serum cholesterol varies within an individual with increasing age. This may not be physiological, as South African bushmen on a traditional low fat diet do not show the typical rise in later years demonstrated by those who adopt a more European diet.

Serum cholesterol is subject to a number of influences and these have implications in planning cut-off points for screening programmes and in assessing responses to treatment.

Biological variation

Cholesterol levels vary normally from day to day, week to week and year to year. In a cohort of 14 600 people with repeat cholesterol measurements, the within-person coefficient of variation after one year was 7.4 per cent. A person with a mean value of 6.5 mmol/L would thus have a within-person variation of 7.4 per cent $\times$ 6.5 = about 0.5 mmol/L, i.e. for most of the time the cholesterol level will fluctuate 0.5 mmol/L either side of 6.5 mmol/L. If several readings are taken (cf. the taking of several readings in the diagnosis of hypertension), the effect of within-person variation is much reduced.

Variation in women

Lipid concentrations vary during the menstrual cycle; both cholesterol and triglycerides tend to peak mid-cycle then fall away towards menstruation. Pregnancy also causes a progressive rise in total cholesterol, HDL cholesterol and triglycerides, being maximal just before delivery. Serum cholesterol may rise by 1 mmol/L.

Seasonal variation

Serum cholesterol concentrations are highest in the winter and lowest in the summer, varying by 0.5–0.8 mmol/L. This is probably caused by seasonal changes in diet and body weight.

Illness

Illnesses (both major and minor), operations and trauma share the effect of reducing serum cholesterol and raising triglycerides. This effect can be profound and rapid – certainly within 48 hours. Even minor illness, such as upper respiratory infection, can produce a fall that takes 3 weeks to restore. After major illness or operations, serum cholesterol takes up to 3 months to return to previous levels. Reduced cholesterol synthesis is involved and presumably the changes are mediated by catecholamines and corticosteroids. The dangerous significance of this phenomenon lies in misinterpretation of serum cholesterol levels after myocardial infarction or revascularization operations. Blood taken within 24 hours of the event may reflect pre-event levels but sometimes pre-infarction syndromes are operative and the timing of the event is imprecise.

Several drugs influence lipid levels and they are considered in Chapter 8 and page 70.

LABORATORY VARIATION AND SAMPLING ERRORS

It is clear that both normal variation and the timing of testing in relation to illness can reduce the interpretive value of serum cholesterol readings. Sampling errors and inaccuracies in laboratory technique can further compound this.

When blood is taken, the subject should be sitting or lying, preferably after 10 minutes of rest. Venous blood should be taken, avoiding haemostasis (preferably not using a tourniquet) and avoiding haemolysis (cholesterol leaks from ruptured red cell membranes).

Nowadays, laboratories use automated enzymic methods for lipid estimations. Figure 4.3 shows the measurement variation related to different coefficients of variation for a given level of serum cholesterol. Modern laboratories should achieve coefficients of variation less than 3 per cent and many approach 2 per cent. This measurement variation emphasizes the need for repeated testing, particularly in the diagnostic and assessment settings and conflicts with those laboratories that report serum cholesterol levels to two decimal places.

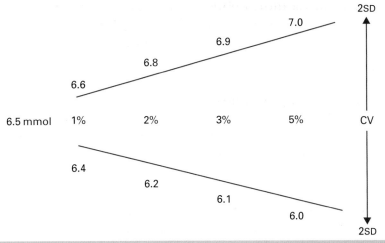

FIGURE **4.3** • Measurement variation related to different coefficients of variation (CV) for a given level of serum cholesterol.

Triglyceride levels are even more inaccurate, being subject to wider natural variation within individuals and of course being affected by the timing of the last meal. HDL cholesterol levels have also been subject to variation in the past, particularly as different laboratories have tended to use different measurement kits.

Clearly, if the basic elements of the lipid profile are so variable, it follows that calculated elements such as LDL cholesterol and ratios involving HDL cholesterol are also affected. The inaccuracies surrounding HDL cholesterol measurement have cast doubt on the usefulness of ratios, particularly when values of HDL cholesterol are low. Ratios are, however, incorporated into modern risk assessment programmes and are helpful in the assessment of menopausal women where HDL cholesterol values are often high.

NEAR SITE TESTING

The feasibility of mass near site testing increased with the development of compact measurement machines such as the Reflotron or the Lipotrend C. Being expensive and weighing 5.5 kg, they were no rivals to the sphygmomanometer as a cheap and convenient instrument. Both machines used a dry reagent strip with a drop of venous or capillary blood. The value was read by reflectance photometry and took 5 minutes to complete, allowing perhaps 50 tests in a day. Quality control was achieved using strips to check the optical system and external assessment using control sera was available. In 1989, Broughton estimated the coefficient of variation in three surveys to be 5.5 per cent, worsening with poor technique (e.g. not allowing alcohol from the swab to dry). Unfortunately, this meant it was impossible to distinguish between serum cholesterol samples as far apart as 5.2–6.5 mmol/L.

Nowadays, devices such as the Cholestech L.D.X.® Lipid Testing System are capable of measuring total cholesterol, HDL cholesterol, triglycerides and glucose with a degree of accuracy equating to the clinical laboratory. LDL cholesterol and the Framingham risk function can be calculated to enhance the usefulness of the assessment.

The clinician can be forgiven for feeling downhearted about the validity of serum cholesterol readings. As with any diagnostic technology, the problem is one of balancing false positives (initiating treatment unnecessarily) and false negatives (patients receiving false reassurance). Only repeated testing and careful consideration in the assessment phase (Chapter 5) can mitigate this.

Screening for familial hypercholesterolaemia

The tragedy of undetected cases of FH is all too common and affected men often die from atherosclerotic heart disease before the age of 50 or even younger. These deaths are all the more tragic because treatment is both safe and effective. To compound the tragedy, screening is often not extended to other, asymptomatic family members who may also be affected. In the UK, Durrington and colleagues tested all first-degree relatives of 200 index cases and found another 121 patients; 60 000 tests would have been required to detect this number of cases by conventional screening. In the Netherlands, Kastelein's group screened all 5442 relatives of 237 people with FH but made the screening more sophisticated by adding LDL-receptor gene mutation analysis. DNA testing enabled 2039 further individuals to be diagnosed with heterozygous FH and an additional finding was that 18 per cent of these would have been misdiagnosed by cholesterol testing alone. After 1 year, the proportion of affected patients receiving lipid-lowering medication had risen from 39 per cent to 93 per cent.

DNA testing may be less feasible in countries with a wider variety of LDL-receptor mutations and there are ethical, psychological and cost implications. Screening based on cholesterol testing is likely to remain and in the UK the Family Heart Association has embarked on a nurse-led, cascade, family tracking screening project based on serum cholesterol.

REFERENCES AND FURTHER READING

Bhatnagar, D., Morgan, J., Siddiq, S. *et al.* (2000) Outcome of case finding among relatives of patients with known heterozygous familial hypercholesterolaemia. *Br Med J* **321**, 1497–500.

Neil, H.A.W., Hammond, T., Huxley, R. *et al.* (2000) Extent of underdiagnosis of familial hypercholesterolaemia in routine practice: prospective registry study. *Br Med J* **321**, 148.

Umans-Eckenhausen, M.A.W., Defesche, J.C., Sijbrands, E.J.G. *et al.* (2001) Review of first 5 years of screening for familial hypercholesterolaemia in the Netherlands. *Lancet* **357**, 165–8.

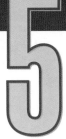

RISK FACTORS AND THEIR ASSESSMENT

We have seen how the risk factor concept evolved in the 1960s from the evaluation of long-term epidemiological studies in which individual characteristics were related to the subsequent incidence of CHD. More than 280 such associations have been published, ranging from the established major risk factors of dyslipidaemia, hypertension and smoking to less plausible characteristics including snoring, the speed of beard growth and even lack of attendance at church. In the field of infectious disease, the possession of the LP 'Judy Garland – Live at the Carnegie Hall' is positively associated with acquired immunodeficiency syndrome (AIDS), but no one would suggest a causative role!

The process of attributing a causative effect to an association must therefore be governed by guideline criteria:

- The association must be strong and consistent in different studies and populations.
- The association should be independent, graded and continuous – the incidence of the disease relating to levels of the risk factor.
- Prospective studies should establish an appropriate temporal sequence (the factor should precede the disease).
- The association should be plausible in terms of biological studies, clinical observations and controlled trials of risk factor reduction.

Using these criteria, the major risk factors for CHD all qualify as causal risks. The major risk factors are common and their influence on risk is powerful, particularly when acting in concert. Modifiable risk factors are amenable to prevention or treatment.

RISK FACTORS FOR CHD

The major risk factors for CHD are listed according to their potential for modification in Table 5.1.

TABLE **5.1** • Risk factors for CHD

Non-modifiable	Modifiable
Age	**Plasma lipids**
Sex	(Especially high total cholesterol, high LDL-C,
Family history of CHD	low HDL-C and high TG/low HDL-C)
Personal history of atherosclerosis (CHD,	**Hypertension**
peripheral or cerebrovascular disease)	**Smoking**
Ethnic origin	Diabetes and impaired glucose tolerance
	Obesity
	Physical inactivity
	Thrombogenic factors
	Psychosocial factors
	Homocysteinaemia

'Western' diet with its high positive energy balance, high content of saturated fats and dietary cholesterol and high sugar, sodium and alcohol intake is a necessary precondition for a high population rate of CHD. Diet mediates its effects through several risk factors and is discussed in Chapter 7. Inappropriate diet and physical inactivity, expressed as dyslipidaemia, high blood pressure and high BMI, together with smoking, explain at least 75 per cent of new cardiovascular disease.

Risk factors seldom occur in isolation and tend to 'cluster' in individuals. For example, individuals with low HDL cholesterol and high triglyceride may also have truncal obesity, hypertension and impaired glucose tolerance with hyperinsulinaemia, the so-called insulin resistance syndrome (page 120). Even without glucose intolerance, patients with hypertension tend to have above-average cholesterol levels.

When risk factors coincide, it is well known that their effect is often multiplicative rather than additive. Using the MRFIT data, a smoker with a cholesterol level of 6.2 mmol/L and with a diastolic blood pressure of 90 mmHg has, over a 6-year period, a 14-fold greater CHD mortality than a non-smoker with cholesterol and diastolic pressure below these limits.

For several risk factors there are no clearly defined threshold levels at which increased risk begins. This is particularly the case for serum cholesterol and blood pressure, and dichotomous thinking that suggests an individual either has or does not have one of these risk factors is inappropriate. Whilst an individual may be either of male sex or not, the contribution from risk factors that are distributed across a range will be a question of degree.

It is important to assess the global risk of CHD for an individual to predict a prognosis, choose intervention options if necessary and select therapeutic targets. Cholesterol levels must be interpreted and treated only in the light of their clinical and biochemical context, i.e. on the basis of the global risk. Global risk is increased by:

■ the presence of pre-existing atherosclerosis (CHD, PAD, etc.);
■ the presence of two or more risk factors;
■ the presence of a single, severe risk factor.

NON-MODIFIABLE RISK FACTORS

AGE

The risk of CHD increases exponentially with age. Three in four of the deaths from CHD occur after the age of 65. Framingham data demonstrate that a 60-year-old man with no risk factors at all has the same CHD mortality risk as a 45-year-old smoker with hypertension and hypercholesterolaemia.

Coronary atherosclerosis is noted in 60 per cent of autopsies performed on individuals aged over 65. Much of the disease must be asymptomatic, as only 20 per cent volunteer CHD symptoms. As 40 per cent are clear of lesions, CHD should not be considered as an inevitable consequence of ageing.

There has been a dearth of observational studies and clinical trials focusing on the elderly, yet despite inadequate data, it seems that the classical CHD risk factors still operate in the elderly, albeit at reduced relative risk. An example is seen in Doll's British Doctors study where the relative risk of smoking is reduced in the elderly, prompting the explanation of selective survival. Small increases in relative risk nevertheless translate into large increases in absolute risk, where disease rates are high. The rate of cardiovascular disease is so high in the elderly that the possible benefits of preventative programmes to stop smoking, lower blood pressure and cholesterol are likely to be high.

SEX

The male preponderance of CHD mortality around the world is remarkably consistent with an overall male:female sex ratio of between 3 and 4 (see Figure 2.2). This finding is all the more remarkable when one considers the variation between countries with different lifestyles, risk factor profiles and CHD rates. The ratio decreases with age but does not disappear even in old age (Table 5.2). Although after the menopause the rate of CHD increases to approach that of men, women appear to lag 10 years behind men in the first presentation of CHD. The implication is that an intrinsic gender-mediated factor is active, protecting women, and much speculation has centred on oestrogen.

When the other risk factors are examined, women tend to have higher cholesterol levels (see Figure 2.11), blood pressure and fibrinogen levels, are more obese and have more diabetes than men. Favourable factors include higher HDL cholesterol levels (throughout

TABLE **5.2** • CHD mortality: sex ratios and age

Age	Sex ratio CHD death male : female
35–44	6.8
45–54	5.3
55–64	3.3
65–74	2.3
75+	1.6

life), lower triglyceride levels, less central obesity and lower rates of smoking. Diabetes is the only common condition that equalizes the difference between the sexes. The different CHD rates and the factors responsible are considered in detail in Chapter 11.

FAMILY HISTORY OF CHD

It is the everyday experience of clinicians that CHD is seen to cluster in some families. Family history reflects the dual influences of genetic factors and shared family environment, particularly dietary and social habits. It has proved difficult to differentiate the relative contributions of genetic and environmental factors because of the complexity of their interactions. Nevertheless, twin studies show increased rates of CHD in the siblings of affected twins, albeit that the effect diminishes with age. Other observational studies establish a family history of CHD as an independent risk factor. Framingham data show that siblings of a brother with CHD have more than double the risk of a CHD event themselves, even after controlling for cholesterol, hypertension and smoking. A history of CHD in parents is associated with a 30 per cent increased risk. At an individual level, there is great variation in susceptibility to a risk factor and again both genetic and environmental factors must be active.

Recently, there has been interest in the possibility that intrauterine and perinatal experiences may exert a programming effect on the future handling of risk factors and hence provide an alternative explanation to variations in susceptibility (see page 57, 'From womb to tomb').

Clear contributions are made by family history in the assessment of patients with genetic hyperlipidaemias, such as FH, with its pattern of autosomal dominant inheritance.

When taking a family history of cardiovascular disease, the interviewer needs to ascertain:

- the pedigree of blood relatives – index patient, parents, siblings, children (first-degree relatives), grandparents, aunts and uncles (second-degree relatives);
- the number and proportion of affected relatives;
- the closeness of affected relatives to the index patient;
- the current age and state of health of relatives if alive;
- the age and cause of death if dead;
- the age of onset of disease in the affected relatives (especially if <55 years);
- whether the affected relatives had other risk factors (such as smoking, hypertension or diabetes).

A PERSONAL HISTORY OF ATHEROSCLEROSIS

Patients with a history of CHD are at increased risk of further events. American Heart Association statistics show that 21 per cent of male and 33 per cent of female MI survivors suffer a further MI within 6 years. Although the historical fact of a personal history of CHD is non-modifiable, the same risk factors associated with the initial development of CHD continue to contribute to disease progression and govern the likelihood of recurrence. In 1990, Pekkanen *et al.* showed that the risk of dying of a further MI was

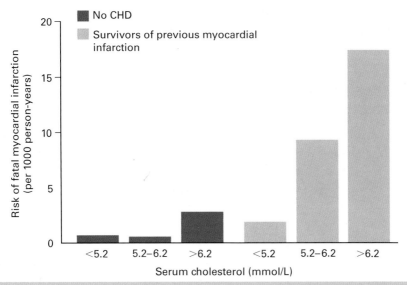

FIGURE 5.1 • The risk of subsequent fatal myocardial infarction in survivors of myocardial infarction and in those without clinically evident CHD, according to serum cholesterol. Data from Pekkanen, J., Linn, S., Heiss, G. *et al.* (1990) *N Engl J Med* **322**, 1700–7.

greatly increased in men with previous myocardial infarction when serum cholesterol remained raised (Figure 5.1). The positive results of numerous secondary prevention trials now highlight such high-risk patients as priorities for intervention.

Atherosclerosis is a generalized disease and this means that individuals with symptomatic arterial disease elsewhere are also at risk from CHD. Ten per cent of stroke survivors suffer an MI in the first year and 40 per cent of these are fatal. Fifteen per cent of claudicants will suffer a non-fatal coronary event within 6 years and ultimately more than 50 per cent will die of CHD. It is increasingly recognized that it is necessary to look more broadly at individuals with non-coronary atherosclerosis and intervene appropriately.

ETHNIC ORIGIN

Different CHD rates are commonly observed between immigrant groups and the norm for their adoptive country. The reasons for this are discussed in Chapter 2.

MODIFIABLE RISK FACTORS

SUMMARY OF THE EVIDENCE FOR THE POSITIVE RELATIONSHIP BETWEEN LIPIDS AND CHD

LDL cholesterol

Epidemiological evidence

- Studies between countries, e.g. the Seven Countries Study
- Migration studies, e.g. Ni Hon San
- Studies within countries, e.g. MRFIT, Framingham and BRHS

The positive relationship between CHD and cholesterol levels is strong, continuous, graded and curvilinear. This applies to both sexes and whether or not an individual already has established CHD. The risk becomes increasingly steep as cholesterol concentration increases and is considerably modified by the presence of other risk factors.

Clinical studies

Genetic disorders such as familial hypercholesterolaemia confirm the relationship between high LDL cholesterol levels and premature CHD.

Experimental studies

Animal studies link hypercholesterolaemia with premature atherosclerosis and studies on the mechanisms of atherogenesis *in vitro* confirm the causative link with LDL cholesterol.

Clinical trial evidence

Cholesterol lowering by diet or drug therapy is associated with a reduction in CHD. Reducing LDL cholesterol by 25–35 per cent has been the focus of treatment in the six major statin trials and the beneficial outcomes mandate implementation into everyday practice according to baseline risk.

HDL cholesterol

We have seen from Framingham data that HDL cholesterol is also a powerful and independent predictor of CHD (Table 5.3). The relationship is inverse, low levels of HDL cholesterol being associated with an increased risk of CHD. This relationship is particularly important in women. Low levels of HDL cholesterol often reflect obesity, smoking, lack of exercise or impaired glucose tolerance but genetic influences may also be responsible. Epidemiological studies, such as PROCAM, have shown that a combination of triglyceride elevation (>2.0 mmol/L) and low HDL cholesterol (<1.0 mmol/L) predict high CHD risk, particularly if the cholesterol to HDL cholesterol ratio is greater than five. Levels <0.9 mmol/L in a man and <1.1 mmol/L in a woman are negative risk factors whereas levels >1.5 mmol/L in a man and >1.7 mmol/L in a woman appear to be protective. Patients with low HDL cholesterol levels are not rare and a recent

TABLE **5.3** • HDL-C and CHD rates (Framingham)

HDL (mmol/L)	CHD rate/1000 population
<0.65	177
0.65–1.38	103
1.40–1.64	54
1.65–1.90	25

estimate suggests there are 16 million individuals with HDL cholesterol <0.9 mmol/L in the USA.

Several mechanisms appear to explain the beneficial actions of HDL cholesterol:

- reverse cholesterol transport.
- antioxidant effects. HDL cholesterol seems to protect LDL cholesterol from oxidative modification, probably through the effect of paraoxonase (PON 1), an enzyme closely associated with HDL cholesterol, which hydrolyses oxidized phospholipids.
- anti-thrombotic effects. Effects on blood viscosity, thrombin generation, platelet activity and fibrinolysis are all described.
- effects on monocyte adhesion proteins [e.g. reduced vascular cell adhesion molecule 1 (VCAM-1) expression].
- effects on endothelial activity.

No prospective trial has been targeted specifically at HDL cholesterol to determine whether increasing HDL cholesterol can reduce CHD events. However, in some drug trials, particularly those using fibrates, a rise in HDL cholesterol appears to contribute to CHD risk reduction. Concomitant HDL cholesterol elevations of 5–8 per cent in the six major statin trials are often overlooked but are likely to have contributed to the favourable outcomes. The Air Force/Texas Coronary Atherosclerosis Prevention Study (AFCAPS/TexCAPS) was conducted in a low-risk population with average cholesterol levels but below average HDL cholesterol (0.94 mmol/L in men and 1.03 mmol/L in women) and resulted in a 37 per cent reduced risk of a first major coronary event.

Triglycerides

Whilst the dominant roles of LDL cholesterol and HDL cholesterol in the development and prevention of CHD are wholly accepted, debate continues about whether hyper-triglyceridaemia constitutes an independent risk factor. Studies incorporating triglyceride measurement are subject to its greater measurement variability compared with other lipids, due to both laboratory factors and greater short-term biological variation. Despite this, uni-variate statistical analyses of numerous epidemiological studies have tended to suggest that triglycerides up to a level of about 5.0 mmol/L predict the risk of CHD and that the relationship is strongest for women and younger individuals. In 1993, the NIH Consensus Development Conference showed that the relationship between plasma triglyceride levels and CHD was lost when other risk factors, particularly HDL cholesterol, were taken into account by multivariate analysis. This is because the metabolisms of triglyceride and HDL cholesterol are inextricably linked, resulting in a strong inverse correlation, such that increased triglycerides are associated with reduced levels of HDL cholesterol.

Perhaps the strongest evidence of a link between triglycerides and CHD to date comes from Hokanson and Austin's meta-analysis of six cohorts (including Framingham and PROCAM). Multivariate analysis of 46 000 men and 10 000 women showed that, without adjustment for HDL cholesterol, for every 1 mmol/L increase in triglyceride level there was a 76 per cent increase risk of CHD in women and a 32 per cent increased risk in men. When adjusted for HDL cholesterol, the risks remained significant at 37 per cent and 14 per cent respectively.

Another reason for confusion is that not all triglyceride-carrying particles are atherogenic. This means measurements of whole plasma triglyceride levels do not necessarily reflect atherosclerotic potential. Whilst triglycerides are carried by all lipoproteins, chylomicrons, synthesized in the small intestine and VLDLs, synthesized in the liver, are the most triglyceride-rich. These large triglyceride-rich lipoproteins are generally cleared more quickly from the circulation than smaller particles, which can complete the metabolic cascade and produce more atherogenic species (small forms of VLDL, IDL and LDL cholesterol). Severe levels of hypertriglyceridaemia are found in familial hypertriglyceridaemia where chylomicrons and large forms of VLDL predominate. The risk to the patient is of pancreatitis, not CHD, because the lipoprotein particles are too large to enter the vessel wall. By contrast, small forms of VLDL, IDL and LDL cholesterol may rapidly penetrate endothelium and are highly atherogenic.

The atherogenic changes accompanying hypertriglyceridaemia can be summarized as:

- low HDL cholesterol
- increased VLDL
- increased small, dense LDL cholesterol
- postprandial lipaemia
- coagulation changes.

The combination of low HDL cholesterol and high triglycerides is often seen in conjunction with elevated levels of small, dense LDL cholesterol, which is the most readily oxidized and atherogenic of the lipoproteins. This profile is commonly seen in diabetic patients and those of South Asian extraction. It is an important feature of the insulin resistance syndrome, which is associated with both groups and contributes to their excess cardiovascular mortality. Small, dense LDL cholesterol particles tend to predominate at triglyceride levels in excess of 1.4–1.6 mmol/L and experts have begun to review what is considered an acceptable upper limit for triglycerides. Currently this is set at 2.3 mmol/L but the increased risk associated with triglyceride levels extends to less than half this level. A recent consensus statement for diabetics recommended a desirable level of <1.5 mmol/L.

Post-prandial triglyceride concentrations have also been shown to be an independent risk factor for CHD. Even healthy humans spend the majority of their time in the post-prandial state as triglyceride levels are increased in the plasma after a fatty meal for approximately 8 hours. The extended postprandial lipaemia that accompanies hyper-triglyceridaemia appears to reduce the protective effect of HDL cholesterol as well as increasing the uptake of VLDL into endothelial cells.

The role of haemostasis in atherosclerotic plaque evolution and event precipitation is increasingly recognized. Triglyceride-rich lipoproteins appear to be important in determining the mass and reactivity of coagulation factor VII. Increased factor VII activity generates increased thrombin at sites where tissue factor is expressed. PAI-1 is a fast acting inhibitor of tissue-type plasminogen activation and is the major determinant of fibrinolytic activity in plasma. Triglyceride-rich lipoproteins have been shown to increase secretion of PAI-1 from endothelial and liver cells, reducing fibrinolytic capacity.

There are no intervention trials specifically targeting triglyceride reduction but the closest answer as to whether triglyceride lowering is worthwhile comes from clinical trial data from studies of fibrates, which primarily lower triglyceride. Subgroup analysis of the Helsinki Heart Study (HHS) suggests gemfibrozil exerts its most beneficial effect on the cohort with moderate hypertriglyceridaemia and an LDL cholesterol:HDL cholesterol ratio >5. The VA-HIT also studied gemfibrozil in recruits with either isolated low HDL cholesterol or low HDL cholesterol associated with hypertriglyceridaemia. The combination of lowering triglycerides by 24 per cent, increasing HDL cholesterol by 7.5 per cent, without changing LDL cholesterol was associated with a 22 per cent decreased incidence of CHD.

Considering the greater accuracy in measurement and predictive capacity of serum cholesterol and HDL cholesterol, the usefulness of triglyceride levels may evolve as a marker for atherogenic patterns. Estimation of fasting triglyceride level remains essential for the identification of those patients whose hypertriglyceridaemia exposes them to the risk of pancreatitis and, until direct LDL cholesterol measurement arrives, for LDL cholesterol calculation.

Apolipoprotein B

Apolipoprotein B is the major protein component of LDL cholesterol, IDL, VLDL and chylomicrons and one molecule is present in each lipoprotein particle. In the fasting state, chylomicrons are absent and therefore Apo B can be seen as a measure of the atherogenic lipoproteins and a good indicator of the risk of atherosclerosis.

Lipoprotein(a)

Some studies have suggested that raised levels of lipoprotein(a) are associated with increased risk of CHD, post-angioplasty restenosis and cerebrovascular disease. The findings are not always consistent, with problems with study design and measurement technicalities. The role of lipoprotein(a) is, however, biologically plausible, as it contains an apolipoprotein that has a structural homology with plasminogen. By acting as a competitive inhibitor of plasminogen it reduces fibrinolytic activity. Unfortunately, standard lipid-lowering drugs do not modify concentrations and only oestrogens in postmenopausal women and high-dose nicotinic acid have any significant impact.

NON-LIPID MODIFIABLE RISK FACTORS

HYPERTENSION

Hypertension is established as one of the major independent risk factors for CHD and satisfies the criteria suggesting a causal relationship. Most population-based studies confirm that hypertension increases an individual's risk of a cardiovascular event two- to

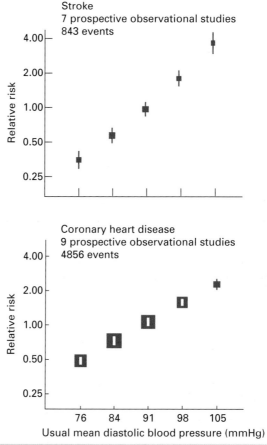

FIGURE 5.2 • Risk of stroke and coronary heart disease associated with hypertension.
Source: MacMahon, S., Peto, R., Cutler, J. et al. (1990) Lancet **335**, 765–74.

threefold and it is implicated in 35 per cent of all atherosclerotic cardiovascular events. The major causes of death attributable to hypertension are cerebrovascular disease (stroke) and CHD and the relative incidence of these varies around the world according to the impact of other risk factors (see Table 2.3). The consequences of hypertension are:

- stroke (embolic, thrombotic, haemorrhagic and multi-infarct damage including dementia);
- coronary heart disease;
- left ventricular hypertrophy;
- heart failure;
- reno-vascular disease;
- peripheral vascular disease (including aortic dissection).

There is a strong, continuous, graded, near linear relationship between both systolic and diastolic blood pressure and subsequent atherosclerotic events. This is illustrated in Figure 5.2, the size of the squares being proportional to the number of events and the vertical lines representing 95 per cent confidence intervals.

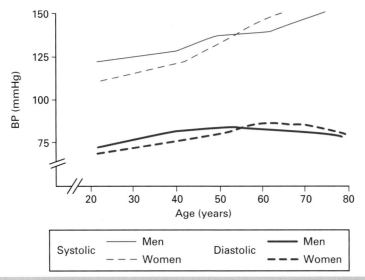

FIGURE **5.3** • Changes in systolic and diastolic pressure with age. Source: Acheson, R.M. (1973) *Int J Epidemiol* **2**, 293–301.

It can be seen that the majority of strokes and CHD events occur in 'normotensives' (i.e. individuals whose blood pressure levels would not normally warrant treatment). We have seen the same phenomenon with cholesterol (see Figure 4.2) and interaction with other risk factors is responsible. Lipid risk factors coexist in the hypertensive individual more often than by chance even when confounding variables such as obesity, drug side-effects and alcohol consumption are taken into account. Nutritional influences, genetic factors and the insulin resistance syndrome may provide unifying explanations for the relationship.

The definition of hypertension is consequently much debated but remains arbitrary due to the continuous and graded relationship of blood pressure to cardiovascular risk. There is no point at which blood pressure is 'safe' or suddenly becomes 'dangerous'. The World Health Organization-International Society of Hypertension (WHO-ISH) definition of 140/90 mmHg or greater takes into account the point at which the attributable risk starts to become significant as well as acknowledging the results of clinical trials that aim to explore the lowest point to which treatment benefits can be ascribed.

From middle age onwards, systolic blood pressure is a greater predictor of CHD events than diastolic blood pressure. Systolic pressure tends to rise throughout life but diastolic pressure peaks at about 60 years and then declines (Figure 5.3). This rise is not observed in primitive societies and it cannot therefore be viewed as part of normal ageing.

The risks of blood pressure are much higher once hypertension has induced target organ damage. Left ventricular hypertrophy (LVH) is easily recognized on an ECG and is a powerful predictor of CHD events, carrying a poor prognosis if untreated. The relative risk of LVH is 2.7 in men and 2.0 in women, rising to 5.8 and 2.5 if LVH is accompanied by repolarization changes (strain) on the ECG. The discovery of target organ damage or the presence of other severe CHD risk factors, such as diabetes, should invoke a lower threshold for antihypertensive intervention and a more stringent target level.

Clinical trials of blood pressure lowering offer convincing evidence of reduction in strokes and heart failure but reduction in CHD is more modest than predicted. The possible reasons for this are discussed in Chapter 6. Interestingly, although not designed for the purpose, clinical trials of lipid lowering are associated with a small reduction in blood pressure. Explanations include improved endothelial and smooth muscle function, facilitating normal vasodilatation responses in vascular beds beyond the coronary circulation. It is possible that small changes in blood pressure contribute to the reduction in vascular risk seen with lipid lowering but the magnitude of the effect is impossible to quantify.

SMOKING

The tobacco plant, *Nicotiana tabacum*, is indigenous to North America and came to Europe following Christopher Columbus's voyages of exploration. For hundreds of years, North American Indians had either smoked or chewed leaves for narcotic, medicinal, religious or social purposes. Sir Walter Raleigh introduced tobacco to Britain during Elizabeth I's reign and almost immediately her government imposed a tobacco tax of two pence in the pound, recognizing an early potential for revenue generation. In 1604, James I described tobacco as 'hateful to the nose, harmful to the brain and dangerous to the lungs'. Even by then, duty had risen to six shillings and eight pence in the pound.

Over the next three centuries, tobacco was smoked in pipes, chewed or taken as snuff. In the early nineteenth century the first cigars were made but the development of the cigarette in the latter half of the same century provided the springboard for the huge worldwide growth in smoking behaviour. At first cigarettes were crude and hand rolled but manufacturing processes improved and the first cigarette factory in England opened in London in 1856. With the help of many additives, the smoke of the cigarette was made more pleasant and before long the cigarette evolved into the wonderfully efficient delivery device we recognize today, capable of the rapid conveyance of nicotine to the dependent brain.

Cigarette smoking dramatically increased amongst men in the UK, North America and Western Europe in the decade before the First World War and rates in women soon began to increase as well.

Smoking around the world

Current estimates identify 1.1 billion smokers world wide, representing about a third of the world's population over 15 years old. They smoke a total of 6.05 trillion cigarettes each year and this equates to a tobacco consumption of 1.9 kg/person over 15. More men smoke than women and although there are wide variations, women account for a third of smokers in developed countries but only one-eighth in undeveloped countries. Developed countries have cut consumption by 17 per cent over the last decade but this is more than offset by a corresponding increase in developing countries. Eighty per cent of cigarettes are now smoked in low- and middle-income countries and Chinese men now smoke nearly 30 per cent of the world's cigarettes. Mounting mortality from smoking-related diseases can be expected on a global scale. In 1998, it is estimated that smoking killed 4 million people. This contrasts with 0.2 million deaths in 1950 and projections of 10 million for 2030 and means that smoking represents the most important preventable cause of death in the world today.

Smoking in the UK

Smoking prevalence for men in the UK peaked just after the Second World War (65 per cent in 1948) but the peak for women was in the 1970s (50 per cent). Over the last 10 years rates have dropped significantly and the latest figures show that 29 per cent of men and 28 per cent of women smoked in 1996. The figures disguise high rates in certain sub-groups – for example, in young women aged 20–24 years, 36 per cent were smokers in 1996. Smoking behaviour in different socioeconomic groups has polarized since 1960, when there was an even spread and in 1996, 12 per cent of social class I males smoked compared with 41 per cent of social class V. Fewer than 5 per cent of British GPs now smoke. There are, however, still 14 million smokers in the UK and it is estimated that at least 111 000 people are killed by their habit each year.

Smoking in Europe

It is estimated that each year about a million European men and 200 000 European women will die as a result of smoking. The prevalence of smoking is generally higher in Southern, Central and Eastern Europe but wide variations are seen. In Turkey, 63 per cent of men smoke compared with 17 per cent in Sweden. In Norway, 33 per cent of women smoke but only 5 per cent of women in Belarus smoke.

Smoking in the USA

Between 1990 and 1994, 430 700 Americans died each year from smoking-related illnesses. Although smoking has declined by 42 per cent since 1965, current estimates suggest that 26.7 per cent of men and 22.8 per cent of women still smoke.

Smoking in young people

Children who smoke are influenced by the habits of their peers, parents and siblings and there is good evidence that they smoke the most heavily advertised brands. Seventy-five per cent of smokers start before the age of 15, 90 per cent before 21. In 1994, more than one in four 15-year-old English schoolchildren smoked cigarettes regularly (Figure 5.4). Interestingly, this figure has now begun to fall, leading investigators to speculate whether the increasing attraction of mobile telephones is responsible. Whether or not this is true, their statement that 'the mobile phone is an effective competitor to cigarettes in the market for products that offer teenagers adult style, individuality, sociability, rebellion, peer group bonding and adult aspirations' beautifully summarizes the dilemmas facing young people.

In the USA, it is estimated that 6000 people try a cigarette each day and 3000 initiate the habit. Between 1980 and 1997, 39.2 per cent of male high school seniors, but only 5.4 per cent of girls, smoked.

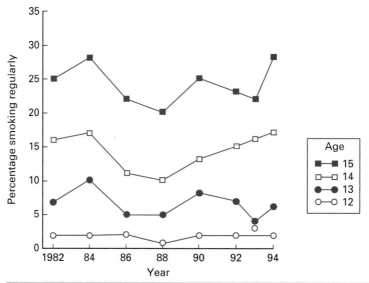

FIGURE 5.4 • Percentage of English schoolchildren (by age) smoking regularly. Source: *OPCS Survey of Smoking among Secondary Schoolchildren, 1982–94.*

In 1994, the UK government was estimated to receive £108 million in tax from cigarettes sold illegally to children under 16. Total revenue in this year from tobacco taxation was £8463 million with a taxation rate now at 80 per cent.

Consequences of cigarette smoking

In 1951, shortly after establishing the relationship between smoking and lung cancer, Doll and Hill set up the British Doctors Study. A 40-year follow-up (Doll *et al.*, 1994) is now available on 34 439 British male doctors and it is clear that half of all regular smokers are eventually killed by their habit. Of the excess deaths in the smoking group, 31 per cent succumbed to CHD and 21 per cent to other cardiovascular diseases, including stroke.

Overall, about a fifth of cardiovascular deaths and about a quarter of all deaths are directly attributable to smoking. The relative risk of smoking for cardiovascular disease is 1.4 for men and somewhat greater, 2.2, for women. Primary pipe or cigar smokers have almost the risk of non-smokers but those who switch from cigarette smoking appear to receive little benefit.

The consequences of cigarette smoking are:

- reduced lifespan;
- coronary heart disease;
- peripheral vascular disease, aneurysm;
- cerebrovascular disease (particularly in women using oral contraception);
- venous thrombosis;
- cardiac arrhythmias;

TABLE **5.4** • The life expectancy of smokers and non-smokers in years at 35 and 65

Age (years)	Male non-smoker	Male smoker	Female non-smoker	Female smoker
35	45	38	48	42
65	16	10	18	13

- increased perioperative mortality;
- cancer of lung, larynx, oesophagus, mouth, tongue, bladder, kidney, pancreas and cervix;
- chronic obstructive airways disease;
- peptic ulcer;
- low birth weight infants, premature birth, miscarriage;
- Crohn's disease;
- osteoporosis;
- passive smoking effects – asthma in infants, lung cancer, CHD;
- economic penalties.

The reduced life expectancy of smokers is shown in Table 5.4.

It has been calculated from Richard Doll's data that each cigarette smoked reduces life expectancy by 11 minutes.

Amongst cigarette smokers, risk is increased by the number of cigarettes smoked, the amount of inhalation, the age of starting, the number of years of smoking and the tar yield of the preferred cigarette. Increasing numbers of cigarettes smoked increases mortality in a near linear fashion (Figure 5.5).

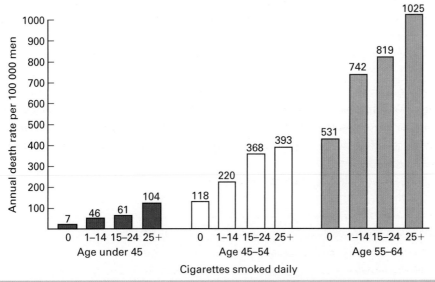

FIGURE **5.5** • CHD mortality in male British doctors by age and smoking habit. Source: Doll, R. and Peto, R. (1976) *Br Med J* **4**, 1525.

Passive smoking

For a non-smoker, the environmental exposure to tobacco smoke (e.g. from a smoking spouse) is only about 1 per cent that of smoking itself. Lung cancer is a well-known hazard of passive smoking but epidemiological studies have also consistently suggested a much greater risk of CHD in non-smokers who live with smokers than this figure might suggest.

In 1997, Law *et al.* comprehensively examined the CHD risk of passive smoking and the findings are summarized below.

- A meta-analysis of the 19 acceptable published studies identifying CHD in lifelong non-smokers who live with a smoker, showed that the increased relative risk of CHD is 1.30 ($P < 0.001$).
- An analysis of the dose–response relationship for the numbers of cigarettes smoked from five large cohort studies (including the British Doctors Study) was used to identify the calculated risk of smoking one cigarette per day at the age of 65. The relative risk of CHD in this case is 1.39, comparable to the risk of passive smoking.
- The diet of both smokers and the non-smokers who live with them shows a lower consumption of fruit and vegetables. This means a lower consumption of nutrients that protect against CHD such as folic acid, potassium, linoleic acid and antioxidants. The authors estimate the increased risk of a less cardioprotective diet to be 6 per cent and this confounding effect reduces the relative risk of CHD due to passive smoking from 1.30 to 1.23.

The Caerphilly Collaborative Heart Disease study showed a linear relationship between increasing CHD risk and increasing platelet aggregation. Laboratory studies show that even single environmental exposure to tobacco smoke results in an immediate increase in platelet aggregation. This finding may provide a plausible explanation for the low-dose effect. The effect of environmental tobacco smoke is not trivial and the hazard both in public places and in the home requires greater public education so that smokers recognize their responsibilities to others.

Mechanisms of damage

Cigarette smoke contains 3000–4000 different components and each puff contains 10^{13} free radicals. Studies in rats have demonstrated endothelial cell changes as a result of injury, and enhanced deposition of fibrinogen and lipids contributes to atherogenesis. Fibrinogen levels and platelet aggregation are increased, leading to increased blood coagulability and viscosity. Smoking appears to reduce HDL cholesterol and increase triglycerides. By sympathoadrenal stimulation, nicotine reduces coronary blood flow – most markedly in areas already compromised by ischaemic damage – and this may precipitate arrhythmias or angina, potentially resulting in the observed increased risk of sudden death among smokers.

Reducing the risk

Many attempts have been made over the last 30 years to reduce the emission levels of tar, carbon monoxide and nicotine from cigarettes. Ninety-two per cent of men and 97 per cent of women use filters, and low tar cigarettes (5–15 mg per cigarette) are associated with slightly reduced mortality. By January 2004, the tar content of European cigarettes will be reduced from 12 mg/cigarette to 10 mg, with a ceiling of 1 mg for nicotine. The regulatory systems for tobacco products, however, are weak and ineffectual. Export products, such as Chesterfield cigarettes in the Philippines, have a tar content of 31 mg. Unfortunately, smokers smoke in ways to achieve desired nicotine levels in order to avoid the symptoms of nicotine withdrawal. There is evidence, that when switching to lower-tar brands, smokers compensate by smoking more aggressively. New evidence from the Netherlands has linked the use of low-tar, filter cigarettes with a rising incidence of, and poorer survival from, lung adenocarcinoma. From September 2003, descriptions such as 'low tar', 'light' or 'mild' will be banned by the European Union and health promotion messages on packs will be increased.

There is little doubt that stopping smoking can reduce CHD risk. The Oslo study (page 243) provides convincing evidence, as does a study from Sweden which showed 85 per cent survival at 5 years in a group of non-smoking female MI survivors compared with 73 per cent survival in the group who continued to smoke.

Doubt, however, exists as to how quickly the benefits of cessation are achieved. Here surveys vary; in the BRHS, the risk for heavy smokers remained increased for more than 20 years after stopping, whereas the Framingham data suggest a much swifter effect. Changes in coagulation and rheological (flow) factors are improved within 48 hours of cessation and it may be that the benefits are more rapid than was previously thought.

DIABETES AND IMPAIRED GLUCOSE TOLERANCE

Most health professionals and an increasing number of patients appreciate that both major types of diabetes mellitus, type 1 (insulin-dependent) diabetes and type 2 (non-insulin-dependent) diabetes are associated with a markedly increased risk of cardiovascular disease.

Diabetes is one of the most common chronic diseases in the world, affecting about 8 per cent of Western populations and with more than 175 million cases world wide. Type 2 diabetes predominates, accounting for about 90 per cent of all cases. The prevalence of diabetes has always varied widely between ethnic groups and countries, ranging from <2 per cent in rural Bantu to nearly 50 per cent in American Pima Indians and South Pacific Naurauns. 'Transplanted' populations such as Asians in Europe and African Americans are also vulnerable to the development of type 2 diabetes, particularly when exposed to 'westernized' diet and lifestyle habits with attendant obesity.

Diabetes is projected to increase dramatically world wide due to population ageing and growth, as well as from rising levels of obesity and the adoption of unhealthy diets and the sedentary lifestyles associated with urbanization and industrialization (Table 5.5).

An enormous world-wide public health challenge is thus presented which will tax the health-care systems of industrialized countries and strain the health economies of many poorer nations. In many African countries the cost of one vial of insulin may be the equivalent of a month's salary.

Type 1 diabetes generally starts in younger individuals, is more common in northern Europeans and is the result of absolute insulin deficiency due to autoimmune destruction

TABLE **5.5** • Projection of the number of individuals with diabetes by 2010 (millions)

	1994	2000	2010
Type 1	11.5	18.1	23.7
Type 2	98.9	157.3	215.6

TABLE **5.6** • The diagnosis of diabetes and impaired glucose tolerance

Diabetes

With symptoms (polyuria, polydipsia, unexplained weight loss):
- Random plasma glucose: >11.1 mmol/L
- Fasting plasma glucose: >7.0 mmol/L
- Plasma glucose: >11.1 mmol/L 2 hours after 75 g oral glucose load in oral glucose tolerance test (OGTT)

With no symptoms:
- Diagnosis should not be made on a single determination
- Test again on another day to the same criteria

Impaired glucose tolerance (IGT)
- Fasting plasma glucose <7.0 mmol/L and OGTT 2-hour value >7.8 mmol/L but <11.1 mmol/L

Impaired fasting glycaemia
- Covers individuals with fasting plasma glucose 6.1–6.9 mmol/L
- Such patients should all have OGTT to exclude diabetes or IGT

World Health Organization. 'Definition, Diagnosis and Classification of Diabetes Mellitus and its Complications.' WHO/NCD/NCS 99.2; 1–58.

of pancreatic beta cells. Most type 2 diabetes is preceded by a symptom-free period of impaired glucose tolerance wherein the criteria for a diagnosis of diabetes are not met but there is an abnormal response to an oral glucose challenge (see Table 5.6). Impaired glucose tolerance is common, with a prevalence ratio to type 2 diabetes of 1.5:1. Estimates in the UK suggest that 17 per cent of the population aged 40–65 years and 11 per cent in the USA (20–74 years) have impaired glucose tolerance. The significance of impaired glucose tolerance is that there is a doubling of the CHD rate and this has been studied in the UK Whitehall population and the Paris Prospective study. In addition, progression from impaired glucose tolerance to type 2 diabetes appears to occur at a rate of between 2 and 5 per cent per annum. Type 2 diabetes develops when underlying insulin resistance, associated with impaired glucose tolerance, is compounded by failing insulin secretion from functionally compromised beta cells.

The cardiovascular risk of diabetes and impaired glucose tolerance

Diabetics have an increased all cause mortality of ×2–3 compared to age-matched non-diabetic controls and their life expectancy is reduced by 5–10 years. This is largely promoted by increased cardiovascular mortality of ×3–6 and increased CHD mortality of ×2–4. To make matters worse, when patients with diabetes develop cardiovascular disease, they sustain a worse prognosis for survival than similar patients without diabetes. The relative risk is consistently greater for women than for men and diabetic women essentially lose most of the inherent cardiovascular protection conferred by their gender. The outcome of this is that three-quarters of diabetics die from large vessel (macrovascular) disease and half from CHD, with significant contributions from cerebrovascular disease and peripheral vascular disease. The atheromatous plaques of diabetics are similar to those of non-diabetics but their evolution is accelerated and they are more extensive and diffuse compared with non-diabetics.

In 1998, Haffner *et al.* published data from a study cohort of 1059 type 2 diabetic Finnish men and women aged 45–64 and compared the 7-year CHD death or non-fatal MI rates with those of age-matched non-diabetic controls. In the diabetic subjects, the 7-year CHD rates with and without MI were 40.5 per cent and 20.2 per cent, respectively, compared with 18.8 per cent and 3.5 per cent in the non-diabetics. The striking finding is the similarity between the event rates for the diabetic subjects without prior MI and the non-diabetics with prior MI. To date, all consensus guidelines have championed secondary prevention for aggressive intervention but the results of Haffner's work show the risk equivalence of patients with diabetes and the priority need for effective risk reduction. US NCEP ATP III guidelines (see page 152) have officially endorsed this concept suggesting that patients with diabetes should be treated as if they had existing CHD. Other population studies have not suggested such close equivalence with CHD risk (e.g. UKPDS and Tayside UK) but as diabetic patients also show increased case fatality at the time of myocardial infarction and a doubling of long-term mortality thereafter, the American stance seems justified.

The mechanism of increased risk remains controversial. 'Established' risk factors such as hypertension and obesity cluster in diabetic patients but despite their high prevalence, account for no more than half the excess CHD. Insulin resistance provides a unifying hypothesis but other, less well-defined abnormalities are clearly important and chief amongst them are the influences of hyperglycaemia itself and dyslipidaemia.

Hyperglycaemia and CHD

There are clear mechanisms whereby hyperglycaemia might play a role in the pathogenesis of CHD including structural and functional changes in lipoproteins, vessel walls and accelerating the processes of atherosclerosis. However, because there is a poor correlation between the duration of type 2 diabetes and the development of macrovascular disease, it seems that hyperglycaemia does not play a major role. This is supported by the findings of the United Kingdom Prospective Diabetes Study (UKPDS) in which improved glycaemic control (represented by a 0.9 per cent reduction in Hb A_{1C}) reduced microvascular outcomes but failed to achieve a significant reduction in CHD.

Despite the lack of data to support a relationship between the degree of hyperglycaemia and CHD in type 2 diabetes, there is evidence linking glycaemia and coronary risk in populations in which most people are not diabetic. Khaw *et al.* have shown that glycosylated haemoglobin levels are positively associated with future CHD in a linear, stepwise fashion independent of other risk factors. It may be that, as with other risk factors, the risk associated with glucose intolerance may be continuous and graded and therefore incompatible with the artificial categorization that the current WHO classification imposes.

Insulin resistance

When insulin binds to cellular insulin receptors, it triggers the activation of intracellular metabolic mechanisms to regulate glucose homeostasis. Insulin resistance describes the subnormal response of tissues (chiefly skeletal muscle) to insulin, resulting in reduced uptake of glucose. Where pancreatic beta cell function is intact, the physiological response to this is to increase insulin secretion and create a compensatory hyperinsulinaemia. When beta cells cannot meet the extra demand for insulin, hyperglycaemia and diabetes mellitus result (Figure 5.6).

The entity of insulin resistance was first described in 1988 by Reaven who observed the common clustering of a number of atherogenic risk factors, including diabetes or impaired glucose tolerance, hyperinsulinaemia, central obesity, hypertension and a dyslipidaemia characterized by low HDL and raised triglycerides. He used the term 'Syndrome X' to describe the pattern, which was unfortunate, as the term had already been coined to describe angiographically negative patients with angina (microvascular angina). Ironically, many patients with cardiac Syndrome X display features of the insulin resistance syndrome.

Hyperuricaemia is also a feature of the insulin resistance syndrome although the exact relationship is not clear. Uric acid correlates with hypertension, glucose intolerance and dyslipidaemia and is a marker for CHD. Plasminogen activator inhibitor 1 (PAI-1) is a similar marker and is also elevated in insulin-resistant states. As an inhibitor of tissue-plasminogen activator, the principal mediator of clot lysis, it plays an important role in fibrinolytic activity. Elevated levels are associated with a prothrombotic state.

Much work remains to be done to find out the causes of insulin resistance. Major contributory factors include genetic abnormalities, obesity, physical inactivity and advancing

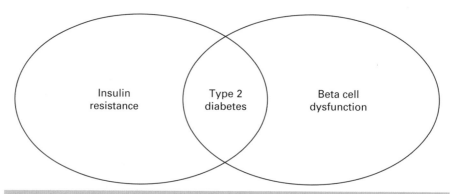

FIGURE **5.6** • Schematic representation of the origins of type 2 diabetes mellitus.

age. Rare genetic defects of the insulin receptor have been identified but most defects are active at the post-receptor level and candidate genes await elucidation. The role of intrauterine malnutrition and fetal programming may be important. The mechanism behind the association between central obesity and insulin resistance is poorly explained but it may be that the high levels of free fatty acids found in obese people reduce glucose utilization in muscle, causing a rise in circulating glucose. In the liver, high free fatty acid levels promote gluconeogenesis, further elevating blood glucose. That physical inactivity is a factor is evidenced by the fact that increased physical activity improves insulin sensitivity, independent of weight loss.

Circulating levels of adrenaline, growth hormone and cortisol antagonize the actions of insulin and can be active during stress or disease. Drugs such as corticosteroids, thiazides and beta-blockers also antagonize peripheral insulin action. Insulin resistance is also an important characteristic of polycystic ovary syndrome.

The relationship between insulin resistance and hypertension is also complex. Insulin does not cause hypertension directly but may contribute to hypertension by stimulating renal reabsorption of sodium and by sympathetic nervous system stimulation.

The relationships of insulin resistance and hyperinsulinaemia to cardiovascular risk factors are shown in Figure 5.7.

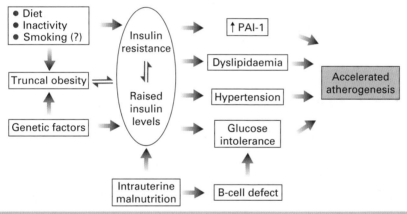

FIGURE 5.7 • Relationships of insulin resistance and hyperinsulinaemia to cardiovascular risk factors.

Diabetic dyslipidaemia

Although virtually every lipid and lipoprotein is affected by insulin resistance and diabetes mellitus, hypertriglyceridaemia is the dominant feature. Hypertriglyceridaemia arises as a consequence of the increased production and reduced catabolism of triglyceride-rich lipoproteins.

■ Insulin is normally secreted postprandially and decreases VLDL secretion from the liver. This promotes triglyceride storage at a time when triglyceride-rich lipoprotein production is high. Triglyceride catabolic pathways are also freed to deal with remnants and IDL and prevent their accumulation. When insulin levels fall later, VLDL secretion increases and hepatic triglyceride is mobilized. In situations of insulin deficiency or resistance there is impaired suppression of postprandial VLDL secretion and persistence of relatively atherogenic remnant and IDL particles. As most people eat regularly and therefore spend more hours in the postprandial state this may enhance cardiovascular risk.

■ Obese individuals secrete more free fatty acids from their adipocytes. Increased free fatty acids arriving at the liver increase hepatic triglyceride synthesis. Increased free fatty acids also reach the liver as a result of the activation of hormone-sensitive lipase, the enzyme in adipocytes that hydrolyses their stored triglycerides. Insulin normally inhibits this enzyme but insulin deficiency or resistance activates it.

■ Lipoprotein lipase, normally activated by insulin, leads to reduced breakdown of triglycerides in insulin deficiency or insulin resistant states and occasionally very high levels of triglycerides can be seen.

The resulting hypertriglyceridaemia changes the composition of all lipoproteins, enriching them with triglyceride and making them better substrates for hepatic lipase, whose activity is increased. This leads to decreased levels of HDL cholesterol and smaller, denser LDL cholesterol particles, which penetrate the arterial wall more easily and are more susceptible to oxidative modification. As triglyceride levels increase, abnormalities in HDL cholesterol and LDL cholesterol become more apparent. When triglyceride levels are more than 2.3 mmol/L, 90 per cent of LDL cholesterol particles will be of the small, dense variety.

Most patients with diabetes do not have marked elevations of LDL cholesterol. LDL cholesterol remains, however, a common risk factor for diabetics and subgroup analysis of the major statin studies shows that reducing it is effective.

Summary

It is clear that hyperglycaemia does not play a major role in the development of macrovascular disease. Haffner has said that 'the clock starts ticking for macrovascular disease in diabetes' long before the appearance of hyperglycaemia. The metabolic abnormalities that characterize the asymptomatic, prodromal period of insulin resistance, prior to developing diabetes, predispose to the development of macrovascular disease. Quantitative and qualitative abnormalities in lipoproteins contribute substantially to the increased risk.

Diabetic nephropathy

Diabetic nephropathy has four distinct phases:

■ microalbuminuria (urine albumin 30–300 mg/day);
■ macroalbuminuria (>300 mg/day);
■ nephrotic syndrome (urine protein >3 g/day);
■ chronic renal failure.

The progression of diabetic renal disease is associated with an incremental risk of cardiovascular disease. In the WHO Multinational Study of Vascular Disease in Diabetes, the presence of proteinuria increased the risk of death three to four times. In type 2 diabetics, microalbuminuria has emerged as a powerful risk factor for both total and cardiovascular mortality. A multivariate analysis of CHD in type 2 diabetes found microalbuminuria to be the leading predictor [odds ratio (OR) 10.02], ahead of smoking, diastolic blood pressure and serum cholesterol.

Macroalbuminuria usually denotes significant nephropathy and heralds declining glomerular function. When nephrotic syndrome develops, patients usually develop nephrotic dyslipidaemia, characterized by high cholesterol levels. Finally, progressive renal insufficiency ensues and the need for dialysis and transplantation to support survival.

CAN TYPE 2 DIABETES BE PREVENTED?

At current rates of projection, analysts predict that by 2025 the number of people with diabetes world wide could reach 300 million. The disease is progressive and places an enormous burden on individuals and society in terms of death, reduced quality of life and adverse social and economic consequences. Major lifestyle changes resulting from industrialization, such as changing dietary patterns, becoming overweight and reduced physical activity mean that diabetes will increase disproportionately, favouring industrializing countries. Treatments are effective in reducing the complications of diabetes but are underused and expensive. The idea of preventing type 2 diabetes by modifying lifestyle factors is therefore very germane.

Several studies have examined this question. Most have looked at the effect of lifestyle interventions on 'at-risk' patients, namely those with impaired glucose tolerance (IGT). The Malmo Study is investigating diet and exercise modification in male subjects with IGT. Results to date are impressive with more than 50 per cent achieving normal glucose control and concomitant benefits in blood pressure and lipid profiles. The Chinese Da Qing Study randomized 577 IGT subjects to one of four groups: control, dietary intervention, exercise or diet plus exercise. After 6 years, the intervention groups were respectively associated with a 31 per cent, 46 per cent and 42 per cent reduction in the risk of developing diabetes.

By far the most impressive evidence, however, comes from a newly published randomized trial from Finland, where Tuomilehto et al. (2001) reduced the progression to diabetes in 522 middle-aged, overweight subjects with IGT, by 58 per cent over 4 years. The intervention comprised individual counselling to lose weight, reduce total and saturated fat and increase dietary fibre and physical activity. Effectively, one case of diabetes was prevented for every five subjects treated over 5 years.

Implementing such programmes represents an enormous organizational challenge and spreads beyond the clinical forum to involve public health and community-based strategies. The alternative, an increasingly complex and expensive medical organization to control diabetes and its consequences is far more daunting.

CAN TYPE 2 DIABETES BE PREVENTED?

OBESITY

Ever since Hippocrates noted that 'sudden death is more common in those who are naturally fat, rather than those who are lean', numerous long-term prospective studies have consistently shown that excess body fat is related to increased levels of cardiovascular disease. The Center for Disease Control and Prevention estimates that obesity causes 300 000 deaths per year in the USA (second only to smoking), at a cost of 8 per cent of the health-care budget and up to US$100 million in indirect costs.

Obesity is the result of positive energy balance. Typically, an obese individual will have gained about 20 kg over 10 years. This derives from a daily energy excess of only 30–40 kcal, an amount corresponding to half a plain biscuit or moderate intensity exercise lasting half an hour, and over the long time scale of obesity development such small amounts are easy to overlook. Genetic factors are active and the heritability of obesity is at least as strong as it is for hypertension, alcoholism and schizophrenia. Several genes involved in energy regulation have now been identified and there is much interest in leptin, a protein produced by adipose tissue, that signals satiety to the hypothalamus.

Measurement of obesity

The **body mass index** (BMI) or Quetelet's index is the scale employed most often to define obesity (see Figure 7.1). It is calculated by using the equation:

$$BMI \ (kg/m^2) = Weight \ (kg)/Height \ (m^2)$$

The WHO classification of overweight and obesity in adults is shown in Table 5.7 with each category's attendant co-morbidity risk.

A BMI of 25–28.9 kg/m^2 has been associated with a twofold increase in cardiovascular disease rising to nearly fourfold once BMI exceeds 29 kg/m^2.

Exactly where healthy weight ends and unhealthy weight begins has been a matter of debate. In a study of 14 077 apparently healthy European women, Ashton *et al.* (2001) found that as BMI increased from <20 to >30, blood pressure, total and LDL cholesterol, apolipoprotein B, fasting triglycerides and fasting blood glucose also increased significantly. In addition, HDL cholesterol and Apo A-I decreased. When the Framingham risk function was used to estimate 10-year CHD risk, that also increased in a linear fashion

TABLE **5.7** • World Health Organization classification of overweight and obesity in adults

Category	BMI (kg/m^2)	Risk for co-morbidities
Underweight	<18.5	Low
Normal weight	18.5–24.9	Average
Overweight	>25	
Pre-obese	25.0–29.9	Increased
Obese class 1	30.0–34.9	Moderate
Obese class 2	35.0–39.9	Severe
Obese class 3	>40	Very severe

across the range. In a study of 100 000 American nurses aged 30–55 the relative risk of CHD compared to those with BMI <21 was 1.19 for women with BMI 21–22.9, 1.46 for women with BMI 23–24.9 and 2.06 for women with BMI 25–28.9. Taken together, these data suggest that risk is increased at BMI values even in the so-called 'healthy' range.

Whilst it is recognized that individuals with high BMI, as a group, have more complications, it is also clear that the risk of complications is not the same in all those with similar BMIs. Raised BMI can result from a large mass of muscle or bone and does not automatically reflect a high degree of adiposity. The distribution of adiposity also seems to be important and we have known for over 40 years that that those with central obesity have a higher risk of diabetes and cardiovascular disease than those with a peripheral distribution. Central, abdominal, truncal, visceral or android obesity is commonly seen in men whose 'pot bellies' make them look 'apple-shaped'. A thick waist and a propensity for fat deposition around the buttocks and hips producing a 'pear shape', characterize peripheral, gluteo-femoral, or gynaecoid obesity. This is more common in women but the patterns are not gender specific; indeed, central obesity for women confers significant CHD risk (Figure 5.8).

The pattern of central obesity is commonly seen in those of South Asian extraction and is associated with the insulin resistance syndrome and the development of type 2 diabetes (up to 75 per cent of patients with type 2 diabetes are reported to be obese). The mechanisms predisposing to this type of fat distribution are poorly understood but, although central adiposity accounts for only 6–20 per cent of total adipose tissue volume, it exerts a profound influence through adverse effects on hepatic lipid and insulin metabolism.

Although precise methods for measuring the distribution of body fat, such as computerized tomography and magnetic resonance imaging, are available, clinicians need simpler tools. **The waist hip ratio** (WHR), ideally measured after an overnight fast, is the waist measurement (half way between the lower costal margin and the iliac crest) divided by the hip circumference (as measured over the widest part of the gluteal region). WHR should not exceed 1.0 in men and 0.85 in women. The problem with WHR measurements is that they can conceal considerable total body fat increases if fat deposition increases both waist and hip circumferences to the same degree, such that the ratio remains the same. In addition, the advent of more sophisticated scanning showed that **waist circumference** by itself was the best correlate of visceral adipose tissue. Table 5.8 shows the risk of obesity-associated complications by waist circumference in Caucasians.

Despres has argued for the recognition of the 'hypertriglyceridaemic waist phenotype' on the basis that 80 per cent of men with waist circumference >90 cm and hypertriglyceridaemia >2.0 mmol/L have metabolic disturbances which include hyperinsulinaemia, increased Apo B, increased small, dense LDL cholesterol and their attendant cardiovascular risks.

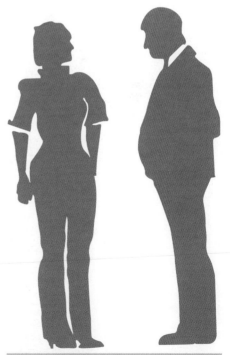

FIGURE **5.8** • Obesity distribution: 'pear' and 'apple' body shapes.

TABLE **5.8** • The risk of obesity-associated complications by waist circumferences (WC)

Risk of complications	Male WC (cm/in)	Female WC (cm/in)
Increased	>94 (>90 Asian origin)/37	>80/32
Substantially increased	>102/40	>88/35

Obesity as a risk factor

It is clear that many of the effects of obesity are mediated through increases in other parameters and this has led to debate concerning the independence of obesity as a risk factor. Obesity is associated with hypertension, increased total cholesterol and triglycerides and reduced HDL cholesterol (Figure 5.9).

There is also associated insulin resistance with increased glucose and insulin levels and increased rates of type 2 diabetes. When studies such as the Seven Countries Study correct for these factors, obesity does not emerge as an independent risk factor, but some investigators, using the same data, have drawn different conclusions. Research from Framingham also supports independence, particularly in the under 50s and where central

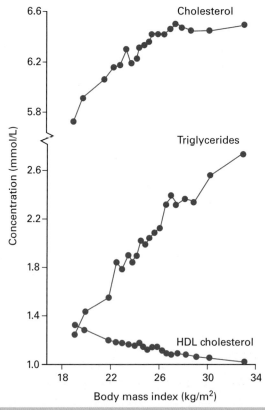

FIGURE **5.9** • The effect of increasing degrees of obesity on serum lipids and HDL cholesterol. Reproduced with permission from BMJ Publishing Group from Thelle, D.S., Shaper, A.G., Whitehead, T.P., Bullock, D.G., Ashby, D. and Patel, I. (1983) *Br Heart J* **49**, 205–13.

obesity is present. Whether obesity is an independent risk factor or merely a 'marker' for others is, in practice, an unnecessary distinction as it certainly represents a readily identifiable and potentially modifiable risk factor.

Consequences of obesity

The consequences of obesity are:

- coronary heart disease
- hypertension
- cerebrovascular disease
- type 2 diabetes mellitus
- musculoskeletal disease and reduced exercise tolerance
- breathlessness and heartburn
- sleep apnoea
- venous thromboembolism
- psychological distress and social dysfunction
- gallstones
- infertility and pregnancy-related problems
- problems with surgery and anaesthesia
- cancer of the colon, breast, endometrium, kidney and oesophagus. Adipose tissue contains aromatase, which converts androgens to oestrogens, contributing to both fertility problems and sex-hormone-sensitive cancers.

Prevalence of obesity

The prevalence of obesity has increased dramatically in both developed and developing countries. Half of European and 61 per cent of American adults are now overweight and the situation continues to deteriorate. As the gene pool is relatively stable and there has been an overall reduction in saturated fat consumption, the explanation must lie in an increased intake of total calories, coupled with reduced physical activity.

The UK has the fastest growing rate of obesity in Europe, almost trebling in the last two decades (Table 5.9).

Countries such as the UK, France and Germany each have 5–10 million inhabitants who are obese and need treatment. Apart from treating a few prioritized individuals at highest risk, the task is beyond the resources of each country's health-care system to manage and therefore the focus must be on prevention.

TABLE **5.9** • Increasing prevalence of obesity in UK (% total male/female pupulation, respectively)

BMI (mg/kg^2)	1980		1994		1997	
	Male	**Female**	**Male**	**Female**	**Male**	**Female**
25–30	33	24	43	29	45	33
>30	6	8	13	16	17	20

The intense relationship with socioeconomic status has already been noted (Table 2.6). The relationship is, however, inconsistent, as in developed countries poverty is associated with increased obesity prevalence (particularly in women) whereas in developing countries, it is relative affluence that carries the greater risk. In the USA, the African and Mexican American minorities are most affected. Developing countries are now seeing serious increases in obesity, for example, in the Caribbean, South America and South East Asia. Prevalences of up to 80 per cent have been recorded in Australian aborigines and Polynesian islanders.

The Pima Indian experience highlights that it takes 15–20 years before increased body weight leads to diabetes and another 5–15 years before morbidity and mortality consequences impact on health-care systems. Effectively the 'time bomb' of obesity is already ticking.

FATNESS OR FITNESS?

Amongst the earliest characteristics we notice about other people are the observations that unfit people are often fat and that fat people are rarely fit. Inactivity is linked to loss of cardiorespiratory capacity and loss of muscle mass and tone. This frequently leads to weight gain, mostly as fat and a decrease in an individual's power to weight ratio such that physical activity becomes more difficult, heralding a further tightening of the vicious circle that accelerates into further weight gain and inactivity. Even Falstaff, in *Henry IV*, acknowledged that: 'Eight yards of uneven ground is three score and ten miles a-foot with me.'

Claims have been made that it is not obesity *per se* that produces ill health but lack of physical fitness. Moreover, by achieving physical fitness, overweight individuals can reduce both future cardiovascular disease and type 2 diabetes.

Professor Steve Blair, from Dallas, is the leading proponent of the 'fat can be fit' debate and his analysis of the follow-up of 25000 men in the Aerobics Center Longitudinal Study is shown in Figure 5.10. Cardiorespiratory fitness was measured by maximal exercise treadmill testing and just as in other studies, levels of activity correlate well with cardiovascular outcomes (greater levels of activity being associated with lower risks of death). As the risk ratio has been set at unity for each of the low-risk groups, the effect of obesity is obscured. However, the death rates in the low-activity groups by increasing BMI were 52.1, 49.1 and 62.1 per 10000 person-years respectively. In the high-fit groups the death rates were 20.0, 19.7 and 18.0.

Blair's hypothesis rests on the comparison between the two extreme groups wherein:

■ the death rate of unfit men with low BMI was 52.1 per 10000 man-years compared with only 18.0 in highly fit men with BMI $> 30 \, kg/m^2$.

The same database also shows that the incidence of type 2 diabetes mellitus in highly fit men with BMI $> 27 \, kg/m^2$ is also reduced below the level seen in unfit men with BMI $< 27 \, kg/m^2$.

It seems that physical activity can lead to improved outcome independent of

FATNESS OR FITNESS?

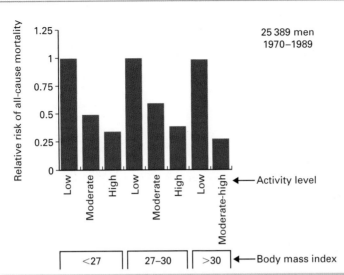

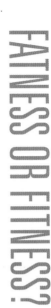

FIGURE 5.10 • All-cause mortality versus fatness and fitness. Aerobics Center Longitudinal Study. Adapted from Barlow, C.E., Koh, H.W., Gibbons, L.W. *et al.* (1995) *Int J Obes* **19**(Suppl. 4), S41–4.

achieving weight loss. The greatest benefit seems to derive from moving people from low levels of activity to moderate activity and as high levels of fitness are an impossible goal for many, the best strategies are probably to encourage moderate activity, and at all costs to avoid inactivity.

PHYSICAL INACTIVITY

Lack of exercise is also difficult to categorize as an independent risk factor because of the positive effects of exercise on other characteristics. 'Exercisers' tend to lead healthier lifestyles and, because of the absence of randomized controlled trials, the data are mostly epidemiological. Nevertheless, in nearly 50 epidemiological studies, none has shown higher risks of CHD in physically active men. The relative risk of CHD for physical inactivity ranges between 1.5 and 2.4, an increase in risk that is comparable to those associated with high cholesterol, high blood pressure or cigarette smoking. The link between coronary mortality and different levels of fitness is summarized in Figure 5.11.

Typical of the epidemiological studies is the Harvard Alumni study wherein the rate of myocardial infarction was 64 per cent higher in graduates who expended less than 2000 kcal/week on exercise compared with classmates with higher levels of activity.

Occupational exercise was neatly investigated when London double-decker bus conductors were found to have half the incidence of CHD compared with their driver colleagues. The question of self-selection arose when it was pointed out that conductors were of slimmer build than drivers and that perhaps conductors were innately healthier and able to choose more active jobs. When the trouser band width of their uniforms (a surrogate for central obesity?) was related to the rates of CHD, it was shown that whatever the size of the conductor – slim, normal or overweight – their rates were still half those of drivers.

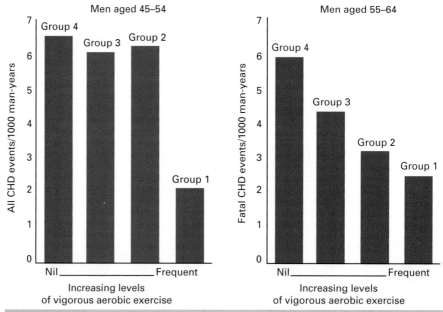

FIGURE **5.11** • Incidence of CHD events by level of vigorous aerobic exercise.

Similar findings were reported in San Francisco dockworkers where those with sedentary occupations had an 80 per cent excess risk of fatal CHD compared with the stevedores.

As the number of heavy jobs in industrialized societies diminishes, more exercise will need to be taken in leisure time.

Benefits of exercise

Exercise causes slight reduction in blood pressure, definite reduction in weight, improved glucose tolerance and coagulation profiles, reduced myocardial oxygen consumption and psychological and social benefits. HDL cholesterol is increased and LDL cholesterol and triglycerides reduced. A study in overweight men showed that jogging an average 11.7 miles/week produced a 10.4 per cent increase in HDL cholesterol. Similarly, in middle-aged women, 2.5 hours brisk walking per week improved HDL cholesterol by 27 per cent. Meta-analyses of cardiac rehabilitation programmes that include exercise regimens for post-MI patients have shown 20–25 per cent reduction in overall and cardiac mortality.

There has been a shift away from recommendations that advise vigorous exercise towards those advising exercise of moderate intensity. This coincides with the appearance of evidence of effectiveness from studies of moderate activity, particularly walking and the realization that targeting sedentary people with a more achievable intervention is more likely to be effective. There is evidence from Harvard, that walking 9 miles per week produces a 21 per cent reduction in death rate. In the British Regional Heart Study, 40–60 minutes of walking per day was again associated with reduced risk. Moderate activity is defined as achieving 40–60 per cent of VO_{2max}. It makes you feel warm and slightly out of breath and can be achieved by brisk walking (3–4 mph), cycling, swimming, dancing, golf (carrying clubs), vigorous housework and gardening.

Death during recreational exercise is uncommon (4.46 deaths/100 000 men in Rhode Island) but unaccustomed strenuous exercise is to be avoided.

Prevalence of physical inactivity

Twenty-five per cent of Americans report no leisure time physical activity and only 37 per cent are active enough to give themselves some protection against CHD. The figures are worse in the UK with only 30 per cent of men and 20 per cent of women reaching desirable levels. Inactivity increases with age and is also more prevalent in women, the less educated and certain ethnic groups (African and Hispanic Americans and South Asian British).

THROMBOGENIC FACTORS

Although a thrombotic component was recognized as long ago as 1912, in Herrick's description of coronary thrombosis, the role of thrombogenic factors in the development of unstable angina, myocardial infarction and sudden death was not established until the early 1980s. Now it is clear that several components of the coagulation and fibrinolytic systems (fibrinogen, factor VII, von Willebrand factor, tissue-type plasminogen activator and PAI-1) are correlated with CHD.

Fibrinogen is a large molecule that increases blood viscosity and platelet aggregation, leading to a hypercoagulable state favouring plaque thrombosis. It also has a role in atherogenesis by fibrin deposition in vessel walls and may promote smooth muscle migration and proliferation. From the early 1980s, Meade began to demonstrate an independent, positive relationship between fibrinogen and CHD (Table 5.10).

TABLE **5.10** • The relationship between fibrinogen and CHD

Factor	MI	Angina	CHD	No CHD
Number in study	38	33	71	1350
Fibrinogen (g/L)	3.24	3.21	3.22	2.91

Source: Meade, T., Mellows, S., Brozovic, M. *et al.* (1986) Haemostatic function and ischaemic heart disease: principal results of the Northwick Park Heart Study. *Lancet* **2**, 533–7.

A fibrinogen level in the upper third of the population increased the risk of CHD threefold over those in the lower third of the population. This level of increased relative risk has been replicated in other studies and a meta-analysis by Ernst and Resch in 1993 concluded that high fibrinogen levels independently predicted a 2.3-fold increase in CHD risk, a predictive power comparable to that of elevated cholesterol itself. Fibrinogen is also a powerful predictor for stroke and peripheral vascular disease.

Despite the strength of its apparent predictive capacity, fibrinogen is not often measured in clinical practice. The development of fibrinogen as a CHD predictor has been hampered by the lack of consensus agreement as to which assay technique should be standard. In addition, assays can be difficult to interpret, as there is only a small difference between levels that are considered normal and those that are considered pathological.

High fibrinogen levels are most common in smokers where levels are increased by up to 10 per cent, the rise being proportional to the number of cigarettes smoked. It is interesting that in the WHO clofibrate trial, most of the reduction in CHD was in the heavy smoking group (clofibrate also reduces fibrinogen).

The list of situations where fibrinogen is increased reads like a list of CHD risk factors:

- **smoking**
- increasing age
- heredity, e.g. polymorphisms of beta fibrinogen gene
- obesity
- oral contraception
- diabetes/insulin resistance
- hypertension
- peripheral vascular disease
- 'stress'
- high LDL cholesterol and triglycerides
- low HDL cholesterol
- physical inactivity
- menopause and pregnancy
- season (winter)
- infection.

This is hardly surprising as fibrinogen is an acute phase protein, whose synthesis is increased in response to virtually any pro-inflammatory stimulus. Some observers think fibrinogen is a marker for the inflammatory process associated with atherosclerosis rather than a causal factor, where it would play a more direct role.

Apart from smoking cessation, moderate alcohol intake, physical activity and weight loss, fibrinogen levels can be lowered by fibrates (except gemfibrozil) and oestrogens in postmenopausal women. N-3 fatty acids and beta-blockers also have fibrinogen-lowering activity in addition to their principal effects. After stopping smoking, there are differences in fibrinogen levels within 2 days but the return to non-smoker levels is very slow and may take 5–20 years.

Subgroup analyses of studies like the Bezafibrate Infarction Prevention (BIP) study suggest that treatment of raised fibrinogen levels, in parallel with lipid lowering, may be beneficial in the secondary prevention of CHD, but further studies are needed.

The evidence of a relationship between **factor VII** and CHD risk is weaker than that for fibrinogen. Two studies have provided evidence of the existence of such a relationship but PROCAM did not. Elevated levels of **plasminogen activator inhibitor 1 (PAI-1)** have been noted to be associated with an increased risk of recurrent myocardial infarction and higher levels have been reported in patients with unstable angina.

Increased activation and aggregation of **platelets** are associated with an increased risk of clinical CHD. Platelet activation involves increased surface glycoprotein (GP) IIb/IIIa receptor expression such that when fibrinogen molecules bind to these receptors, aggregation is induced. Antiplatelet drugs such as aspirin, clopidogrel and GP-IIb/IIIa receptor antagonists interfere with platelet metabolism and compelling evidence underwrites their use in acute coronary syndromes, established cardiovascular disease and percutaneous interventions.

PSYCHOSOCIAL FACTORS

If the relatives of a victim of CHD are asked for antecedent factors, it is inevitable that 'stress' will figure prominently. The evidence, however, is limited, not only because stress is difficult to define and measure, but also because there is great individual variation of response. A few retrospective studies have examined life events before myocardial infarction but there is no predictive link. There is a lack of studies looking at the acute crisis situation where the reaction is probably neurohumoral.

In 1959, Friedman and Rosenman linked type A personality (competitive, aggressive, time urgent) with increased CHD, when compared with the more passive type B personality. In the Whitehall study of British civil servants, men of the lowest working grades (messengers, office support staff and the like) had three times the CHD rate of workers in the highest grades (the senior administrators). The inverse social gradient of CHD has been noted before (see Chapter 2) but it was surprising in the Whitehall study that a social gradient was maintained within a much narrower social group. Although the highest grades had the lowest rates for CHD, they also included more type A individuals and this weakened the personality theory. Differences in traditional risk factors also failed to completely explain the findings and the conclusion was reached that an individual's position within a hierarchy is important. This is reflected in an animal model where lower-order monkeys on a high fat diet developed the most atherosclerosis.

Much of the inverse social gradient in CHD incidence can be attributed to differences in the psychosocial work environment. A particularly stressful work environment is characterized by high demand and time pressure, with low control and decision latitude. The situation is compounded by inadequate reward for effort expended, boring monotonous tasks, poor working conditions and under-use of skills. Individual behavioural responses include hostility, depression, anxiety, hopelessness and the adoption of unhealthy lifestyles including smoking, poor diet and lack of activity. Further negative influences have been identified as unemployment, poverty, poor social support, lower educational attainment and insufficient health-care utilization.

The relationship between psychosocial factors and CHD has important implications for managers, as attention is necessary to each individual's work situation, social environment and emotional reactions as well as lifestyle and health habits. Comprehensive behaviour modification programmes, such as the Lifestyle Heart Trial, show relatively promising results and may increase the effectiveness of conventional risk factor management.

Psychosocial factors may exert their effects alone or in clusters and may be active at different stages in the life course. Their main mechanisms of action are interrelated and include:

■ an adverse effect on health-related behaviours – smoking, diet, alcohol consumption and physical activity.

- a direct acute or chronic effect on pathophysiological processes – one study has linked a boring job with high fibrinogen levels.
- an adverse influence on the uptake of health-care provision.

HOMOCYSTEINE

Homocysteine is a sulphur amino acid produced by demethylation of the essential amino acid, methionine. If plasma homocysteine concentrations are sufficiently high, urinary excretion occurs and the disulphide homocystine can be detected in the urine. It has been known since 1969 that patients with the homozygous form of the autosomal recessive condition, homocystinuria (classically deficiency of the breakdown enzyme, cystathionine beta-synthetase), often die before the age of 30 from premature atherothrombotic disease. The upper limit of normal for plasma homocysteine is generally considered to be 12–15 μmol/L but in homocystinuria, levels exceed 30 μmol/L and sometimes more than 100 μmol/L. Although there is no evidence of a threshold effect, homocysteine levels exceeding 15 μmol/L are common and are found in up to 30 per cent of patients with vascular disease and possibly more with venous thromboembolism.

A plethora of observational studies have established, with reasonable consistency, that raised plasma homocysteine levels constitute a risk factor for coronary, cerebral and peripheral atherosclerosis. Boushey *et al.*'s meta-analysis in 1995 of 27 studies indicated that raised homocysteine levels were associated with increased CHD ($\times 1.7$), cerebrovascular disease ($\times 2.5$) and peripheral vascular disease ($\times 6.8$). Boushey estimated that a 5 μmol/L increase in homocysteine increased vascular risk by about one-third, which is similar to an increase in plasma cholesterol of about 0.5 mmol/L. Since 1995, more than 40 studies have supported these findings. The large European Collaborative Study showed a similar relative risk increase for vascular disease of 35 per cent for men and 42 per cent for women for each 5 μmol/L increment of homocysteine.

The mechanism whereby homocysteine may exert its action is not clear but experimental evidence points to its ability to induce endothelial dysfunction, to affect platelet function and coagulation factors and to promote LDL cholesterol oxidation, monocyte adhesion and smooth muscle proliferation. Interaction with other conventional risk factors, particularly smoking, hypertension and hyperlipidaemia, further increases risk.

Vitamins B6, B12 and folic acid all act as co-factors in homocysteine metabolism and nutritional deficiencies of both B12 and folate importantly relate to increased homocysteine levels. Renal impairment is also associated with increased levels as the kidney is the route of excretion for homocysteine. Mutations of the gene that codes the enzyme methylene tetrahydrofolate reductase (especially *MTHFR 677T*) can also cause modest rises of up to 50 per cent in homocysteine levels but, surprisingly, studies have not correlated the presence of this common genetic defect with increased vascular risk. *MTHFR 677T* is common, affecting up to 40 per cent of the Caucasian population. It is thought that the effects of the mutation are expressed only when dietary folate is low. Similar mutations affecting the influence of B12 on methionine synthetase are also described.

Plasma concentrations of homocysteine are higher in South Asian populations. The frequency of *MTHFR* mutations, however, is reduced and the explanation probably lies in nutritional B12 and folate deficiencies or an increased prevalence of renal impairment.

Whatever the specific cause of hyperhomocysteinaemia, more than 90 per cent of subjects respond to vitamin treatment within 2–6 weeks. Folic acid is the single most effective therapy and dietary supplementation reduces plasma homocysteine by about 25 per cent and offers the potential for therapy. The minimum effective daily dose appears to be 400 µg and except in renal failure, larger doses do not seem to confer extra benefit. Adding vitamin B12 (mean 0.5 mg/day) is associated with an additional reduction of 7 per cent but adding B6 has no further effect. Folic acid supplementation is an integral recommendation for the prevention of neural tube defect and the health benefits of fortifying flour with folic acid are being discussed.

Although the observational data for the establishment of raised homocysteine levels as an independent risk factor are strong, the possibilities of bias and the presence of confounding factors mean that the case is not proven. Confounding factors include age, sex, smoking, physical activity and coffee drinking. The possibility remains that raised homocysteine is simply a marker for a poor diet, deficient in fruit and vegetables, B vitamins and other cardioprotective micronutrients. Ultimately, the case will depend on the outcome of at least nine controlled trials that are in progress to evaluate the potential of homocysteine reduction. One of the first to publish, from Schnyder *et al.* (2001), examined the effect of a combination of folic acid (1 mg), vitamin B12 (400 µg) and pyridoxine (10 mg) versus placebo in 205 coronary angioplasty patients. Homocysteine levels were reduced from 11.1 ($\pm$4.3) to 7.2 ($\pm$2.4) µmol/L and after 6 months there were significant differences in minimal luminal diameter and a most impressive reduction in the restenosis rate (19.6 per cent versus 37.6 per cent).

INFLAMMATORY MARKERS

Although Virchow postulated over 100 years ago that atherosclerosis was inflammatory in nature, it is only in the last two decades that studies have convincingly demonstrated the significant role played by inflammation in both the initiation and progression of arterial disease. The concept that a systemic, low-grade inflammatory response is an integral part of the atherosclerotic process has been suggested by detailed investigations of vulnerable plaques and by the associations of levels of various markers of inflammation with the future risk of events.

Characteristically, activated macrophages and T-cell lymphocytes actively congregate in the shoulders of vulnerable plaques about to erode or fissure. The inflammatory cells, together with altered endothelial cells, secrete pro-inflammatory cytokines, growth factors, leucocyte chemo-attractant and adhesion molecules and collagen-degrading metalloproteinases. The net result of all this activity is a decrease in the integrity of the plaque cap, potentially triggering an acute event. The inflammatory process at this juncture is so intense that it has been equated to that found in the synovium of patients with acute rheumatoid arthritis. As atherosclerosis is a generalized disorder and plaques are multiple, sufficient inflammatory markers are expressed to allow measurement in the laboratory and subsequent correlation with events. Table 5.11 lists inflammatory markers that have potential to predict CHD.

Inflammatory mediators are released by a variety of acute stimuli including extreme exercise, acute infection, temperature change and acute psychological stress. All of these

TABLE **5.11** • Systemic inflammatory markers in patients with CHD

Inflammatory mediators
- High pro-inflammatory cytokines, e.g. interleukin-1beta (IL-1β), IL-6, IL-8, tumour necrosis factor alpha (TNF-α) and interferon-gamma (IFN-γ)
- Increased monocyte adhesion molecules, e.g. soluble intercellular circulating adhesion molecule 1 (ICAM-1), soluble vascular circulating adhesion molecule (VCAM-1) and E-selectin
- Activated nuclear factor-kappa B (NF-κB)

Acute phase proteins
- High C-reactive protein
- High serum amyloid A protein
- High fibrinogen

Other
- Raised erythrocyte sedimentation rate
- Raised white blood cell count
- Reduced serum albumin
- Increased macrophage neopterin

can precipitate an acute coronary event. In chronic terms, the most important triggers are oxidized LDL cholesterol and smoking. Released cytokines activate endothelial cells, stimulating the production of adhesion molecules and thrombogenic factors. The function of circulating adhesion molecules (CAMs) is to allow circulating leucocytes to adhere to and enter the endothelium. Monocyte-transformed macrophages then incorporate oxidized LDL cholesterol, stimulate fibroblast and smooth muscle proliferation and orchestrate a wide range of pro-atherosclerotic activities. In addition, cytokines [particularly interleukin 6 (IL-6)] also stimulate the production of acute phase proteins from the liver.

One such acute phase reactant is **C-reactive protein** (CRP). First discovered in 1930, CRP is synthesized by the liver after induction by cytokines, in response to tissue injury, infection or inflammation. It has no diagnostic specificity, being a general marker of inflammation, and can increase from baseline levels 10 000-fold as part of an acute phase response. High sensitivity assays can now detect levels of low-grade inflammation (<10 mg/L) that would previously have been unnoticed. This has opened up the possibility of using the measurement of CRP, originating from the chronic inflammatory processes of atherosclerosis, as a predictor of CHD risk.

In the general population, individuals with baseline levels in the top third (mean CRP level 2.4 mg/L) have twice the future risk of CHD events than those in the bottom third (mean CRP 1.0 mg/L). This is similar to the risk attributed to elevated fibrinogen. Other epidemiological studies have demonstrated similar associations with stroke and peripheral vascular disease. Smoking and being overweight are known to increase CRP levels, but the relationship holds even when these confounding factors are adjusted for. Adipose tissue is a strong source of IL-6 and this may explain the association with obesity. In higher-risk populations, elevated CRP has been shown to predict future events in patients with stable and unstable angina and post-myocardial infarction. Interest in CRP has been heightened by the recent finding that statins reduce CRP levels, although it is not known whether this represents a primary or secondary effect.

Several mechanisms have been described whereby CRP can exert direct harm. In the plaque, CRP binds to oxidized LDL cholesterol and, by activating complement, mediates tissue damage. In MI, increased complement activity is associated with larger infarct size. In addition, CRP releases increased tissue factor, which can trigger thrombosis.

Erythrocyte sedimentation rate (ESR), raised white blood cell count and serum albumin also correlate with increased risk of CHD but, at 1.3, 1.5 and 1.5, respectively, the risk ratios represent weaker associations.

Another possible cause of the release of inflammatory mediators is low-grade infection and biochemical, histopathological, epidemiological and clinical studies have all provided evidence that chronic infections may contribute to atherosclerosis and acute coronary events. The idea that infection could be a causal factor is not new as it was proposed by Osler and others as long ago as 1908. In 1989, a clear relationship was described between poor dental health and CHD but it is unlikely that the relationship is causal as lifestyle factors such as diet and smoking are clearly active. The specific infective agents, cytomegalovirus, *Helicobacter pylori* and *Chlamydia pneumoniae*, have come under close scrutiny, with perhaps more positive associations being described for the latter.

Rabbits inoculated nasally with *C. pneumoniae* develop extensive atherosclerosis. In addition, *C. pneumoniae* particles are found in post-mortem and atherectomy samples but not normal arteries. Two small antibiotic trials using azithromycin and roxithromycin in CHD patients have suggested clinical benefits, sparking much interest that antibiotics could be the panacea for atherosclerosis and a plethora of large randomized trials designed to give the answer.

Two recent analyses by Wald and Danesh carefully allowed for confounding factors and found no significant association between *C. pneumoniae* serology and the incidence of CHD. These data do not totally exclude a weak association and the possibility of an acute infection triggering a CHD event means the results of the antibiotic trials are still eagerly awaited.

Alcohol as a risk factor

More than 60 prospective studies have shown that people who drink small amounts of alcohol have lower rates of CHD than those who drink heavily or not at all. The U-shaped relationship between overall mortality and the consumption of alcohol was first described by Pearl as long ago as 1926 but the possibility that alcohol in moderation might actually be beneficial was largely ignored by the medical profession for many years. Moderate alcohol consumption, meaning one to two drinks per day, appears to be associated with a relative risk reduction in CHD mortality of about one-third and the relationship holds even when confounding variables are accounted for (Figure 5.12). As vascular disease is such an important cause of death in middle and old age, a reduction in CHD produces a parallel reduction in total mortality. People who do not drink alcohol form a composite group including those who have never drunk

ALCOHOL & CHD

ALCOHOL & CHD

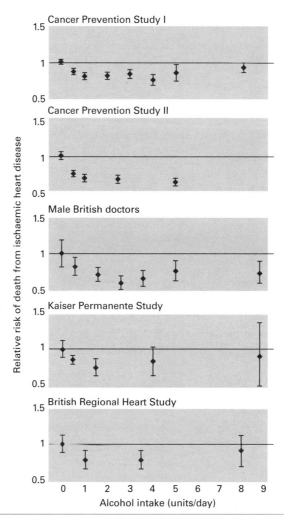

FIGURE **5.12** • The relative risk of CHD death according to alcohol consumption in the five largest cohort studies. Reproduced with permission from BMJ Publishing Group from Law, M. and Wald, N. (1999) *Br Med J* **318**, 1471–80.

alcohol ('never drinkers') and those who have had to give up alcohol because of some other health problem ('sick quitters'). Studies that distinguish 'never drinkers' and 'sick quitters' confirm the validity of the U-shaped curve.

Alcohol consumption is traditionally measured in 'units' and the number of

'units' that can be safely consumed in a week is often defined in lifestyle recommendations. Unfortunately, there is no standardization between countries of what a 'unit' means. In the UK, units are defined as 8 g ethanol, but a unit in Austria is 6.3 g, in Japan, 19.75 g and in the USA, 12 or 14 g. This should be taken into account when advising patients and one to two drinks in the USA would be the equivalent of two to three in the UK. In practice, few individuals measure their consumption precisely. People do not stick to standard measures and because different types of beer, wine and spirits contain different amounts of alcohol, it is difficult to work out the total consumed. Where consumption can be compared to sales figures, surveys consistently show individuals underestimate their intake by 30–80 per cent.

Most studies show little further benefit when consumption exceeds one to two drinks per day. With increasing consumption, the benefits of moderate intake are outweighed by rises in hepatic cirrhosis, hypertension, haemorrhagic stroke, various cancers, cardiomyopathy, arrhythmias, accidents and violent death. Under the age of 40, any alcohol consumption is associated with increased mortality because CHD rates are low and the risk of death by injury is relatively high. This means recommendations to drink alcohol for its cardioprotective benefits should not be applied to the young. The CHD benefits begin to accrue in men over the age of 40 and women over 50 and continue into old age. Patterns of drinking may also be important. There is some evidence that regular 'binge' drinking may be associated with increased risk and some support for the fact that drinking with meals may be important.

How does alcohol protect against CHD?

It has been estimated that half of the beneficial effect of moderate alcohol consumption is mediated through HDL cholesterol.

Alcohol produces two significant effects on lipids. First, there is a beneficial rise in HDL cholesterol, particularly HDL_3 cholesterol and to a lesser extent, the more cardioprotective HDL_2 cholesterol. One to two drinks a day increase HDL cholesterol by an average of 12 per cent. With increasing liver cell damage, the pattern changes and HDL_2 cholesterol becomes more dominant until ultimately, HDL cholesterol levels reduce markedly. Second, like any other source of carbohydrates, alcohol produces a concomitant rise in triglyceride production and VLDL secretion. Unfortunately the beneficial effects of increased HDL cholesterol are offset by the rise in triglycerides and VLDL as consumption increases. If the assembly and secretion of VLDL fails to keep pace with triglyceride production, a fatty liver ensues. Usually a type IV hyperlipidaemia is seen, but some individuals, with impaired triglyceride catabolism, can produce a type V pattern with very high triglyceride levels. The association with pancreatitis, particularly with levels above 20 mmol/L, is well known.

Alcohol also seems to have significant antithrombotic actions, the benefits of which have been compared to those of aspirin. Fibrinogen and tissue factor are reduced and there are beneficial influences on platelet aggregation and plasminogen activation.

In 1999, Rimm et al. attempted to quantify the potential reduction in CHD associated with the intake of 30 g ethanol per day by extrapolating data from 42 experimental studies. After adjusting for intra-individual variability, he attributed a reduction in CHD of 16.8 per cent to a rise

ALCOHOL & CHD

in HDL cholesterol and a reduction of 12.5 per cent to the drop in fibrinogen. An overall 24.7 per cent reduction was associated with this consumption of alcohol when the negative, 4.6 per cent impact of the rise in triglycerides was taken into account.

More than 60 studies, from a range of populations, have described the link between alcohol consumption and hypertension. In the Kaiser Permanente study, the blood pressure of men and women drinking six to eight drinks per day was 9.1/5.6 mmHg higher than that of non-drinkers. After heavy drinking, a transient rise in blood pressure has been described and this takes several days of abstention to settle.

What type of alcohol is the best?

Apart from the issue of optimal alcohol intake, there has also been much debate over which type of alcoholic beverage is most cardioprotective. In the late 1970s, Cochrane's analysis of the social and environmental determinants of CHD in 18 countries suggested that the contribution of alcohol to reduced CHD risk was almost entirely explained by wine drinking. Although aware of confounding influences,

Cochrane's findings triggered tremendous speculation that wine might contain constituents, other than alcohol, that might confer cardioprotective benefits. Cochrane himself expressed some regret about the possibility as he felt it would 'almost be a sacrilege' as 'the medicine was already in a highly palatable form'. It is hardly surprising that the endorsement of wine drinking captured the imagination of health professionals and their patients and that recommendations to drink alcohol, particularly as red wine, are still commonplace.

In the event, other studies showed similar risk reductions for CHD associated with alcohol in countries where grape wine drinking is unusual. The same benefits are seen wherever spirits, beer or other forms of alcoholic beverage predominate. Across the totality of studies, no evidence exists to show that any particular alcoholic drink has a greater effect on blood constituents or blood pressure than any other with the same amount of ethanol. It is the alcohol that matters. The idea that constituent antioxidants or flavonoids or any other substance confers additional benefits remains seductive but entirely speculative.

ASSESSING CARDIOVASCULAR RISK

We have seen that it is an individual's overall, 'global' risk of CHD that determines the benefit of an intervention such as cholesterol lowering and that cholesterol cannot be considered in isolation from the other risk factors.

Whilst the primary prevention of CHD, driven by public health measures, individual risk assessments and personal responsibility, is the ultimate goal for a population, there is a logistical problem due to the sheer numbers of people involved. All modern guidelines for the prevention of CHD therefore recommend that priority for treatment should be given to patients at high absolute risk of developing CHD over a specified time period. This means targeting people with established cardiovascular disease first

TABLE **5.12** • Population burden of primary preventation at different 10-year CHD risks

10-year CHD risk (%)	Percentage of population exceeding threshold
6 (AFCAPS/TexCAPS equivalent)	32.9
15 (WOSCOPS equivalent)	9.7
20 (European Societies Joint Task Force)	5.4
30 (UK National Service Framework CHD)	1.5

Source: Haq, I., Ramsay, L., Wallis, E. *et al.* (2001) *Heart* **86**, 289–95.

(secondary prevention) and subsequently, people without cardiovascular disease, whose absolute risk exceeds an intervention threshold commensurate with the logistical and financial resources available. An idea of what this means for a country with a high rate of CHD has been recently published using data from the Scottish Health Survey 1995. In a cohort of 3963 subjects aged 35–64 years, 8.5 per cent were identified as needing secondary prevention. In addition, the percentages crossing different 10-year CHD risk thresholds, requiring interventions for primary prevention, are shown in Table 5.12.

When the burden of secondary prevention is added, it can be seen that intervening at the lowest absolute risk threshold would, although evidence-based, involve over 40 per cent of this cohort. Even initiating primary prevention interventions at the highest threshold, overall this means treatment for one in ten people.

Whatever CHD risk threshold is chosen, cardiovascular disease registers and risk assessment tools are required to facilitate the identification and assessment of people at high risk. Risk assessment tools should not be used for people with established cardiovascular disease who are already at high risk of a further event (their 10-year CHD risk usually exceeds 30 per cent) and qualify anyway for secondary prevention interventions.

Most relevant interventions, such as lipid-lowering therapy, blood pressure lowering and smoking cessation reduce the risk of both CHD and stroke. There is a strong correlation between CHD and cardiovascular disease and multiplying coronary risk by 4/3 will give a reasonable estimate of cardiovascular risk.

Understanding risk

Relative risk is defined as the number of times an event is more or less likely to occur in one group compared with another.

Absolute risk is defined as the probability that an individual will experience a specified event during a specified period.

Many clinical studies present the benefits of interventions to reduce serious events in terms of relative risk reduction. If, however, the absolute rate of the serious event is low to begin with, then many people would need to be given the intervention for only a few to benefit. Small benefits in terms of absolute risk may not justify changes in clinical practice that would seem appropriate if only relative risk is considered. In risk assessment, absolute risk takes into account the complex and synergistic nature of risk factors, rather than placing an undue emphasis on just one of them. Geoffrey Rose said: 'All policy decisions should be based on absolute measures of risk; relative risk is strictly for researchers only.'

Assessing an individual's absolute cardiovascular risk is difficult without using some form of risk assessment tool. Health professionals using an intuitive approach are inconsistent and the reader is invited to attempt to calculate the absolute 10-year CHD risks of the four individuals in the table below. The answer can be found at the end of the chapter on page 155.

	Ian	Bob	Sue	Ann
Age	65	56	60	38
BP (mmHg)	176/96	140/80	156/92	170/102
Smoker	Yes	No	Yes	Yes
TC (mmol/L)	6.2	5.4	7.8	6.0
HDL cholesterol (mmol/L)	1.2	0.6	1.4	1.5
Diabetes	No	Yes	No	No
Per cent 10-year risk?				

Cardiovascular risk assessment tools

Support tools to assess CHD risk have been available since the 1970s and invariably use multiple logistic equations derived from the Framingham Heart Study. The equations were based on the collection of risk factor data during the follow-up of, ultimately, more than 10 000 residents of Framingham, Massachusetts and are presented as printed tables or computer programs.

The examples in common use include:

- The Joint British Societies Coronary Risk Prediction Chart or the associated computer program (Figure 5.13).
- The European Coronary Risk Chart (Figure 5.14).
- The New Zealand Cardiovascular Risk Prediction Charts (Figure 5.15).
- The Sheffield Risk Table (Figure 5.16).
- The Framingham Point Score (US Adult Treatment Panel III) (Figure 5.17).

The Framingham equations can be used to predict risk of different outcomes, such as fatal and non-fatal CHD, stroke and total cardiovascular disease, including congestive heart failure and peripheral arterial disease. The predictions can range over 1, 5 or 10 years. Britain and the USA have adopted 10-year CHD risk, meaning non-fatal MI and CHD death. The European Joint Task Force also recommends 10-year risk but defines it as risk of non-fatal CHD and CHD death. The New Zealand charts assess total cardiovascular risk over 5 years, claiming better patient comprehension and closer alignment to the standard duration of clinical intervention trials. To make matters more confusing, the Framingham function itself actually predicts a very much wider endpoint: CHD death,

Joint British Societies Coronary Risk Prediction Charts

THESE CHARTS ARE FOR ESTIMATING CHD RISK FOR INDIVIDUALS WHO HAVE **NOT DEVELOPED** SYMPTOMATIC CHD OR OTHER MAJOR ATHEROSCLEROTIC DISEASE (PRIMARY PREVENTION)

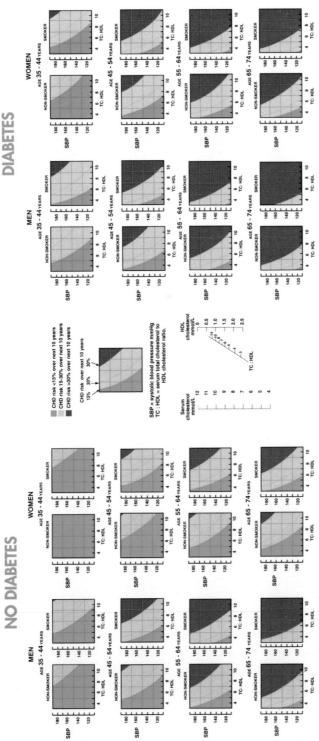

The charts should not be used for patients with:

- Existing CHD or other major atherosclerotic disease
- Systolic BP ≥160mmHg and/or diastolic BP ≥100mmHg
- Familial hypercholesterolaemia
- Diabetes Mellitus with associated target organ damage
- Renal dysfunction.

Drug therapies are required for **all** of these patients as they are already at high risk.

Use charts with caution in ethnic minorities, as they have not been validated in these populations.

Information needed before using the charts:

- Age and gender
- Diabetes status (yes/no)
- Smoking status (reflecting lifetime exposure to tobacco not just use at time of risk assessment)
- Systolic blood pressure (ideally reflecting repeat measurement over a period of time)
- Total cholesterol (TC) to HDL-cholesterol ratio (ideally repeat measurement over a period of time. If no HDL-cholesterol result available, assume this is 1.0 mmol/L).
- To calculate TC:HDL ratio, mark patient's TC and HDL levels on nomogram above. Draw line connecting the two levels. Ratio is point at which line crosses diagonal TC:HDL scale.

How to use the charts:

- Find the chart for the individual's gender, smoking status, age, and diabetes
- Define the level of risk according to the individual's blood pressure and total cholesterol to HDL-cholesterol ratio.

CHD risk is higher than indicated in the charts for:

- Those with a family history of premature atherosclerosis (by a factor of approximately 1.5)
- Patients whose BP or lipid values are already modified by treatment
- Those with raised triglyceride levels
- Non-diabetics with impaired glucose tolerance
- Women with premature menopause
- Patients approaching the next age category.

3412000615a
Date of preparation April 2000

FIGURE 5.13 • Joint British Societies Coronary Risk Prediction Charts. Reproduced and modified with permission from the British Heart Foundation (2000).

Estimate the absolute risk of CHD from the chart to identify individuals at **high multifactorial** risk: an absolute **CHD risk of** ≥ **20%** over 10 years, or >**20%** if projected to age 60 years

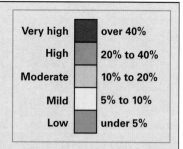

Very high	**over 40%**
High	**20% to 40%**
Moderate	**10% to 20%**
Mild	**5% to 10%**
Low	**under 5%**

How to use the Coronary Risk Charts

1. To estimate a person's absolute 10-year risk of a CHD event find the table for their gender, smoking status and age.

2. Within the table find the cell nearest to the person's systolic blood pressure (mmHg) and total cholesterol (mmol/L or mg/dL).

3. Compare cell colour with the key and read the risk level.

4. The effect of lifetime exposure to risk factors can be seen by following the table upwards.

5. A separate coronary risk chart is shown for diabetics, who are at particularly high risk of CHD.

6. Risk is higher than indicated in the charts in familial hyperlipidaemia, family history of premature cardiovascular disease, HDL, cholesterol < 1.0 mmol/L (40 mg/dL), triglyceride levels > 2.0 mmol/L (180 mg/dL) and as the person approaches the next age category.

(a)

FIGURE 5.14 • Coronary risk chart. (a) Guidance notes.

clinical non-fatal MI, electrocardiographic (silent) MI, physician-assessed angina and coronary insufficiency.

Despite this, the Framingham function performs well, correctly identifying 85 per cent of people who develop CHD with a 30 per cent false-positive rate. It has been shown to give an acceptable prediction of risk in northern European and UK populations but did overestimate risk when compared with the British Regional Heart Study. The equations are more accurate at older than at younger ages, when absolute risk is higher and when HDL cholesterol is incorporated, particularly as the TC:HDL cholesterol ratio. The European charts only include total cholesterol.

Subjects with pre-existing CHD were excluded from the original study and this is why the risk function can only be used for primary prevention. The number and complexity of the variables shown to affect prognosis after MI is great but recently, the Italian GISSI-Prevenzione group have derived a mortality risk chart for assessing the absolute risk of death after MI.

As the study population was mainly Caucasian, the Framingham findings are difficult to extrapolate to other ethnic groups, in particular South Asians. When variables such as blood pressure, cholesterol or BMI are at their extremes, prediction is also unreliable. Family history is not included in the calculations and in people with strong family histories of premature CHD, risks are likely to be greater than predicted. The Joint British

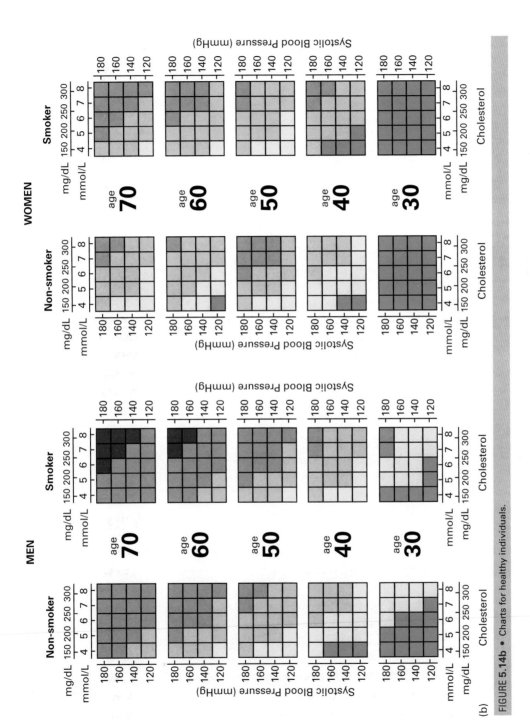

FIGURE **5.14b** • Charts for healthy individuals.

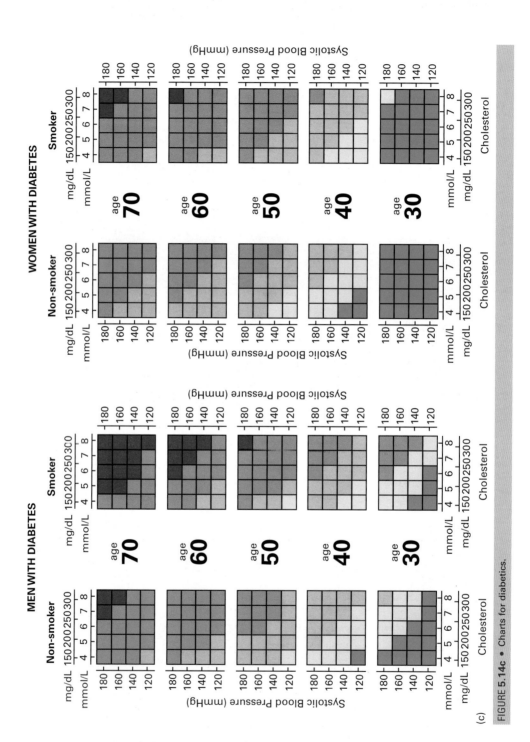

FIGURE **5.14c** • Charts for diabetics.

New Zealand cardiovascular risk prediction charts

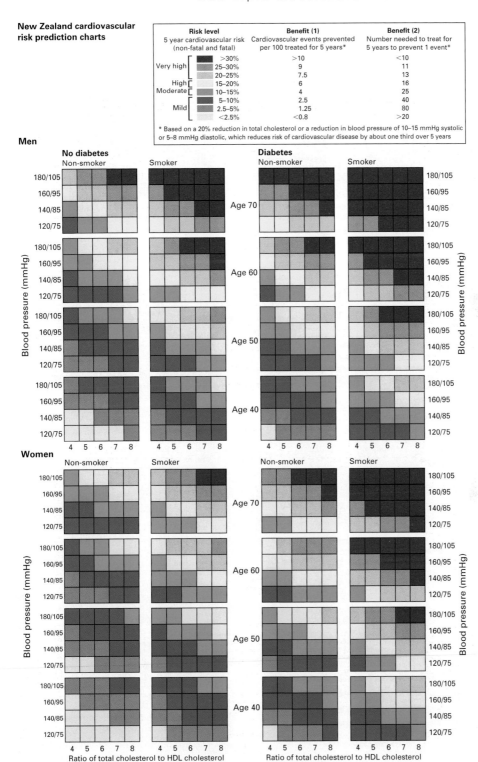

Risk level 5 year cardiovascular risk (non-fatal and fatal)		Benefit (1) Cardiovascular events prevented per 100 treated for 5 years*	Benefit (2) Number needed to treat for 5 years to prevent 1 event*
Very high	>30%	>10	<10
	25–30%	9	11
	20–25%	7.5	13
High	15–20%	6	16
Moderate	10–15%	4	25
	5–10%	2.5	40
Mild	2.5–5%	1.25	80
	<2.5%	<0.8	>20

* Based on a 20% reduction in total cholesterol or a reduction in blood pressure of 10–15 mmHg systolic or 5–8 mmHg diastolic, which reduces risk of cardiovascular disease by about one third over 5 years

FIGURE **5.15** • New Zealand cardiovascular risk prediction charts. Reproduced with permission from BMJ Publishing Group from Jackson, R. (2000) *Br Med J* **320**, 710.

Sheffield table for primary prevention of cardiovascular disease

Showing serum total:HDL cholesterol ratios conferring estimated risk of coronary heart disease events of 15% and 30% over 10 years.

Men — Total:HDL cholesterol ratio

Hypertension	Yes		No		Yes		Yes		No		No		Yes		No	
Smoking	Yes		Yes		Yes		No		Yes		Yes		No		No	
Diabetes	Yes		Yes		No		Yes		No		Yes		No		No	
CHD risk	15%	30%	15%	30%	15%	30%	15%	30%	15%	30%	15%	30%	15%	30%	15%	30%
Age 70	2.0	3.0	2.0	3.6	2.1	3.8	2.4	4.4	2.5	4.6	2.9	5.3	3.1	5.6	3.7	6.7
68	2.0	3.2	2.1	3.8	2.2	4.1	2.6	4.7	2.7	4.8	3.0	5.6	3.3	6.0	3.9	7.1
66	2.0	3.4	2.2	4.0	2.4	4.3	2.7	5.0	2.8	5.2	3.2	5.9	3.5	6.3	4.1	7.6
64	2.0	3.6	2.4	4.3	2.5	4.6	2.9	5.3	3.0	5.5	3.5	6.3	3.7	6.8	4.4	8.1
62	2.1	3.8	2.5	4.6	2.7	4.9	3.1	5.6	3.2	5.9	3.7	6.7	3.9	7.2	4.7	8.6
60	2.2	4.1	2.7	4.9	2.9	5.2	3.3	6.0	3.4	6.3	3.9	7.2	4.2	7.7	5.0	9.2
58	2.4	4.4	2.9	5.3	3.1	5.6	3.5	6.5	3.7	6.7	4.2	7.7	4.5	8.3	5.4	9.9
56	2.6	4.7	3.1	5.7	3.3	6.0	3.8	7.0	4.0	7.2	4.6	8.3	4.9	8.9	5.8	10.6
54	2.8	5.1	3.3	6.1	3.6	6.5	4.1	7.5	4.3	7.8	4.9	9.0	5.2	9.6	6.3	–
52	3.0	5.5	3.6	6.6	3.9	7.0	4.4	8.1	4.6	8.4	5.3	9.7	5.7	10.4	6.8	–
50	3.3	6.0	3.9	7.1	4.2	7.6	4.8	8.8	5.0	9.1	5.7	10.5	6.1	–	7.3	–
48	3.6	6.5	4.3	7.8	4.5	8.3	5.2	9.6	5.4	9.9	6.3	–	6.7	–	8.0	–
46	3.9	7.1	4.6	8.5	5.0	9.1	5.7	10.4	5.9	10.8	6.8	–	7.3	–	8.7	–
44	4.3	7.8	5.1	9.3	5.4	9.9	6.3	–	6.5	–	7.5	–	8.0	–	9.6	–
42	4.7	8.6	5.6	10.2	6.0	10.9	6.9	–	7.2	–	8.2	–	8.8	–	10.5	–
40	2.0	9.5	6.2	–	6.6	–	7.6	–	7.9	–	9.1	–	9.7	–		
38	2.0	10.5	6.9	–	7.3	–	8.5	–	8.8	–	10.1	–	10.8	–		
36	2.0	–	7.7	–	8.2	–	9.5	–	9.8	–						
34	2.0	–	8.6	–	9.2	–	10.6	–								
32	2.1	–	9.8	–	10.5	–										
30	9.4	–														
28	10.8	–														

Women — Total:HDL cholesterol ratio

Hypertension	Yes		No		Yes		Yes		No		No		Yes		No	
Smoking	Yes		Yes		Yes		No		Yes		Yes		No		No	
Diabetes	Yes		Yes		No		Yes		No		Yes		No		No	
CHD risk	15%	30%	15%	30%	15%	30%	15%	30%	15%	30%	15%	30%	15%	30%	15%	30%
Age 70	2.3	4.1	2.7	4.9	3.3	6.1	3.8	7.0	4.0	7.2	4.6	8.3	5.6	10.2	6.7	–
68	2.3	4.2	2.7	5.0	3.4	6.1	3.9	7.0	4.0	7.3	4.6	8.4	5.7	–	6.8	–
66	2.3	4.2	2.8	5.1	3.4	6.2	3.9	7.1	4.1	7.4	4.7	8.5	5.7	–	6.9	–
64	2.4	4.3	2.8	5.2	3.5	6.4	4.0	7.3	4.2	7.6	4.8	8.7	5.9	–	7.0	–
62	2.4	4.4	2.9	5.3	3.6	6.5	4.1	7.5	4.3	7.8	4.9	9.0	6.0	–	7.2	–
60	2.5	4.6	3.0	5.5	3.7	6.7	4.2	7.7	4.4	8.1	5.1	9.3	6.2	–	7.4	–
58	2.6	4.8	3.1	5.7	3.8	7.0	4.4	8.0	4.6	8.4	5.3	9.6	6.5	–	7.8	–
56	2.7	5.0	3.3	6.0	4.0	7.4	4.6	8.4	4.8	8.8	5.5	10.1	6.8	–	8.1	–
54	2.9	5.3	3.5	6.3	4.3	7.8	4.9	8.9	5.1	9.3	5.8	–	7.2	–	8.6	–
52	3.1	5.6	3.7	6.8	4.5	8.3	5.2	9.5	5.4	9.9	6.2	–	7.7	–	9.2	–
50	3.3	6.1	4.0	7.3	4.9	9.0	5.6	–	5.9	–	6.7	–	8.3	–	9.9	–
48	3.6	6.6	4.3	7.9	5.3	9.8	6.1	–	6.4	–	7.3	–	9.0	–		
46	4.0	7.3	4.8	8.8	5.9	–	6.8	–	7.1	–	8.1	–	10.0	–		
44	4.5	8.2	5.4	9.8	6.6	–	7.6	–	7.9	–	9.1	–				
42	5.1	9.4	6.1	–	7.5	–	8.6	–	9.0	–	10.3	–				
40	5.9	–	7.1	–	8.7	–	10.0	–								
38	7.0	–	8.4	–												
36	8.5	–	10.2	–												

Read before using table

- **Do not use for secondary prevention:** patients with MI, angina, PVD, non-haemorrhagic stroke, TIA, or diabetes with microvascular complications have high CHD risk. Treat mild hypertension: treat with aspirin; and treat with statin if serum cholesterol ≥ 5.0 mmol/L
- **Treat hypertension above mild range** (average ≥160 or ≥100)
- **Treat mild hypertension** (140–159 or 90–99) with **target organ damage** (LVH, proteinuria, renal impairment) or with **diabetes** (type 1 or 2)
- Consider drug treatment only **after** 6 months of appropriate advice on smoking, diet and repeated BP measurements
- Use **average** of repeated total:HDL-C measurements. If HDL-C not available, assume 1.2 mmol/L
- Those with total:HDL-C ratio ≥ 8.0 may have **familial hyperlipidaemia**
- The table **underestimates** CHD risk in
  - LVH on ECG (risk doubled – add 20 years to age)
  - family history of premature CHD (add 6 years)
  - familial hyperlipidaemia
  - British Asians

Instructions

- Choose table for men or women
- **Hypertension** means SBP ≥ 140 or DBP ≥ 90 or on antihypertensive treatment
- Identify correct column for hypertension, smoking, and diabetes
- Identify row showing age
- Read off total:HDL-C ratios at intersection of column and row. If there is an entry, **measure serum cholesterol:HDL ratio**. If no entry, lipids need not be measured unless familial hyperlipidaemia suspected
- If total:HDL-C ratio confers CHD risk of 15%, consider treatment of **mild hypertension** (SBP 140–159 or DBP 90–99) and with **aspirin**
- If total:HDL-C ratio confers CHD risk of 30%, consider **statin** if serum cholesterol ≥ 5.0 mmol/L
- Decisions on statin at CHD risk between 15%–30% depend on local policy
- The table can be used to assess CHD risk at an older age

FIGURE **5.16** • Sheffield table for primary prevention of cardiovascular disease. Showing serum total:HDL cholesterol ratios conferring estimated risk of coronary heart disease events of 15 per cent and 30 per cent over 10 years. Reproduced with permission from BMJ Publishing Group from Wallis, E.J., Ramsay, L.E., Ul Haq, I. *et al.* (2000) *Br Med J* **320**, 672.

Men
Estimate of 10-Year Risk for Men

(Framingham Point Scores)

Age	Points
20–34	−9
35–39	−4
40–44	0
45–49	3
50–54	6
55–59	8
60–64	10
65–69	11
70–74	12
75–79	13

Total cholesterol	Points				
	Age 20–39	Age 40–49	Age 50–59	Age 60–69	Age 70–79
<160	0	0	0	0	0
160–199	4	3	2	1	0
200–239	7	5	3	1	0
240–279	9	6	4	2	1
≥280	11	8	5	3	1

	Points				
	Age 20–39	Age 40–49	Age 50–59	Age 60–69	Age 70–79
Non-smoker	0	0	0	0	0
Smoker	8	5	3	1	1

HDL (mg/dL)	Points
≥60	−1
50–59	0
40–49	1
<40	2

Systolic BP (mmHg)	If untreated	If treated
<120	0	0
120–129	0	1
130–139	1	2
140–159	1	2
≥160	2	3

Point total	10-Year risk%
<0	<1
0	1
1	1
2	1
3	1
4	1
5	2
6	2
7	3
8	4
9	5
10	6
11	8
12	10
13	12
14	16
15	20
16	25
≥17	≥30

10-Year risk_____%

Women
Estimate of 10-Year Risk for Women

(Framingham Point Scores)

Age	Points
20–34	−7
35–39	−3
40–44	0
45–49	3
50–54	6
55–59	8
60–64	10
65–69	12
70–74	14
75–79	16

Total cholesterol	Points				
	Age 20–39	Age 40–49	Age 50–59	Age 60–69	Age 70–79
<160	0	0	0	0	0
160–199	4	3	2	1	1
200–239	8	6	4	2	1
240–279	11	8	5	3	2
≥280	13	10	7	4	2

	Points				
	Age 20–39	Age 40–49	Age 50–59	Age 60–69	Age 70–79
Non-smoker	0	0	0	0	0
Smoker	9	7	4	2	1

HDL (mg/dL)	Points
≥60	−1
50–59	0
40–49	1
<40	2

Systolic BP (mmHg)	If untreated	If treated
<120	0	0
120–129	1	3
130–139	2	4
140–159	3	5
≥160	4	6

Point total	10-Year risk%
<9	<1
9	1
10	1
11	1
12	1
13	2
14	2
15	3
16	4
17	5
18	6
19	8
20	11
21	14
22	17
23	22
24	27
≥25	≥30

10-Year risk_____%

U.S. DEPARTMENT OF HEALTH AND HUMAN SERVICES
Public Health Service
National Institutes of Health
National Heart, Lung, and Blood Institute

NIH Publication No. 01-3305
May 2001

FIGURE 5.17 • Framingham point scores. Source: NIH publication no. 01-3305, 2001; Anonymous (2001).

Societies state that a family history of premature CHD increases the CHD event risk by a factor of approximately 1.5 and the Sheffield tables suggest adding 6 years to the assessment. Families with FH or other genetic dyslipidaemias should not be assessed using Framingham-based tools.

The translation of continuous variables such as age, blood pressure, total and HDL cholesterol into charts inevitably leads to some approximation. A patient's age, for example, may lie at any point within a 2, 5 or 10-year band. Computer programs, which can calculate risk for the exact value of continuous variables, clearly increase precision.

Some factors in risk assessment are treated dichotomously. For example, no risk assessment tool recognizes the dose dependency of smoking and the position of a lifelong smoker who has just stopped is not clear. The CHD risk of a diabetic with microalbuminuria is considerably enhanced and yet diabetes is a dichotomous variable. The Sheffield tables, which were designed to facilitate decisions on cholesterol screening, typify this inflexibility, treating diabetes, hypertension and smoking as dichotomous variables. Using two thresholds of 15 per cent and 30 per cent over 10 years, these charts identify the TC:HDL cholesterol ratio needed to reach each threshold.

The major risk assessment tools described here are all designed to predict CHD risk over a period of 5–10 years. Atherosclerosis is a lifelong disease and modelling of lifetime risk suggests that many individuals will have accumulated most of their risk before they become eligible for treatment. The European charts recognize this and allow projection of current risk factor profiles to age 60 to ascertain CHD risk. Mathematical models using lifetime risk calculations can be used to predict an age at which starting treatment will provide maximum benefit, but these are in their infancy.

In summary, despite their apparent sophistication, being population-based, risk assessment tools are not comprehensive and do not cater for the needs of every individual. The experienced clinician who knows the patient and the family involved can still modify the conclusions.

Guidelines for preventing CHD in clinical practice

Several consensus groups have produced guidelines for the primary and secondary prevention of CHD. Recent years have seen increasing collaboration between groups with a common interest in reducing the burden of cardiovascular disease, in the hope that a more unified and therefore, effective approach to prevention will emerge. The reader is particularly recommended to study:

■ The Recommendations of the Second Joint Task Force of European and other Societies on Coronary Prevention (Anonymous, 1998b).
■ The Joint British recommendations on prevention of coronary heart disease in clinical practice (Anonymous, 1998a).
■ The Third Report of the National Cholesterol Education Program (NCEP) Expert Panel on Detection, Evaluation and Treatment of High Blood Cholesterol in Adults (Adult Treatment Panel III) (Anonymous, 2001).

SUMMARY OF THE JOINT BRITISH RECOMMENDATIONS ▬▬▬

PRIORITIES FOR DRUG INTERVENTION

1 Patients with existing CHD or other major atherosclerotic disease – secondary prevention.

2 Other high-risk individuals without clinically overt CHD or other major atherosclerotic disease – primary prevention.

Primary prevention

Absolute risk assessment is a minimum care standard for people with:

- hypertension
- dyslipidaemia
- diabetes mellitus
- family history of premature CHD (males <55 years, females <65 years).

Lifestyle advice and management should be considered in all patients, regardless of level of risk. All clinicians should consider management of all CHD risk factors, rather than viewing single factors in isolation.

Audit of CHD measures should be undertaken routinely.

RECOMMENDED TREATMENT TARGETS

1 Cholesterol (all patients suitable for treatment): total cholesterol <5.0 mmol/L; LDL cholesterol <3.0 mmol/L (or 33 per cent reduction from baseline, whichever is lowest).

2 Blood pressure: non-diabetics, <140/85 mmHg; diabetics, <130/80 mmHg.

MANAGEMENT SUMMARIES

1 **All patients with CHD/existing atherosclerotic disease,** e.g. MI, angina, ischaemic stroke, TIA, peripheral arterial disease:
   (a) Cholesterol: reduce to recommended targets. Initiate statin therapy in patients up to 75 years at doses prescribed in clinical trials.
   (b) Blood pressure: reduce to recommended targets.
   (c) Diabetes: rigorous glucose control, use insulin post-MI.
   (d) Aspirin: 75 mg in all patients where tolerated.

   Additional therapy for post-MI patients:
   (e) Beta-blockers: for at least 3 years.
   (f) ACE inhibitors: heart failure at time of MI or persistent left ventricular systolic dysfunction (ejection fraction < 40 per cent).

2 **Patients at high risk of CHD/atherosclerotic disease,** e.g. hypertension, dyslipidaemia, diabetes mellitus or a combination of these and other risk factors:
   (a) Cholesterol: treat according to CHD risk calculated using the risk assessment charts. Upper age for statin initiation 69 years. Treat all patients with >30 per cent 10-year CHD risk to recommended targets. Treat patients with 15–30 per cent risk progressively, as resources allow. If risk <15 per cent, treat as if patients have severe hypertension (>160/100 mmHg) or diabetes with associated target organ damage or inherited dyslipidaemia.
   (b) Blood pressure: treat regardless of CHD risk if SBP >160 mmHg or DBP >100 mmHg. If SBP 140–159 mmHg and/or DBP 90–99 mmHg, treat if CHD risk >15 per cent or patient has target organ damage.
   (c) Aspirin: use 75 mg in patients aged >50 years with well-controlled hypertension or a CHD risk of >15 per cent.

SUMMARY OF THE JOINT EUROPEAN SOCIETIES RECOMMENDATIONS

In essence, the European recommendations are extremely similar to the British guidelines. There are slight differences in the treatment of raised blood pressure but the recommendations for cholesterol management and lipid targets are the same. The most important difference is the choice of initiation threshold for lipid lowering which is set at a 10-year absolute CHD risk of 20 per cent. In addition, clinicians can extrapolate a patient's current risk profile to the age of 60 to initiate treatment if it is clear the 20 per cent level will be exceeded.

SUMMARY OF THE NCEP ADULT TREATMENT PANEL III RECOMMENDATIONS

The third report of the Adult Treatment Panel maintains the focus on patients with CHD but includes primary prevention in patients with multiple risk factors. LDL cholesterol remains the primary target of therapy and goals are expressed in terms of LDL cholesterol figures.

New features include:

- raising patients with diabetes to the level of a CHD risk equivalent (as with non-coronary atherosclerosis);
- using Framingham 10-year risk projections in primary prevention;
- identifying those with metabolic syndrome as candidates for more intensive therapy;
- making optimal LDL cholesterol <100 mg/dL;
- redefining low HDL cholesterol as <40 mg/dL;
- reducing triglyceride cutpoints and recommending treatment beyond LDL cholesterol lowering in patients with levels over 200 mg/dL;

TABLE **5.13** • Classification of total cholesterol, LDL-C, HDL-C and triglycerides (mg/dL)

Total cholesterol

<200	Desirable
200–239	Borderline high
>240	High

HDL-C

<40	Low
>60	High

LDL-C

<100	Optimal
100–129	Near/above optimal
130–159	Borderline high
160–189	High
>190	Very high

Triglycerides

<150	Normal
150–199	Borderline
200–499	High
>500	Very high

- recommending the full profile for screening in all adults over 20 years, every 5 years;
- encouraging the use of plant sterols/stanols and soluble fibre as part of the cardioprotective diet;
- promoting therapeutic lifestyle changes.

Major risk factors (other than LDL cholesterol) that modify LDL goals are:

- cigarette smoking
- BP <140/90 or on antihypertensive medication
- low HDL cholesterol (<40 mg/dL); >60 mg/dL is protective
- family history of premature CHD in male first-degree relative <55 years; female <65 years
- age (men >45 years, women >55 years).

If 2+ risk factors (other than LDL cholesterol) are present without CHD or CHD risk equivalent, the 10-year CHD risk is assessed using the Framingham Point Score tables. The risk category then determines the LDL cholesterol level at which to initiate therapeutic lifestyle changes (TLC) and drug therapy and the LDL cholesterol goal to be attained.

The finding that triglyceride-rich lipoproteins are atherogenic is recognized by ATP III which includes the sum of VLDL-C and LDL-C (i.e. non-HDL cholesterol) as a secondary target in persons with high triglycerides (>200 mg/dL). The goal for non-HDL cholesterol can be set at 30 mg/dL higher than that for LDL cholesterol, shown in Table 5.14.

TABLE **5.14** • LDL-C goals and cut-points for therapeutic lifestyle changes (TLC) and drug therapy in different risk categories

Risk category	LDL-C goal	TLC initiation	Drug therapy initiation
CHD or CHD risk equivalents (10-year risk >20%)	<100	>100	>130 (100–129 optional)
2+ risk factors (10-year risk <20%)	<130	>130	>130 (risk 10–20%); >160 (risk <10%)
0–1 risk factors	<160	>160	>190 (160–189 optional)

LDL-C in mg/dL.

ATP III recognizes the role of life habit risk factors, such as obesity, physical inactivity and atherogenic diet and also, emerging risk factors, such as lipoprotein(a), homocysteine, prothrombotic and pro-inflammatory factors and impaired fasting glucose. As these can contribute to CHD risk to varying degrees, their presence can modulate clinical judgement when making clinical decisions.

REFERENCES AND FURTHER READING

Anonymous (1998a) Joint British recommendations on prevention of coronary heart disease in clinical practice. *Heart* **80**(Suppl. 2), 1S–29S.

Anonymous (1998b) Prevention of coronary heart disease in clinical practice. Recommendations of the Second joint Task force of the European and other Societies on Coronary Prevention. *Eur Heart J* **19**, 1434–503.

Anonymous (2001) Executive Summary Third Report of the National Cholesterol Education Program (NCEP) Expert Panel on Detection, Evaluation and Treatment of High Blood Cholesterol in Adults (Adult Treatment Panel III). *J Am Med Assoc* **285**, 2486–97.

Ashton, W.D., Nanchahal, K. and Wood, D.A. (2001) Body mass index and metabolic risk factors for coronary heart disease in women. *Eur Heart J* **22**, 46–55.

Assman, G. (1996) High-density lipoprotein cholesterol as a predictor of coronary heart disease risk. The PROCAM experience and pathophysiological implications for reverse cholesterol transport. *Atherosclerosis* **124**(Suppl.), 11–20.

Boushey, C.J., Beresford, S.A., Omenn, G.S. *et al.* (1995) A quantitative assessment of plasma homocysteine as a risk factor for vascular disease. Probable benefits of increasing folic acid intakes. *J Am Med Assoc* **274**, 1049–57.

Doll, R., Peto, R., Wheatley, K. *et al.* (1994) Mortality in relation to smoking: 40 years' observations on male British doctors. *Br Med J* **309**, 901–11.

Fowler, G. (1993) The Indians' Revenge. *Br J Gen Pract* **43**, 78–81.

Haffner, S.M., Lehto, S., Ronnemaa, T. *et al.* (1998) Mortality from coronary heart disease in subjects with type 2 diabetes and in non-diabetic subjects with and without prior myocardial infarction. *N Engl J Med* **339**, 229–34.

Hokanson, J.E. and Austin, M.A. (1996) Plasma triglyceride level is a risk factor for cardiovascular disease independent of high-density lipoprotein cholesterol level: a meta-analysis of population-based prospective studies. *J Cardiovasc Risk* **3**, 213–19.

Law, M.R., Morris, J.K. and Wald, N.J. (1997) Environmental tobacco smoke exposure and ischaemic heart disease: an evaluation of the evidence. *Br Med J* **315**, 973–80.

Rimm, E.B., Williams, P., Fosher, K. *et al.* (1999) Moderate alcohol intake and lower risk of coronary heart disease: meta-analysis of effects on lipids and haemostatic factors. *Br Med J* **319**, 1523–8.

Schnyder, G., Roffi, M., Pin, R. *et al.* (2001) Decreased rate of coronary restenosis after lowering of plasma homocysteine levels. *N Engl J Med* **345**, 1593–600.

Tuomilehto, J., Lindstorm, J., Eriksson, J.G. *et al.* for the Finnish Diabetes Prevention Study Group (2001) Prevention of type 2 diabetes mellitus by changes in lifestyle among subjects with impaired glucose tolerance. *N Engl J Med* **333**, 1343–50.

Answers to problems posed on page 142

	Ian	Bob	Sue	Ann
Age	65	56	60	38
BP (mmHg)	176/96	140/80	156/92	170/102
Smoker	Yes	No	Yes	Yes
TC (mmol/L)	6.2	5.4	7.8	6.0
HDL cholesterol (mmol/L)	1.2	0.6	1.4	1.5
Diabetes	No	Yes	No	No
Per cent 10-year risk?	34.6	30.2	20.4	4.1

Calculations made using Joint British Societies Cardiac Risk Assessor Computer Program.

PART THREE

INTERVENTION

NON-LIPID RISK FACTOR MODIFICATION

C H A P T E R

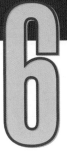

We have seen that the aetiology and assessment of CHD risk are multifactorial. Modification of single risk factors to the exclusion of others is also inappropriate when it comes to treatment options.

Intervention strategies must include attention to lifestyle factors (smoking habit, exercise, obesity and alcohol) and the appropriate chronic management of hypertension and diabetes, as well as lipid modification with diet and drugs. The management of the overweight patient is discussed in Chapter 7.

The Lifestyle Heart Trial (see page 255) demonstrated coronary plaque regression (−1.75 per cent) and a reduction in the number of anginal episodes at one year in a small group of 28 subjects with CHD who were able to make a comprehensive range of lifestyle changes. Participants ate a 10 per cent fat, vegetarian diet, undertook moderate aerobic exercise, stopped smoking and received intensive group psychosocial support. Despite not using lipid-lowering drugs, a 37.2 per cent reduction in LDL cholesterol was achieved. After 5 years, 20 of the original study group, who had sustained their efforts, were re-examined and increased regression (−3.1 per cent) was found in contrast to controls, where stenoses had continued to progress (+11.8 per cent) and events were nearly twice as common.

CHANGING PEOPLE'S HABITS

As health professionals begin to incorporate a preventive approach to their traditional curative and treatment roles, it becomes apparent that there is a requirement for new communication skills. Health promotion has moved on from the days when health professionals gave information, explanations of risk and paternalistic recommendations and expected their patients to comply. In 1968, Davis demonstrated that patients only complied with 55 per cent of their physician's advice. A greater understanding of the processes of change allows health professionals to achieve much higher success rates, particularly if they assess the state of readiness of an individual to commit to the change process.

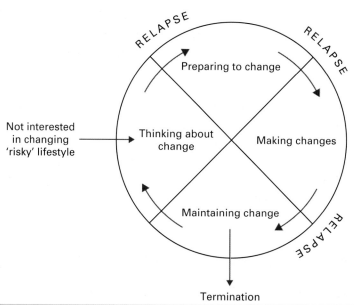

FIGURE **6.1** • Stages of change. Adapted from Prochaska, J.O. and DiClemente, C.C. (1984) *Prog Clin Biol Res* **156**, 131–40.

DiClemente *et al.* (1991) have proposed a 'stages of change' model of behaviour change that is becoming increasingly popular (Figure 6.1). The model divides the process of change into five stages:

- *Pre-contemplation*. Individuals do not intend to change their high-risk behaviour in the immediate future. They may be unaware of the risks or disbelieve them. They are discouraged about their ability to change in the context of their own lives. The task here is to establish the patient's attitude and level of knowledge. The challenge is to facilitate movement to the next stage.
- *Contemplation*. Here, individuals evaluate the pros and cons of their behaviour, but as they are about equal, there is ambivalence about changing. There is a dissonance between actual and ideal behaviour and the task is to reinforce the dissonance and the rationale of change.
- *Preparation*. In this stage there are intentional and behavioural criteria. There is an intention to take action and plans are made. The task is to commit the individual to action, believe change is possible, identify changes, give support and information, enlist the support of family and friends, set stop dates and realistic goals.
- *Action*. Visible change in behaviour begins. This is the most unstable phase with the greatest risk of relapse. The task is to provide positive, motivational support.
- *Maintenance*. Here individuals work hard to prevent relapse. The task is to use helping relationships to increase confidence using behavioural techniques such as stimulus control, counter-conditioning and contingency management.

It is important to realize that the stages of change are cyclical. Patients move back and forth within the cycle and success is not guaranteed. Relapses are common and should not be regarded as failure, rather an indication that the patient has to start again earlier in the cycle. Smokers, for example, may travel the cycle many times, regressing to all stages (including exiting the cycle), before ultimately succeeding. Recognizing the stage the patient has reached allows the health professional to vary advice appropriately. Intervening at the stage of preparation is much more likely to be effective than during the previous stages.

Throughout the counselling process, the techniques of motivational interviewing enhance the chances of success. It is important to foster individual responsibility and allow the individual to retain control. The counsellor should be non-judgemental, positive and encouraging, elicit and reinforce self-motivating statements, help individuals devise or choose their own solutions and emphasize the benefits of success.

CESSATION OF SMOKING

Surveys have shown that more than two-thirds of smokers would like to give up their habit but less than 3 per cent succeed unaided, most failing in the first week. Stopping smoking is complex and difficult because the addiction is both pharmacological and psychological and as strong as the addiction to cocaine or heroin.

The most common reason cited for giving up is 'my doctor told me to' and yet only 22 per cent of smokers recall their doctor advising them about their smoking habit. Whilst the momentum is high at the time of a cardiovascular event, 90 per cent of health contacts are in primary care and many opportunities are lost to engage patients with even brief enquiries.

In 1979, Russell showed that with firm advice to stop smoking, a leaflet and a warning of follow-up, 5.1 per cent of smokers had stopped after one year. The success of this sort of brief intervention has been confirmed on many occasions since. Higher rates have been recorded in specialist smoking centres where support and follow-up are much more intensive and the recruitment of very highly motivated patients may inflate their success. A review of 28 trials of anti-smoking advice from North American physicians showed cessation rates of 3–13 per cent from brief interventions and 19–38 per cent from more intensive strategies. In the British Family Heart Study, a smoking cessation rate of only 5 per cent was recorded in men and in the Oxford Prevention of Heart Attack and Stroke Project (OXCHECK) 4-year results there was no significant reduction.

It is hardly surprising that, with a failure rate of nearly 95 per cent, primary healthcare teams feel despondent about smoking cessation and only 3 per cent of general practitioners feel they are successful in helping patients to stop smoking. A 5 per cent rate applied to all smokers, however, would result in considerable health gain.

NICOTINE REPLACEMENT THERAPY

The evidence that nicotine is the principal addictive component of tobacco smoke is overwhelming and this represents the basis for nicotine replacement therapy (NRT) to aid cessation. Developed in Sweden in the 1970s, a range of delivery devices are now available including chewing gum, skin patches, sublingual tablets, a buccal inhalator and a nasal spray.

A review of over 80 clinical trials identifies a 12-month cessation rate of 18 per cent, compared to an 11 per cent placebo (advice only) rate. No differences are identified between the different delivery systems and ideally choice should rest with the individual, who should be able to try each before deciding which to use. One problem with NRT is that inevitably, lower peak nicotine concentrations are delivered at a slower pace to the bloodstream and the addicted brain than produced by the cigarette, which is a 'wonderfully efficient delivery device'. Some evidence is accruing that using a combination of delivery systems, such as a patch plus a flexible delivery system, may be effective in the highly dependent patient, especially during the first 3 weeks. Another drawback is that patients often discontinue NRT too quickly – at least 2–3 months is recommended.

NRT is one of the most cost-effective interventions a health professional can make. Estimates per life year gained vary from £212 to £873 at 1996 prices. Puska describes an initiative in North Karelia where 3000 individuals who wished to stop smoking were given brief advice and randomized to receive 30 pieces of nicotine gum, seven patches or nothing. After 12 months, 5.7 per cent, 7.0 per cent and 3.8 per cent, respectively, had stopped smoking. This is a good example of a very cost-effective, minimal-intervention strategy in which NRT approximately doubled the quit rate.

Cardiovascular diseases such as angina are often quoted as contraindications to nicotine replacement but this is unwarranted as cigarette smoking itself is more detrimental. It is not advisable to use nicotine replacement in pregnancy. Patches do cause itching and erythema and this can contribute to the sleep and mood disturbance associated with the process of withdrawal. Many young women are deterred from stopping by the average 4 kg weight gain that occurs on cessation. In terms of risk, continuing to smoke is, of course, far more dangerous.

OTHER MEASURES

Acupuncture, hypnosis, relaxation training and meditation are all useful adjuncts, in some individuals, to aid smoking cessation. Effectiveness studies, however, unfortunately suffer from methodological problems.

Bupropion is a new addition to the anti-smoking armamentarium. Originally developed as an antidepressant, its mechanism of action is probably to exploit the neurobiological origin of nicotine addiction, whereby nicotine activates a dopaminergic pathway in the mesolimbic system of the brain, resulting in pleasurable feelings and immediate positive reinforcement. Compared with NRT, there is little published evidence of efficacy but the original study for smokers taking 300 mg sustained release bupropion for 7 weeks showed a 12-month quit rate of 23.1 per cent compared with 12.4 per cent for placebo. A second study compared 150 mg slow-release bupropion twice daily with nicotine patches and placebo and found 12-month quit rates of 5.6 per cent for placebo, 9.8 per cent for patches (lower than normally seen), 18.4 per cent for bupropion and

22.5 per cent for the combination. The main side-effects of bupropion are dry mouth and insomnia and the prescriber is referred to the contraindications, precautions and interactions that, with cost issues, potentially constrain the use of this drug. In particular, the epileptogenic potential of bupropion limits its use in susceptible patients with up to one patient per thousand experiencing an epileptic fit.

Public health measures, including the provision of information and education, health warnings, bans on smoking in public places and reducing the tar content of cigarettes, are effective. More resources are needed for smoking cessation resources. Smoking rates have flattened off in some countries, such as the UK and Australia, but continue to decline in others. In California, only 17 per cent of the population still smoke and the rates continue to decline. Every 1 per cent increase in taxation produces a 0.5 per cent drop in tobacco consumption and as a response to increased tobacco taxation in Massachusetts, the annual prevalence of smoking in adults has fallen by 0.43 per cent per year since 1992 compared with an annual rise of 0.03 per cent in comparison states.

The sale of tobacco to children under 16 is banned in the UK, but this is hard to enforce. Most smokers start in adolescence and educational measures are of limited success in the face of the powerful role models provided by adult smokers. Tobacco advertising and promotion are powerful and millions are spent on campaigns, particularly in undeveloped nations, often linking smoking with sport and a glamorous lifestyle. A complete ban on advertising would potentially cut consumption by 6 per cent.

THE RECALCITRANT SMOKER

If individuals must smoke, advice should concentrate on harm reduction. They might be persuaded to smoke a lower tar cigarette and leave a longer butt. They might envisage non-smoking periods or locations – for example, not in front of children or in the car, etc. They may also be counselled to avoid situations they would naturally associate with smoking. Many smokers make several attempts before giving up, and continued encouragement and support will promote success.

- ASK about smoking at every opportunity
- ADVISE all smokers to stop
- ASSIST the smoker to stop
- ARRANGE follow-up

IMPROVING EXERCISE

The majority of men and women exercise insufficiently to gain health benefits. Those who do exercise generally have healthier lifestyles, eat better, are slimmer and smoke less. The health benefits of exercise are multiple and the cardiovascular benefits are shown in Figure 6.2.

Aerobic exercise involves the repetitive movements of large muscle groups to induce cardiorespiratory training. Jogging, swimming, skiing, tennis, skipping, cycling and

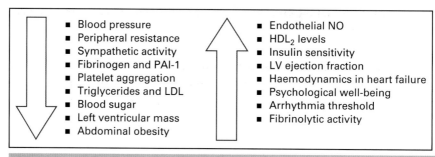

Decreased:
- Blood pressure
- Peripheral resistance
- Sympathetic activity
- Fibrinogen and PAI-1
- Platelet aggregation
- Triglycerides and LDL
- Blood sugar
- Left ventricular mass
- Abdominal obesity

Increased:
- Endothelial NO
- HDL$_2$ levels
- Insulin sensitivity
- LV ejection fraction
- Haemodynamics in heart failure
- Psychological well-being
- Arrhythmia threshold
- Fibrinolytic activity

FIGURE **6.2** • The cardiovascular benefits of exercise.

dancing will achieve this as well as fashionable exercise regimens. As an unsupervised exercise, particularly in older people, brisk walking will achieve adequate thresholds in up to two-thirds of patients. Exercise needs to be a lifelong pattern, enjoyable and convenient. If there is a social element, it is more likely to be repeated.

Exercise is monitored by heart rate. Ideally exercise should achieve 75 per cent of a patient's maximum heart rate over 20–30 minutes if repeated four to five times per week, or over 45–60 minutes if repeated two to three times per week. Exercise sessions should be preceded by 5–10 minutes of 'warm up' and followed by 5–10 minutes of 'cool down'. American Heart Association (AHA) consensus recommendations suggest 30 minutes of moderate activity, preferably every day. Maximum heart rate is best estimated by exercise ECG testing but this is impractical and European Atherosclerosis Society (EAS) guidelines are shown in Table 6.1.

TABLE **6.1** • EAS guidelines to exercise

Age	20–29	30–39	40–49	50–59	60–69
Target rate	115–145	110–140	105–130	100–125	95–120

Recent studies from Boston have shown that individuals who expend 1000 kcal of energy per week on exercise have a 20 per cent reduction in the risk of CHD compared with those who don't. Even those who expend 500–999 kcal per week show a 10 per cent benefit. The studies also confirm the gradual appreciation that the effect of short, sharp periods of exercise within the day can be cumulative, as long as the weekly energy expenditure is sufficient.

Primary care doctors are often asked about the safety of exercise, particularly in those with pre-existing disease. Indeed, sanctioning of exercise by certification is often requested. An exercise ECG may be necessary for some patients to attest their fitness to exercise. Unlike isometric exercise, which can produce large rises in blood pressure, aerobic exercises are positively indicated for those with CHD provided a few simple rules are considered. For example, the dangers of exercise may be enhanced:

- in cold weather or after meals;
- with intercurrent illness, e.g. uncontrolled hypertension, viral infection;

■ if symptoms emerge during exercise – feeling unwell, faint, chest pain, palpitations or excessive fatigue.

All regimens should follow a graded, progressive increase until cardiorespiratory fitness, based on frequency of exercise and pulse monitoring, is achieved. The patient should 'listen to the body' and report any adverse symptoms. Exercise must then be undertaken regularly, as unaccustomed or erratic exercise is hazardous.

SENSIBLE DRINKING

There is increasing consensus agreement that safe daily alcohol consumption should not exceed 10–30 g for men and 10–20 g for women. Where one unit equates to 8 g alcohol, this means that men should drink no more than 21 units of alcohol a week and women no more than 14.

CONTROL OF HYPERTENSION

Part of every general practitioner's daily life involves the management of patients with hypertension in the hope that treatment will prevent or delay the onset of heart disease, stroke and renal impairment.

From the results of meta-analyses of randomized controlled trials it is clear that each reduction of 10–14 mmHg in SBP and 5–6 mmHg in DBP confers about two-fifths less stroke and one-sixth less CHD. Given the central role of hypertension in the pathogenesis of CHD and stroke, the numbers involved and the evidence base for the benefits of interventions, the management of hypertension represents a continuing and increasing challenge for health-care professionals in primary care.

Sadly, surveys of current practice reveal woeful discrepancies in the detection, treatment and control of hypertension. The problem is international (Figure 6.3), but particularly acute in the UK. In addition, even when contemporary treatment is deemed optimal, the survival of treated hypertensives is significantly reduced compared with matched normotensives. The Gothenburg Multifactor Primary Prevention Trial, started in 1970, followed 686 hypertensive men aged 47–55 years for over 20 years in comparison with 6810 non-hypertensive controls. Despite a carefully structured programme achieving good mean blood pressure control (145/89 mmHg), a reduction in smoking from 34 to 17 per cent and a reduction in mean serum cholesterol from 6.6 to 6.1 mmol/L, the hypertensive group showed reduced survival, with deaths from CHD being predominant.

This is not a new finding, as CHD outcomes in randomized controlled trials have consistently failed to match the epidemiological expectations of an equivalent fall in blood pressure. The shortfall is important because numerically CHD events remain the most important outcome of hypertension. There are several explanations for this discrepancy:

■ Cardiovascular disease is multifactorial and only a global risk factor perspective for assessment and treatment will optimize outcomes. In the Gothenburg study, the

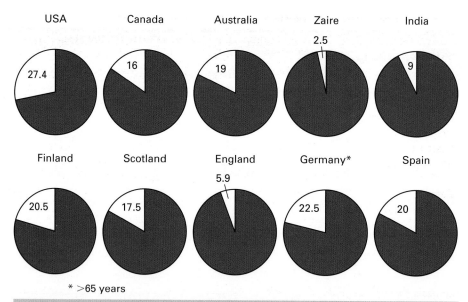

FIGURE **6.3** • Percentage of hypertensive patients (expressed by numbers in each panel) with controlled blood pressure values (<140/90 mmHg) in different countries. Reprinted from *Eur Heart J Suppl*, **1** (Supp L), Mancia, G and Grassi, G. Rationale for the use of a fixed combination in the treatment of hypertension, pp. L14–L19, © 1999, with permission from Elsevier Science.

cardiovascular risk profile of the hypertensive group at entry was less acceptable than controls. Some individuals already had evidence of target organ damage and, in common with other surveys of hypertensive patients, clustering of risk factors (especially those associated with the insulin resistance syndrome) was more evident.

■ Blood pressure reduction in early randomized controlled trials may have been inadequate to maximize the reduction in cardiovascular events. Recent evidence of the benefits of tighter blood pressure control has now led to a reduction in treatment targets.

■ Antihypertensive drugs themselves may have exerted a deleterious effect on CHD risk reduction. This is discussed in 'The hypertensive patient' (page 324).

The incorporation of global risk strategies, treatment to new targets and the organizational structures involved represent major areas of change in the management of hypertension for primary care professionals.

The acknowledgement of the contribution of other risk factors to overall cardiovascular risk and the endorsement of global risk assessment using Framingham-based risk factor calculators, are major advances and should become routine for every clinician in primary care making decisions about the initiation of antihypertensive and lipid-lowering therapy in primary prevention. For patients in the range 140–159/90–99 mmHg without target organ damage or diabetes, antihypertensive initiation is indicated where the 10-year absolute CHD risk is 15 per cent or greater.

Although there is no direct evidence that reducing blood pressure through lifestyle measures reduces the risk of cardiovascular disease, it is recommended to all patients on

TABLE **6.2** • Effectiveness of lifestyle interventions for lowering blood pressure

Intervention	Mean reduction in SBP/DBP (mmHg)	Number of RCTs	Mean change in risk factor
Weight loss	3/3	18	3–9% of body weight (ideally increments of 5 kg)
Low fat, high fruit and vegetable diet	5.5/3	1	
Exercise	5/3	29	50 min aerobic × 3/week
Salt restriction	4/2	58	118 mmol/day
	2.0/0.5	28	60 mmol/day
Potassium supplementation	4.4/2.5	21	60–100 mmol/day (equivalent to 5 bananas!)
Fish oil supplementation	4.5/2.5	7	3 g/day

the basis that the benefits of antihypertensive treatment are determined *per se* by the blood pressure reduction itself. A summary of the trials of lifestyle interventions is shown in Table 6.2, but it should be noted that all these trials are of short duration.

Smoking cessation is, without doubt, the single most important lifestyle intervention but its benefits are independent of an effect on blood pressure. Similarly, although over 60 population studies demonstrate the almost linear association between alcohol consumption and blood pressure levels, the effects are negligible below a threshold of 2–3 units per day. Trials of alcohol reduction in heavier drinkers (25–50 units/week) are inconclusive.

The majority of hypertensive patients also demonstrate abnormalities of their serum lipids. Although the evidence of benefit using statins extends to a risk as low as 6 per cent over 10 years, current recommendations endorse much higher thresholds in primary prevention, of 20–30 per cent over 10 years. When resources allow (e.g. following patent expiries) a move to a lower threshold is anticipated. For those treated currently, target levels of total cholesterol <5.0 mmol/L and LDL cholesterol <3.0 mmol/L are appropriate.

TREATMENT TO NEW TARGETS

The relationship between cardiovascular risk and blood pressure is continuous, without a lower 'threshold'. Logically, the goal of antihypertensive therapy should therefore be to reduce blood pressure to levels defined as 'normal'.

Expert international panels distil clinical, scientific and statistical evidence into consensus recommendations and, not surprisingly, there are some discrepancies (Table 6.3). It is important to realize that the recommendations are consensus statements and not supported by any individual trial evidence. Data from the Hypertension Optimal Treatment (HOT) trial largely underpin the latest wave of target reductions although it should be noted that in this study there were no significant differences in the risk of

TABLE **6.3** • International target blood pressure recommendations

Guideline	SBP target (mmHg)	DBP target (mmHg)	Target in diabetics (mmHg)
BHS	<140	<85	<140/80
WHO/ISH	<140	<90	<130/80
	(<130 if <60 years)	(<85 if <60 years)	

cardiovascular events between the adjacent target groups (DBP <90, 85 or 80 mmHg). Nevertheless, there was no increase in cardiovascular risk in the lower target group and optimal event reduction was achieved at a DBP of 82.6 mmHg. In diabetic patients, reducing DBP to <80 mmHg dramatically reduced cardiovascular events and more aggressive targets have therefore been evolved for diabetic patients. An aggressive approach to hypertension management in diabetic patients is supported by the United Kingdom Prospective Diabetes Study (UKPDS) 38, where tight blood pressure control (144/82 versus 154/87 mmHg) was associated with significantly reduced risk of both macro- and microvascular disease.

Most drugs from the main classes produce very similar blood pressure reductions. The placebo-adjusted reductions for patients with blood pressure of about 160/95 mmHg are not large and are about 7–13 mmHg SBP and 4–8 mmHg DBP. For many patients these reductions would not achieve target levels. In HOT, where 90 per cent of patients were lowered to <90 mmHg, 70 per cent of participants required combination therapy.

Combinations with additive effects typically achieve reductions of the order of 12–22 mmHg SBP and 7–14 mmHg DBP from a baseline of 160/95 mmHg. The magnitude of the blood pressure reductions achieved in HOT with combination therapy was impressive and it is important to remember that patient acceptability of these aggressive regimens was high.

WHICH DRUG?

Psaty's *et al.*'s meta-analysis of 18 controlled clinical trials in 1997 compared the benefits of first-line therapy with low- and high-dose diuretics and beta-blockers. Both agents significantly reduced the risk of stroke but only low-dose diuretics significantly reduced the risk of CHD.

Collectively, the calcium-antagonist-based studies (Syst-Eur, STONE, Syst-China and HOT) provide evidence that they, too, reduce the risk of stroke and CHD and that the magnitude of this effect appears to be similar to that of diuretic and beta-blocker therapy.

For angiotensin-converting enzyme (ACE) inhibitors, similar benefits were noted between captopril and atenolol in the UKPDS 39 and also, despite randomization failings, between captopril, diuretics and beta-blockers in the Captopril Primary Prevention Project (CAPPP). In the newly published Swedish Trial in Old Patients with Hypertension-2 (STOP-2), 6614 patients aged 70–84 years with hypertension were randomly assigned to a 'conventional' beta-blocker/thiazide regimen or an ACE inhibitor or a calcium antagonist. All three therapies again showed similar efficacy in the prevention of cardiovascular mortality and major morbidity.

A note of caution has emerged with the withdrawal, by the Data Safety Monitoring Board, of doxazosin from the ongoing Antihypertensive and Lipid Lowering Treatment to prevent Heart Attack Trial (ALLHAT). The decision was based on the finding that more patients on doxazosin developed heart failure and therefore that, despite lowering blood pressure, doxazosin may confer significantly fewer benefits than diuretic therapy on a major cardiovascular endpoint.

If all antihypertensive effects are, however, equal, the choice of treatment will thus be related to other factors such as cost, side-effects and coexisting disorders. The guidelines all contain useful tables identifying compelling and possible indications, contraindications and cautions for the major classes of antihypertensive drugs.

PRIORITY PATIENTS

Absolute risk assessment highlights the increased cardiovascular risk of diabetic and elderly patients. In addition, there is accumulating evidence that patients with existing cerebrovascular disease, CHD and renal disease all reduce the likelihood of future disease progression with antihypertensive therapy. Some ethnic groups such as Afro-Caribbeans and South Asians are also at increased risk.

Hypertension is extremely common in the elderly, with more than 50 per cent of the over-60s having isolated systolic hypertension (>160/<90 mmHg). New evidence shows that treatment of hypertension also reduces the risk of developing heart failure and preserves cognitive function. Treatment decisions in the over-80s are difficult but a meta-analysis in 1999 of seven studies provided data on 1670 patients and the results are shown in Table 6.4.

TABLE **6.4** • Percentage of cases prevented and 95% confidence intervals

	CV events	Stroke	Heart failure
Reduction in the morbidity of patients aged 80+ years	22 (2–60)	34 (10–52)	39 (10–60)

Source: Lueyffier, F., Bulpitt, C., Boissel, J. *et al.* (1999) Antihypertensive drugs in very old people: a sub-group meta-analysis of randomized controlled trials *Lancet* 1999; **353**, 793–6.

ORGANIZATIONAL CHANGES

Once diagnosed, the number of patients with uncontrolled hypertension highlights the difficulty of implementing the results of tightly controlled clinical trials and meticulously debated consensus advice. In 1995, Jones *et al.* reported continuation rates of only 40–50 per cent at 6 months for the four classes, diuretics, beta-blockers, calcium antagonists and ACE inhibitors. There is evidence that barriers to persistence with treatment occur early in the therapeutic course and primary care professionals are challenged to form a therapeutic alliance with their patients to maximize the acceptance of treatment regimens. Practitioners need to optimize the use of drugs, set agreed targets, review adverse effects and maximize information and choice for patients.

Patient involvement is the key issue for the future and already, in many countries, the availability of simple electronic home monitors has led to a rise in interest in home monitoring. There is good evidence for high degrees of interest, satisfaction, compliance and reliability of recording amongst patients. The monitors function well and cost a fraction of ambulatory monitoring devices. Both methods of home monitoring facilitate the recognition of 'white coat hypertension' but even when this is excluded, recordings are consistently 10–15/5–10 mmHg lower than office readings. Unfortunately, there is little prospective data relating home readings to events and consequently initiation and treatment guidelines are extrapolations of office-based recommendations. Ongoing studies are forthcoming, but with the European Union's intention to withdraw mercury-containing manometers, all practitioners will themselves eventually need to convert to electronic devices.

Nurse specialists have demonstrated improvements in control and compliance with medication and lifestyle advice when compared with doctors and, if available, represent a valuable potential resource to the practice. The increasing use of computers in primary care will encourage the construction and use of disease registers and improved protocol adherence and information capture through the use of customized templates for multidisciplinary hypertension management.

Clinical audit is a powerful tool for the generation of change, is facilitated by computerized recording and should become a routine exercise for the primary care team. Subtle differences in methodology and definitions may, however, generate discrepancies in results that can confound comparison of practitioner performance.

CONTROL OF DIABETES

The prevalence of dyslipidaemia and atherosclerosis is increased in diabetics and in type 2 diabetes the risk of myocardial infarction is raised two to six times higher than that of the general population. In diabetic women, the usual protective effect of the female sex is lost. Apart from attention to glycaemic control, the management of hyperlipidaemia in diabetes requires attention to all risk factors and integrated approaches to cessation of smoking, dietary change, increasing exercise and the choice of appropriate antihypertensives when necessary. Combining the results of the UK Prospective Diabetes Study and the Hypertension Optimal Treatment trial suggests that a target blood pressure of 130/80 and an Hb A_{1C} value of <7 per cent is desirable for diabetics in whom the absolute risk of myocardial infarction is >3 per cent per year. The excess risk of dyslipidaemia (often patterns of low HDL cholesterol with raised triglycerides) make lipid lowering with medication more appropriate. The management of diabetic patients is considered in detail in 'The patient with diabetes' in Chapter 11.

REFERENCES AND FURTHER READING

Anderson, O., Almgren, T., Persson, B. *et al.* (1998) Survival in treated hypertension: follow up study after two decades. *Br Med J* **317**, 167–71.

Ashenden, R., Silagy, C. and Weller, D. (1997) A systematic review of the effectiveness of promoting lifestyle change in general practice. *Fam Pract* **14**, 160–76.

Collins, R., Peto, R., MacMahon, S. *et al.* (1990) Blood pressure, stroke and coronary heart disease. Part 2. Short-term reductions in blood pressure: overview of randomized drug trials in the epidemiological context. *Lancet* **335**, 827–38.

Diclemente, C., Prochaska, J., Fairhurst, S.K., Velicer, W.F., Velasquez, M.M. and Rossi, J.S. (1991) The process of smoking cessation: an analysis of precontemplation, contemplation and preparation stages of change. *J Consult Clin Psychol* **59**, 295–304.

Guidelines subcommittee (1999) World Health Organisation–International Society of Hypertension Guidelines for the management of Hypertension. *J Hypertens* **17**, 151–83.

Hansson, L., Zanchetti, A., Carruthers, S.G. *et al.* (1998) Effect of intensive blood pressure lowering and low dose aspirin in patients with hypertension: principal results of the hypertension optimum treatment (HOT) randomized trial. *Lancet* **351**, 1755–62.

Jones, J., Gorkin, L., Lian, J. *et al.* (1995) Discontinuation of and changes in treatment after start of new courses of antihypertensive drugs: a study of a United Kingdom population. *Br Med J* **311**, 293–95.

Lancaster, T., Stead, L., Silagy, C. *et al.* (2000) Effectiveness of interventions to help people stop smoking: findings from the Cochrane library. *Br Med J* **321**, 355–8.

Ornish, D., Scherwitz, L.W., Billings, J.H. *et al.* (1998) Intensive lifestyle changes for reversal of coronary heart disease. *J Am Med Assoc* **280**, 2001–7.

Psaty, B., Smith, N., Siscovick, D. *et al.* (1997) Health outcomes associated with antihypertensive therapies used as first line agents: a systematic review and meta-analysis. *J Am Med Assoc* **277**, 739–45.

United Kingdom Prospective Diabetes Study Group (1998) Efficacy of atenolol and captopril in reducing risk of macrovascular and microvascular complications in type 2 diabetes: UKPDS 39. *Br Med J* **317**, 713–20.

DIET

Earlier chapters have suggested how changes in the current 'Western' diet would confer benefits in CHD prevention at both population and individual levels. These changes can be summarized as:

- attainment of ideal body weight;
- reduction in intake of total fat, saturated fat and cholesterol;
- relative increase in intake of poly- and monounsaturated fats;
- increase in omega-3 polyunsaturated fats;
- increase in intake of unrefined carbohydrate;
- increase in intake of vitamin and mineral antioxidants;
- reduction in dietary sodium with an increase in potassium.

ATTAINMENT OF IDEAL BODY WEIGHT

Body mass index (BMI) is calculated as a person's weight in kilograms divided by their height in metres squared and has become an accepted measure in the assessment of body weight (Figure 7.1). Although optimal BMI is considered to be 18.5–24.9 kg/m^2, in 1997, 45 per cent of UK males and 33 per cent of UK females were overweight (>25 kg/m^2) and 17 per cent and 20 per cent, respectively, were obese (>30 kg/m^2). In common with many other countries, these figures are rising. In the USA, the percentage of the population considered obese rose from 12.3 per cent to 20 per cent in men and from 16.5 per cent to 24.9 per cent in women between 1976–80 and 1988–94.

If an individual is overweight, losing weight produces a drop in total cholesterol and triglyceride levels, and the level of HDL cholesterol tends to rise. The effect is potent and there is no patient with hyperlipidaemia and obesity whose lipid levels would not benefit from weight loss.

In a survey of 20 000 people who lost weight (mean loss 15 kg), 72 per cent achieved their weight loss alone, 20 per cent employed commercial programmes and relatively few

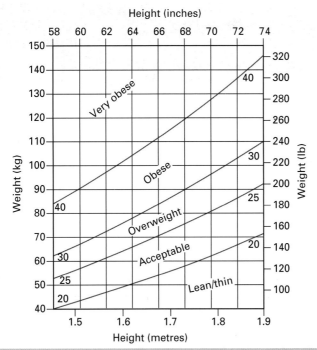

FIGURE **7.1** • Obesity: relationship between height and weight. Adapted from Garrow, J.S. (1981) *Treat Obesity Seriously*. Churchill Livingstone, Edinburgh.

consulted health professionals. Whilst this underlines the fact that the responsibility for weight loss ultimately lies with the individual, health professionals have much to offer in terms of advice, support and encouragement.

■ The **benefits** of weight loss (Table 7.1) can be illustrated in terms of improved appearance, effort tolerance, metabolic change (blood pressure, lipids and glucose), a reduction in sleep apnoea and increased life expectancy. In 1995, Williamson *et al.*

TABLE **7.1** • The effects of a 10 kg weight loss in an individual with a baseline weight of 100 kg and co-morbidities

Mortality	■ >20% fall in total mortality ■ >30% fall in diabetes-related deaths ■ >40% fall in obesity-related cancer deaths
Blood pressure	■ Fall of approximately 10 mmHg SBP and DBP
Diabetes	■ Fall of 50% in fasting glucose
Lipids	■ Fall of 10% in total cholesterol ■ Fall of 15% in LDL-C ■ Fall of 30% in triglycerides ■ Rise of 8% in HDL-C

Adapted from Jung R. (1997) Obesity as a disease. *Br Med Bull* **53**(2), 307–21.

showed that in a group of 15 069 women with BMI >27 and co-morbid conditions, **any** weight loss (0.5–9 kg) was associated with a 20 per cent reduction in all-cause mortality. Weight loss of 5–10 per cent in patients with type 2 diabetes improves blood glucose profile, Hb A_{1C} and reduces the need for medication. In hypertensive, obese patients, weight loss reduces blood pressure by about 1–2 mmHg for every 1 kg fall. The results of a meta-analysis of 70 studies of the effects of intentional weight loss on lipids show that for every 1 kg of weight lost, the serum concentration of LDL cholesterol falls by 0.02 mmol/L, while triglyceride levels fall by 0.015 mmol/L and HDL cholesterol increases by 0.009 mmol/L.

- The **construction of a coherent plan** may involve no more than suggesting a change from inappropriate foods (fatty foods, sugar and alcohol) to more appropriate ones.
- **Specific behaviour modification strategies** are increasingly employed including the promotion of self-monitoring, stress management, stimulus control (cues to overeating), contingency management, cognitive restructuring (especially with body image dissatisfaction) and improved social support.
- An **exercise regimen** can be recommended. The target should be moderate physical activity progressing to 30 minutes on most or all days of the week. Whilst it takes a lot of exercise to lose only a little fat, lean body mass is maintained and there is improved morale and fitness.
- **Targets** can be set, encouraging a specific weight loss over a certain period. If possible, a 10 per cent weight loss over 6 months will maximize health benefits but targets should be flexible, with intermediate levels when attainment of ideal body weight is a remote possibility. A loss of 0.5–1 kg per week is reasonable.
- **Follow-up** (including weighing every 2–4 weeks) is essential to foster compliance and to motivate positively. The rate of weight loss usually declines after 6 months and weight often plateaus. Emphasis may then have to change to weight maintenance rather than continue with increasingly frustrating and futile attempts to lose further weight. There is some evidence that continued contact with a therapist reduces the risk of long-term relapse.

The **calorie-controlled diet** is the commonest weight-reducing strategy. This operates from the observation that excess weight is 75 per cent fat and 25 per cent fat-free tissue and has an energy value of 7000 kcal/kg. Therefore to lose 1 kg/week a person needs 1000 kcal negative balance per day. An average man requires 2500 kcal/day and an average woman 2100 kcal/day; therefore, all obese people should lose weight on a diet of 1000 kcal/day and this is confirmed in controlled metabolic studies. Randomized controlled trials show that diets allowing 1200 kcal/day and behaviour modification produce 8.5 kg weight loss at 20 weeks. The calorie-counting approach is limited by the need for meticulous measurement and recording and the ease of deception when faced with excess food that must be discarded.

'Crash diets' tend to achieve gratifying short-term loss but this is more at the expense of glycogen and water. Losses of greater than 1 kg/week (such as produced by very low calorie diets) tend to lose lean body mass as well as fat. Their use should be confined to periods of less than 4 weeks, their benefit being mainly motivational.

Many patients attend groups where the provision of structured plans, support and competition increases compliance. Simple behaviour modification techniques are used such as learning to eat more slowly or take smaller mouthfuls. Interestingly, men do well (in all-male groups); women often achieve more weight loss with individual attention. For both men and women, 50–60 per cent respond to the group approach, with average weight loss of 6–12 kg.

For some patients a lot of eating is automatic and bypasses critical analysis. For these people, food diaries can provide information on patterns of eating, types of food, quantities and 'danger times' that may respond to modification.

DRUG THERAPY

Drug therapy may be considered for obese and overweight patients with significant co-morbidity or risk factors, in whom diet, exercise and behaviour modification have failed. Their action should be viewed as adjunctive or motivational. Drugs such as diuretics and thyroid hormones have no role in the management of obesity and bulking agents, such as methylcellulose, which claim to induce satiety, lack supportive evidence from randomized trials. The centrally active adrenergic drugs, such as amphetamine, diethylpropion, phentermine and mazindol act by appetite suppression but have prohibitive side-effects and are no longer licensed in many countries.

Orlistat is a potent inhibitor of pancreatic lipase and induces weight loss by reducing fat absorption (25–35 per cent of dietary fat is lost in the faeces). In 1998, Sjöström and colleagues prescribed a reducing diet (600 kcal/day less than calculated requirement) for 743 patients with BMI ranging from 28 to 47. After a 4-week run-in period, during which they lost on average 2 kg, 688 patients compliant with the dietary regimen were randomized to orlistat (120 mg three times daily) or placebo for 12 months. Subjects in the orlistat group lost on average 10.3 kg (10.2 per cent of body weight) whereas subjects in the placebo group lost 6.1 kg (6.1 per cent). In a second 12-month period, subjects were reassigned to orlistat or placebo with a eucaloric, maintenance diet. Patients who continued on orlistat gained 2 kg by the end of year 2 but those switched to placebo gained 4 kg. Patients switched to orlistat from placebo lost an additional 0.9 kg; patients who stayed on placebo regained a mean 2.5 kg (Figure 7.2).

Total cholesterol, LDL cholesterol, and glucose fell dramatically in both groups during the run-in period. These changes persisted in the orlistat group but rebounded, almost to the initial levels, in the placebo group. The main side-effects in the trial reflected orlistat's action, with complaints of oily spotting, flatus with discharge, faecal urgency and oily faeces being common. As these side-effects relate to fat malabsorption, their net effect is probably to improve dietary compliance! Low levels of some fat-soluble vitamins were found in 5.8 per cent of subjects. Orlistat can be used for patients with BMI $>28 \text{ kg/m}^2$ where diet alone produces a weight loss of 2.5 kg or more over 4 weeks and should be discontinued if treatment has not resulted in a >5 per cent weight loss over 12 weeks.

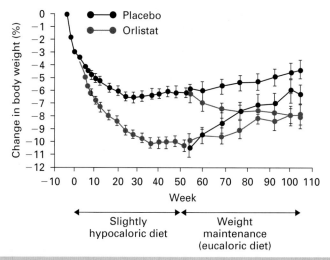

FIGURE **7.2** • Mean percentage change in body weight over 2 years in orlistat versus placebo groups of obese patients. Source: Reproduced (with permission) from Sjöström, L., Rissanen, A., Andersen, T. *et al.* (1998).

After initial first-pass metabolism in the liver, using the cytochrome P450 3A4 system, metabolites of **sibutramine** act centrally, blocking noradrenaline, serotonin and dopamine re-uptake. Taking 15 mg daily has been associated with a modest 7.3 per cent weight loss at one year and with favourable reductions in total cholesterol and LDL cholesterol and a small increase in HDL cholesterol. Weight lost, however, is quickly regained when sibutramine is stopped. Unfortunately, a sympathomimetic action is significant in up to 10 per cent of patients, with small elevations of blood pressure and pulse rate and sleep disturbance. The drug is therefore contraindicated in those with CHD, heart failure and hypertension. The many contraindications, the need for monitoring of pulse and blood pressure, the potential for interaction with other drugs and methodological doubts surrounding the efficacy studies mean that its use is limited.

REDUCTION IN TOTAL FAT

Apart from making food more palatable, fat has physiological roles, contributing to the structure of every cell membrane, to the manufacture of steroids, prostaglandins and bile acids and as a major source of energy provision and storage. Fat is high in calories (9 kcal/g) compared with carbohydrate (4 kcal/g) and this is due to the extra oxygen atoms in carbohydrates and therefore less potential for oxidative respiration. Throughout nature, fat represents a high energy/low weight storage material, for example seed oils, which keep seeds light, thus aiding dispersal.

During the Second World War a deficiency of dietary energy led to a nutritional crisis in some countries. In Finland, Norway and Sweden the shortage of meat, eggs and butter correlated closely with a drop in CHD levels during the war years. In the UK, the pre-war rise in CHD levelled off, then resumed after the war; in the USA, there was no change. High energy fat came to be viewed favourably and the impression that fat was good and carbohydrate bad lingered long after the war had ended. The ingenious variety whereby the food industry now presents us processed fat in multiple disguises, from sausages and pâté, to pastries and cheese, tempts us to choose by flavour rather than by required energy content (Figure 7.3).

It is hardly surprising that, faced with nearly 2000 new products per year, little reduction in the fat content of the UK diet has occurred. In the mid-1970s, the percentage of energy derived from dietary fat in the British diet was 42 per cent, with 46 per cent being derived from carbohydrate and 12 per cent from protein. The figure for 1997 is just over 39 per cent, which corresponds with the average for European Union countries but not with the European average of 32 per cent. In Europe, the proportion of energy derived from fat varies from as much as 43 per cent in Austria to 16 per cent in Georgia. In addition to the slight fall in fat consumption in the UK, the type of fat consumed has changed, with consumption of saturated fats falling from 20.3 per cent to 15.2 per cent. The consumption of polyunsaturated fats has risen from 4.0 per cent to 7.0 per cent

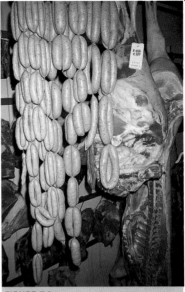

FIGURE **7.3**

but the consumption of monounsaturated fats has stayed more or less the same.

As the total fat content of diet does not reflect its component fatty acid constitution, total fat is not strongly associated with serum cholesterol levels. However, high intakes are often associated with high intakes of saturated fatty acids, which are strongly associated with high total and LDL cholesterol. Total fat does contribute to obesity and factor VII clotting activation.

FATTY ACID BIOCHEMISTRY

Fatty acids are formed from hydrocarbon chains with a **terminal methyl group** (CH_3) at one end and a **carboxyl group** (COOH) at the other. If there are no double bonds (C=C), the fatty acid is described as **saturated**.

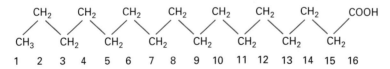

This is palmitic acid. There are 16 carbon atoms and no double bonds. It is noted C16:0.

If double bonds are present, the fatty acid is **unsaturated**. If one is present, it is **monounsaturated**, if more than one, **polyunsaturated**.

This is oleic acid (C18:1), a monounsaturated fatty acid.

TABLE **7.2** • Major dietary fatty acids

Structure	Fatty acid	Melting point (°C)
Saturated		
C 12:0	Lauric acid	44
C 14:0	Myristic acid	54
C 16:0	Palmitic acid	63
C 18:0	Stearic acid	70
Unsaturated		
Omega-9 (N-9)		
C 18:1 *cis*	Oleic acid	11
C 18:1 *trans*	Elaidic acid	45
Omega-6 (N-6)		
C 18:2	Linoleic acid	−5
Omega-3 (N-3)		
C 18:3	Linolenic acid	−11
C 20:5	Eicosapentaenoic acid (EPA)	−50
C 20:6	Docosahexaenoic acid (DHA)	−54

The carbon of the terminal methyl group is called the **omega carbon** and the position of the double bond is counted from this (omega-9, or N-9).

This is eicosapentaenoic acid (EPA) (C20:5), an omega-3 fatty acid. Omega-3 (N-3) describes the position of the double bond nearest the methyl group. Table 7.2 shows the major dietary fatty acids.

The hydrogen atoms bonded to the carbon atoms of the double bonds in unsaturated fatty acids normally lie on the same side of the double bond, forming *cis* **isomers** (Figure 7.4). A kink is imparted to the hydrocarbon chain, which means that unsaturated fatty acids cannot pack closely together. The forces between them are less and their melting points correspondingly lower. This explains why vegetable oils rich in unsaturated fatty acids are liquid at room temperature. Conversely, if the hydrogen atoms are on opposite sides of the double bond, the chains remain straight and *trans* **isomers** are formed (Figure 7.4). Saturated fatty acids are also straight and both they and *trans* fatty acids have higher melting points. This explains why saturated fat is solid at room temperature and so difficult to wash away after the Sunday roast.

Plants and cold-blooded animals can contain only those fatty acids that will remain liquid at the temperature of their habitat. Fish, for example, contain highly polyunsaturated fatty acids such as EPA and DHA (Table 7.2). Warm-blooded animals can tolerate saturated fats unless they live in cold habitats, in which case high levels of polyunsaturates are necessary to maintain fluidity – for example, the blubber of whales.

The percentage pattern of fatty acids in some fats, oils and meat in our diet is shown in Table 7.3. Whilst the proportions of fatty acids vary from food to food, no food is pure in fatty acid composition. Free use of a monounsaturate-predominant vegetable oil, such as olive oil, still adds saturates to the diet and so a reduction in total fat content in the diet is still required as well as a change in pattern.

TABLE **7.3** • Percentage of fatty acids in diet

Source	Saturated (C14–18)	Monounsaturated	Linoleic acid
Butter	69	28	3
Lamb	50	38	4
Beef	48	48	2
Palm oil	45	45	9
Pork	42	50	7
Hard margarine	37	33	12
Chicken	34	45	18
Soft margarine	21	22	52
Olive oil	14	73	11
Sunflower oil	12	33	58
Rapeseed oil	7	62	31

SATURATED FATTY ACIDS (SFA)

Saturated fatty acids (SFA) predominate in meat, butter, lard, hard margarine, suet and palm and coconut oils. They have the most significant effect on lipoproteins, raising total cholesterol, LDL cholesterol and triglyceride. Increased saturated fat intake was associated with increased CHD rates in the Seven Countries Study (page 34).

Whilst C6–20 SFA are found in the diet, C12–18 SFA are the most prevalent: C16 (palmitic acid) is the commonest and C14 (myristic acid) the most hypercholesterolaemic. Short-chain (C10 or less) saturated fatty acids and C18 (stearic acid) seem to have no effect on lipoprotein levels, the latter being converted quickly into oleic acid in humans. This means that only three saturated fatty acids are atherogenic (C12, C14 and C16).

The proportion of dietary polyunsaturates to saturates is often expressed as the **P/S ratio** and used to describe the atherogenicity of a particular diet. As only three saturates are hypercholesterolaemic, this use of the ratio is technically inappropriate.

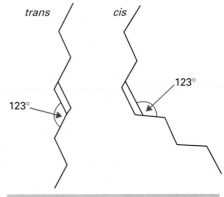

FIGURE **7.4** • *Cis* and *trans* isomers of unsaturated fatty acids.

TRANS FATTY ACIDS (TFA)

Low levels of *trans* unsaturated fatty acids are present naturally in the diet, forming in ruminants and appearing in dairy products. Others are manufactured in the hardening of vegetable oils to produce margarine (hydrogenation). Their straight chains allow them to act like saturated fats and there is some evidence of a link with CHD from the Harvard Study of American Nurses. Metabolic studies show increased LDL cholesterol and decreased HDL cholesterol and most major margarine manufacturers have now reduced the *trans* fatty acid content of their spreads.

DIETARY CHOLESTEROL

Dietary cholesterol is mostly derived from dairy products, particularly eggs, but is also well known to originate from shellfish and avocado pears. It is incompletely absorbed from the gut (30–60 per cent) and only exceeds 500 mg/day in diets already high in saturated fat. Halving this amount would have little impact on total cholesterol reduction (approximately 0.2 mmol/L) and attention to lowering dietary cholesterol is of major importance to few. Nevertheless, advising patients to restrict egg consumption as part of a healthy diet is a widespread practice and most authorities advise an intake of 300 mg/day or less, of dietary cholesterol. As a 50 g egg contains about 213 mg of cholesterol, the question of how many eggs a patient can have is commonly asked.

The link between egg consumption and incident cases of CHD was investigated in a prospective study of 37 851 men from the Health Professionals Follow-up Study over 8 years and 80 082 women from the Nurses' Health Study over 14 years. After multivariate adjustment, no overall significant associations were found between egg consumption and the risk of CHD or stroke. In subgroup analysis, significant associations were found for diabetics consuming more than one egg per day compared with those diabetics eating fewer than one egg per week. Saturated fat intake, rather than dietary cholesterol, provides by far the greatest contribution to an individual's cholesterol level. While rich in cholesterol, eggs contain only about 5 g of fat, two-thirds of which is unsaturated. It is possible that potentially beneficial effects on HDL cholesterol and triglycerides and the effect of other nutrients within the egg, such as antioxidants, folic acid and B vitamins, offset any small adverse effect of the total cholesterol content.

Many products achieve credibility in the eye of the purchaser by being labelled as 'low cholesterol.' This has created a lot of uncertainty, the confusion arising from a failure to understand that the diet to reduce the incidence of CHD is 'cholesterol lowering', not 'low cholesterol'.

MONOUNSATURATED FATTY ACIDS (MUFA)

Monounsaturated fatty acids are found in all animal products and vegetables. Particular sources include olives, rapeseed (canola), avocados, most nuts, meat and peanut oil. The beneficial effects on lipoproteins were first described in 1957 but the observations were neglected for 30 years. When substituted for saturated fatty acids, total cholesterol,

LDL cholesterol and triglyceride are reduced and HDL cholesterol either remains unchanged or slightly increased. The LDL cholesterol produced appears lighter and less susceptible to oxidation.

The use of olive oil in Mediterranean countries over thousands of years provides strong epidemiological support for its use and safety.

POLYUNSATURATED FATTY ACIDS (PUFA)

Polyunsaturated fatty acids can be divided into omega-6 (N-6) and omega-3 (N-3) polyunsaturates. Omega-6 polyunsaturated fatty acids are found in vegetable oils, fish oils, most margarines, nuts and seeds and predominate in sunflower, safflower, corn, sesame, soybean and walnut oils. Coconut and palm oils tend to have more saturated fat than polyunsaturates. Linoleic acid is the commonest PUFA in the diet, being found particularly in PUFA-rich margarines. In countries such as Finland and Scotland, a low intake of linoleic acid (<4 per cent of energy) has been associated with an increased risk of CHD. Where populations have an average intake of 6 per cent there is no association with coronary risk.

When substituting for saturates, PUFAs lower total cholesterol, LDL cholesterol and triglyceride more significantly than do monounsaturates. Unfortunately, they also produce a slight drop in HDL cholesterol. Some polyunsaturates are essential to life as precursors of prostaglandins and prostacyclins.

Recently, some concerns have emerged regarding the safety of polyunsaturates and these explain the switch of focus to monounsaturates as substitutes for saturates:

- No society has consumed high levels of omega-6 PUFAs for long enough to provide reassuring epidemiological evidence of safety.
- The slight reduction in HDL cholesterol may be significant, particularly in women.
- LDL cholesterol from people on a diet rich in linoleic acid seems to be more susceptible to oxidation.
- Animal experiments seem to suggest a decreased resistance to infection or neoplasia. This has not been verified in humans.
- The prevalence of gallstones is increased.
- Repeated reheating of polyunsaturated oil (e.g. a deep fat fryer) increases hydrogenation.

Alpha linolenic acid is the parent compound of the polyunsaturated fatty acids of the omega-3 (N-3) family and is found in certain oils – soybean, flaxseed and rapeseed (canola) – as well as wholemeal bread, fruits and vegetables. The omega-3 polyunsaturates – eicosapentaenoic acid (EPA) and docosahexaenoic acid (DHA) – are found particularly in oily fish such as sardines, pilchards, mackerel, herring, salmon, trout, halibut and tuna (not tinned). For example, 10 ml of cod-liver oil contains about 2 g of omega-3 fatty acids.

In 1927, attention was drawn to the apparently low rates of CHD in fish-eating communities such as Greenland Inuits (Eskimos). In recent years the accuracy of the mortality statistics have been questioned but in 1970 Danish scientists led an investigation into the dietary habits of Inuits. Compared with Danes or Inuits who had migrated to Denmark, native Inuits showed a slight reduction in serum cholesterol but a large (60 per cent) reduction in triglycerides. Dietary analysis, using a double portion technique, led to the discovery that the diet of native Inuits contained five times the level of omega-3 PUFAs than the diet of native Danes. The high levels of omega-3 polyunsaturates found in phytoplankton were being assimilated through the food chain by fish, whales and seals into the Inuit diet. In 1982, similar contrasts were found between Japanese fishermen and inland farmers.

Four prospective studies, including MRFIT, have all demonstrated the protective effect of fish consumption. Interestingly, the findings in these studies also demonstrate the benefit of white fish in the diet. White fish is high in protein, vitamins and minerals and because it is low in fat it can act as a meat substitute.

Much literature on diet and heart disease reports on small feeding trials and there is a dearth of properly conducted randomized controlled trials. The only such trial of fish consumption is the Diet and Reinfarction Trial (DART). In this secondary prevention trial, the study group assigned to eating oily fish twice weekly showed a surprising 29 per cent reduction in all-cause mortality (33 per cent reduction in CHD mortality).

The major effect of ingesting omega-3 fatty acids is on triglyceride levels but at high dose (24 g/day), total cholesterol may fall (10 per cent). At moderate consumption levels, HDL cholesterol may rise. In addition, fish oils have been shown to have antithrombotic, anti-atherosclerotic and anti-arrhythmic actions. EPA displaces arachidonic acid in platelets, reducing thromboxane synthesis and interfering with prostacyclin mechanisms, leading to reduced platelet aggregation. Platelet counts and fibrinogen are also reduced and prolonged bleeding times were confirmed in the Danish study (anecdotally, Inuits were notorious for nosebleeds!). Other effects include reduced monocyte adhesion and migration, reduced expression of endothelial cytokines and improved endothelial function. A meta-analysis of fish oil studies showed a reduction of blood pressure of 3.4/2.0 mmHg with improved blood viscosity and arterial compliance. Reduced heart rate variability has been shown in survivors of myocardial infarction.

The Lyon Diet Heart Study is a randomized, single-blind, secondary prevention trial testing whether a Mediterranean type diet, rich in alpha linolenic acid especially from rapeseed oil, has any advantages over a 'prudent Western diet'. It was originally undertaken to explore the reasons behind the low incidence of CHD in Mediterranean countries compared to those of northern Europe (Table 7.4).

TABLE **7.4** • Key components of a Mediterranean diet

- High intake and variety of fruits, vegetables, legumes and grains – fresh fruit with meals as dessert
- High ratio of MUFA to SFA – olive oil as principal source of fat
- Moderate consumption of milk and dairy products – principally as cheese and yogurt
- Enhanced consumption of fish and poultry
- Low intake of red meat and meat products
- 0–4 egg yolks consumed weekly
- Alcohol consumption at moderate levels – typically wine with meal

Patients suffering a first myocardial infarction, aged less than 70 between March 1988 and March 1992 were randomized with the intention of comparing the different dietary groups over 5 years. In March 1993, the trial was halted when interim results were statistically significant and the findings, at a mean 27 months per patient, were published.

Commentators criticized the findings, citing the small number of events and the wide confidence intervals of the interim analysis and this undermined the impact of the study. For ethical, medical and scientific reasons, all patients were invited for a final visit and by the time they had all been seen, an additional 19 months of analysis per patient became available. The results at 46 months are shown in Table 7.5.

TABLE **7.5** • Findings of the Lyon Diet Heart Study

	Control group (*n*)	Experimental group (*n*)	*P* value
CHD deaths	19	6	0.01
Non-fatal MI	25	8	
All-cause mortality	24	14	0.03
Total primary and secondary endpoints	180	95	0.0002

The inclusion of more events does not weaken the findings of the interim analysis. Furthermore, a comparison of the main risk factors between the groups shows that the differences were achieved without modification of the traditional risk factors such as cholesterol (Table 7.6).

TABLE **7.6** • Main risk factors recorded on the final visit

Risk factor	Control group	Experimental group
Body mass index (kg/m^2)	26.9	26.3
Blood pressure (mmHg)	128/79	128/78
Total cholesterol (mmol/L)	6.18	6.20
HDL-C (mmol/L)	1.28	1.29
LDL-C (mmol/L)	4.23	4.17
Triglycerides (mmol/L)	1.75	1.94
Current smokers (%)	17.9	18.3

Compliance with dietary change has traditionally proved difficult for practical, economic and gastronomic reasons. In this study, even several years after randomization, it is remarkable that most experimental patients were still closely following the Mediterranean diet recommended to them.

Whilst lipid lowering in the secondary prevention of CHD is massively evidence based, relatively simple dietary changes appear to achieve greater reductions in all-cause and CHD mortality. The study does not contradict the importance of lipid lowering, but indicates that there are other powerful risk factors that can be modified by diet that must be considered. If a larger scale trial confirms these findings, traditional CHD prevention diets will need to be reassessed.

The GISSI-Prevenzione trial (GISSI-P) was initiated to explore the benefits of marine N-3 PUFA 1 g daily and vitamin E 300 mg daily, separately and together in comparison with placebo (GISSI-Prevenzione investigators, 1999). Some 11 324 patients with a history of myocardial infarction within the preceding 3 months were enrolled from 172 centres across Italy and randomized to the four groups. At 42 months, four-way intention to treat analysis showed a significant reduction in death, non-fatal MI and stroke of 15 per cent in the group with N-3 PUFA supplementation. Patients receiving vitamin E did not differ from controls except when taking N-3 PUFA in addition and then the effect was consistent with that achieved by taking N-3 PUFA alone. Both N-3 PUFA and vitamin E were well tolerated with low rates of reported side-effects.

The therapeutic effect of fish oil supplements is further considered later.

CARBOHYDRATES

DIETARY FIBRE

In 1975, Burkitt and Trowell presented their 'fibre hypothesis' linking low fibre intake in the diet to numerous Western diseases, including CHD. Interest had been stimulated by epidemiological observations, in this case linking the high fibre diet of Africans (Ugandans eat 150 g/day) and their low rates of CHD. The average fibre consumption in the UK is 20 g/day.

Nowadays the term dietary fibre is misleading, as it does not adequately describe some of the constituent indigestible non-starch carbohydrates, such as gums, that are included in the group. A better term is **non-starch polysaccharides.**

Non-starch polysaccharides (NSPs) can be divided into water-soluble, gel-forming varieties [chiefly pectin, guar gum, ispaghula (psyllium) and oat bran] and insoluble varieties, which are chiefly structural fibres such as cellulose and lignin. Insoluble NSPs, such as bread, pasta, breakfast cereals, brown rice and wheat bran have beneficial effects in preventing constipation and bowel disease, but may only aid CHD prevention by substituting for other more dangerous foods. By contrast, the soluble fraction found in pulses, oats, barley, nuts, seeds, fruit and vegetables excites interest because it has a cholesterol-lowering effect. The DART investigated the effect of dietary fibre as well as fish, but used cereal fibre that was largely wheat based. No benefit was found and a randomized controlled outcome trial of soluble fibre is needed.

Oat bran has been extensively studied and in 1987, a book extolling its virtues, *The Eight Week Cholesterol Cure*, sold 2 million copies. The observation was made that 30–60 g/day of oat bran lowered cholesterol by 10–15 per cent and cereal manufacturers produced heart-shaped bowls to promote their products. Unfortunately, the amounts of cereal needed were large and impractical and required several bowls. Pectin and guar gum also lower cholesterol (guar gum by 15 per cent) but again the amounts used are too large and unpalatable.

Oats contain beta-glucan, which forms a viscous NSP in the gut that delays bile acid reabsorption. This leads to increased bile acid output and colonic bacteria sequester the excess bile acids. The reduction in bile acid reabsorption is barely measurable, but sufficient to reduce serum cholesterol. Some of the effect must involve substitution but it is hard to quantify. If you eat enough oats you will have no room left for your bacon and eggs. It is ironic that the countries with the highest oat consumption in the world are Scotland and Finland, both renowned for their high rates of CHD.

There are many individual trials of dietary fibre and most suggest a significant effect in lowering total serum and LDL cholesterol. There is much debate, however, about the degree of cholesterol reduction produced. Meta-analyses have attempted to quantify this but differences between the studies, such as the dose and type of fibre used, methodological variations, publication bias and confounding variables mean there is no definitive answer. Glore's meta-analysis of 77 studies published in 1994 found that average serum cholesterol reduction from baseline in hypercholesterolaemic subjects was 10.9 per cent (LDL cholesterol 13.6 per cent), although the values were not placebo corrected. A meta-analysis of 22 ispaghula studies showed average placebo-corrected reductions of 3.2 per cent. Brown *et al.*'s (1999) meta-analysis chose studies using a more practical range of fibre (2–10 g/day) and found significant but more modest reductions, LDL cholesterol being reduced by 0.057 mmol/L per gram of fibre. This means an intake of 3 g of soluble fibre, such as would be contained in three apples or three 28 g servings of oatmeal, would reduce LDL cholesterol by 0.13 mmol/L or 2 per cent.

SIMPLE SUGARS

There is little evidence that simple refined carbohydrates such as sucrose directly promote CHD; indeed Cuba, with the highest per capita sucrose consumption in the world, has low rates of CHD. North Americans eat too much food and, in particular, too much refined sugar. Per capita consumption has risen to 152 lb per year – equivalent to 47 teaspoons per person per day and much of this is hidden. The effect on obesity and therefore glycaemic control and lipoprotein profiles will manifest in an increased burden of cardiovascular disease in the near future.

GLYCAEMIC INDEX

Diets low in fat necessarily contain a high proportion of carbohydrates, the effect of which is to reduce not only LDL cholesterol but also HDL cholesterol. Not all carbohydrates act in the same way and carbohydrates with a low glycaemic index may actually raise HDL cholesterol. The glycaemic index is the area of the blood glucose curve produced by a certain food, expressed as a percentage of the area produced by the same amount of carbohydrate eaten as glucose or white bread. It was originally produced to aid diabetics reduce postprandial peaks of glucose but was shown to be positively associated with CHD in the Nurses' Health Study.

TABLE **7.7** • Glycaemic indices relative to white bread (101)

Food	Glycaemic index (%)
Glucose	138
Sucrose	92
Wholemeal bread	99
White rice	81
Baked potato	121
Kidney beans	42
Milk	39
Apples	52

Carbohydrates vary considerably in their glycaemic indices and the results are surprising, as low glycaemic index does not equate to fibre content (Table 7.7). Sucrose has a glycaemic index less than bread and this is because it contains 50 per cent fructose, which has very little effect on postprandial glucose levels. The degree of cooking and whether the food is whole or mashed also influence glycaemic index. Beans, peas, spaghetti, barley and certain fruits have consistently low glycaemic indices.

ANTIOXIDANTS

Respiration depends on oxygen to release energy to drive all bodily functions. The notion that oxygen may be harmful to us is not immediately apparent, but reactive oxygen species, leaking from normal cellular processes or from pollutants such as cigarette smoke, can react with lipids to produce oxidized LDL cholesterol and structural phospholipid damage, with proteins to produce cross-linking and degradation and with DNA to produce errors and deletions. Thus, free radicals may be implicated in the processes of cardiovascular disease, cancer and ageing.

All organisms use enzyme systems, redox pathways and antioxidant vitamins and provitamins to defend themselves against free radical attack and much interest has been generated in the potential of antioxidant supplementation to reduce CHD. Antioxidants exist to trap free radicals and render them inert and many substances have been described. Examples include vitamin E (alpha-tocopherol), vitamin C (ascorbic acid), the carotenes (more than 600 compounds), flavonoids (more than 3000 compounds) ubiquinolone-10, oestrogen and selenium.

Much of the variation in CHD rates between countries cannot be explained in terms of classical risk factors. For example, southern European countries have much lower rates of CHD than northern countries, despite high rates of smoking and similar cholesterol levels. Epidemiological research suggests that differences in antioxidant status could account for the discrepancies. Certainly, nutritional surveys have consistently demonstrated that the consumption of fruit and vegetables, which are excellent sources of antioxidants, correlates well with reduced CHD mortality. In addition, variations in fruit and vegetable consumption parallel the regional differences in CHD rate. Analyses of antioxidant concentrations in plasma and adipose tissue have consistently shown an increased risk of developing CHD at low antioxidant levels and *in vitro* experiments have shown the beneficial effects of antioxidants on the progression of atherosclerosis.

Unfortunately, cohort studies are easily confounded by concomitant behaviour patterns both cardioprotective and paradoxical (where an individual permits adverse habits as a 'trade-off' against those perceived as 'good'). Cohort studies that have analysed individual antioxidant consumption also demonstrate some inconsistencies in their findings and a number of randomized trials have attempted to clarify the situation. Most have focused on **vitamin E**, which is the most abundant antioxidant in plasma, perhaps reflecting its importance. Vitamin E is commonly found in foods high in polyunsaturates and it is the substance in vegetable oil that prevents it oxidizing (going rancid). In 1993, published surveys of American doctors and nurses showed significant reductions in CHD in users of vitamin E supplement (100 mg). As the supplement users may have been generally healthier and health-conscious individuals, the study may have been confounded. The Cambridge Heart Antioxidant Study (CHAOS) was a secondary prevention study of 2002 patients taking high dose vitamin E (400–800 mg) but with only a short follow-up period of 17 months. Non-fatal MI was dramatically reduced by 77 per cent but there was a non-significant increase in overall mortality and fatal MI. Temporarily, there was interest that somehow vitamin E could prevent non-fatal MI but the results of the GISSI-Prevenzione trial, the Primary Prevention Project (PPP), the Heart Outcomes Prevention Evaluation (HOPE) study and the Heart Protection Study (HPS), which examined the effects of vitamin E supplementation, have shown no benefits.

Most recently, the effect of 800 mg supplements was examined in chronic haemodialysis patients, a group notorious for their high cardiovascular mortality (the SPACE trial) (Boaz *et al.*, 2000). Although a small-number study (196 patients), only five patients assigned to vitamin E suffered a myocardial infarction compared to 17 assigned to placebo (RR 0.30, $P = 0.016$). The results may have been confounded by the use of other antioxidants.

A recently published meta-analysis shows quite clearly the difference between observational studies and intervention trials (Figure 7.5). The evidence for vitamin E is therefore inconclusive. It is possible that vitamin E can have pro-oxidant effects and needs to be recycled by vitamin C. The Antioxidant Supplementation in Atherosclerosis (ASAP) study, which is in progress, will attempt to answer this question.

Much of the observational data on **vitamin C** is inconsistent. Twelve-year follow-up of US adults (NHANES 2) found no relationship between serum ascorbic acid quartile and mortality in women but 57 per cent higher mortality for men in the top quartile compared with the bottom. Such analyses are plagued by measurement error. Ascorbic acid is notoriously difficult to assess in dietary analyses, being present in many foods and considerably affected by processing, cooking and storage. Plasma ascorbic acid is representative of dietary intake over the preceding weeks but is technically difficult to measure consistently. The most recent attempt to provide a more rigorous prospective population analysis comes from the UK, one of nine countries involved in the European Prospective Investigation into Cancer and Nutrition (EPIC). EPIC-Norfolk derived

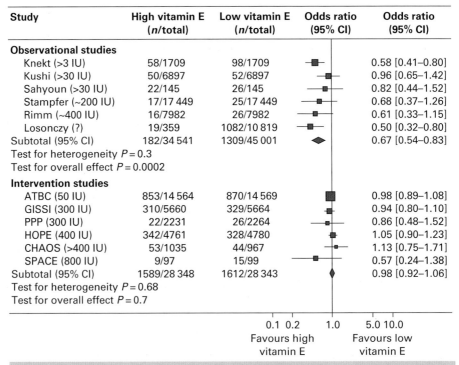

Study	High vitamin E (*n*/total)	Low vitamin E (*n*/total)	Odds ratio (95% CI)	Odds ratio (95% CI)
Observational studies				
Knekt (>3 IU)	58/1709	98/1709		0.58 [0.41–0.80]
Kushi (>30 IU)	50/6897	52/6897		0.96 [0.65–1.42]
Sahyoun (>30 IU)	22/145	26/145		0.82 [0.44–1.52]
Stampfer (~200 IU)	17/17 449	25/17 449		0.68 [0.37–1.26]
Rimm (~400 IU)	16/7982	26/7982		0.61 [0.33–1.15]
Losonczy (?)	19/359	1082/10 819		0.50 [0.32–0.80]
Subtotal (95% CI)	182/34 541	1309/45 001		0.67 [0.54–0.83]
Test for heterogeneity *P* = 0.3				
Test for overall effect *P* = 0.0002				
Intervention studies				
ATBC (50 IU)	853/14 564	870/14 569		0.98 [0.89–1.08]
GISSI (300 IU)	310/5660	329/5664		0.94 [0.80–1.10]
PPP (300 IU)	22/2231	26/2264		0.86 [0.48–1.52]
HOPE (400 IU)	342/4761	328/4780		1.05 [0.90–1.23]
CHAOS (>400 IU)	53/1035	44/967		1.13 [0.75–1.71]
SPACE (800 IU)	9/97	15/99		0.57 [0.24–1.38]
Subtotal (95% CI)	1589/28 348	1612/28 343		0.98 [0.92–1.06]
Test for heterogeneity *P* = 0.68				
Test for overall effect *P* = 0.7				

0.1 0.2   1.0   5.0 10.0
Favours high   Favours low
vitamin E   vitamin E

FIGURE 7.5 • Meta-analysis of effect of high versus low vitamin E intake on cardiovascular mortality for observational and interventional studies. Source: Reproduced from Hooper, L., Ness, A.R. and Smith, G.D. (2001) *Lancet* **357**, 1705–6, with permission from Elsevier Science.

sex-specific quintiles from 19 496 individuals aged 45–79 years, based on a single initial plasma ascorbic acid concentration. After 4 years, after adjustment for age, sex, SBP, BMI, cholesterol, smoking, diabetes and the taking of supplements, all-cause mortality was 20 per cent lower in the top quintile compared with the bottom, with similar significant reductions for cardiovascular disease (30 per cent), CHD (32 per cent) and cancer (15 per cent). It is still possible that other confounders, such as social class and physical activity, could be active but the findings are impressive.

The range of ascorbic acid concentration across the quintiles was only 20 μmol/L. This is equivalent to about 50 g of fruit or vegetable intake or one extra portion. By contrast, no benefit has been found in trials of ascorbic acid supplementation.

Low levels of **beta-carotene** are found in patients with myocardial infarction and in smokers. A small subset of the Physicians Health Study (designed to prevent cancer with beta-carotene) suggested a reduction of CHD events of 44 per cent. The need for caution is highlighted by the finding that beta-carotene supplementation in Finnish smokers increased the risk of lung cancer [Alpha Tocopherol, Beta Carotene Cancer Prevention (ATBC) study group and Beta Carotene and Retinol Efficacy Trial (CARET)].

There has been considerable interest in dietary **flavonoids**, probably due to the fact that apart from being found in fruits, vegetables and tea, red wine is a good source. *In vitro* studies confirm that flavonoids are powerful inhibitors of the oxidation of LDL cholesterol. A 26-year follow-up study from Finland published in 1996 suggests increased levels of CHD where dietary flavonoids are low, the prime sources in Finland being apples and onions. Generally, however, the evidence that flavonoids protect against CHD is inconsistent.

The cocoa bean is another rich source of flavonoid compounds. Cocoa polyphenols impart the characteristic brown colour and bitter flavour to processed cocoa and their antioxidant effect exceeds that of red wine as measured by oxygen radical absorbance capacity. A 50 g bar of dark chocolate contains the antioxidant content of six apples, or seven onions or two glasses of red wine. Further beneficial actions have been shown on platelet activation and function and endothelial effects are being investigated. Most cocoa powder is assimilated into chocolate confectionary where, sadly, the potential health benefits are undermined by its addition to other ingredients, high in saturated fat and calories.

Despite all the inconsistencies of the evidence, vitamin supplementation is common in affluent populations. In the USA, 64 per cent of the population takes vitamins, 34 per cent taking vitamin E. Herbert has said 'Americans excrete the richest urine in the world' and it certainly seems that individuals prefer a pill to nature's packaging. It seems reasonable to increase the consumption of fruit and vegetables, which abound in antioxidants and a recent campaign in the UK extols the virtues of five portions a day (Table 7.8).

Opinions may change with the recent publication of the results of the HPS (see page 275). Here, the effects of a 'cocktail' of three antioxidant supplements (vitamin E 600 mg, vitamin C 250 mg and beta-carotene 20 mg), taken by over 10 000 patients, were compared with placebo. No differences were noted in all-cause or cause-specific mortality and there were no differences in the incidence of major vascular events during the 5.5-year period of the trial. It should be said that the study subjects were all at high risk of vascular events and that perhaps the administration of antioxidants at this stage

TABLE **7.8** • 'Five portions a day': what is a portion?

Type	Example	Portion
Fruit		
Very large	Melon, pineapple	1 large slice
Large	Apple, banana	1 whole
Medium	Plum, kiwi	2 whole
Berries	Raspberries, grapes	1 cupful
Stewed/canned	Stewed apple/tinned peaches	3 serving spoonfuls
Dried	Dried apricots	0.5 serving spoonful
Fruit juice	Orange juice	full wine glass
Vegetables		
Green	Broccoli, spinach	2 serving spoonfuls
Root	Carrots, parsnip	2 serving spoonfuls
Small	Peas, sweetcorn	3 serving spoonfuls
Salad	Lettuce, tomato	1 bowlful
Pulses	Beans	2 serving spoonfuls

is too late in the day. Nevertheless, the HPS deals a body blow to antioxidant supplementation, at least in well-nourished populations.

SODIUM AND POTASSIUM

There is abundant evidence that high dietary sodium and low dietary potassium are causally related to high blood pressure. Blood pressure in Western populations is high and rises with age. In less sophisticated, hunter-gatherer communities such as Soloman Island tribesmen, the rise in blood pressure with age is not seen. In addition, there are obvious differences in the average values of the determinants of blood pressure between the communities (Table 7.9).

A salt intake of 170 mmol/L per day is about 10 g/day and is typical of Western societies. Coastal Soloman Islanders eat more fish and have a salt intake equivalent to Western populations. By extrapolation, it can be estimated that salt intake accounts for 40 per cent of the variability in blood pressure observed between the populations.

The relationship between salt intake and blood pressure depends on age and randomized trials have too often used young (average age 26 years) subjects. In addition, maximum blood pressure reduction is not achieved until salt has been restricted for 1 month and many trials have been of shorter duration.

Observational analysis of 47 000 people allowed estimates of the differences in systolic and diastolic blood pressure to be calculated for a reduction of 100 mmol/L sodium/24 hours according to 10-year age groups and centiles of blood pressure distribution (Table 7.10).

It can be seen that for older age groups the association is large (approximately 10/5 mmHg) and that for those at the highest centile of blood pressure distribution – 'hypertensives' – the estimated difference is 15/7 mmHg.

TABLE **7.9** • Determinants of blood pressure

Age	USA whites Systolic BP (mmHg)	Soloman Islanders Systolic BP (mmHg)
15	113	115
25	123	115
35	126	116
45	132	114
55	139	115
65	147	116
Dietary salt (mmol/L)	170	20
Dietary potassium	+	+++
Body mass index	25.2	21.9
Habitual exercise	+	+++
Alcohol	++	0

+, low; ++, moderate; +++, high.

TABLE **7.10** • Changes in systolic and diastolic blood pressure for three centiles of the population per 100 mmol/24 hour change in sodium intake

Age	SBP (mmHg)			DBP (mmHg)		
	5th	50th	95th	5th	50th	95th
15–19	3	5	7	1	2	3
20–29	2	5	8	1	3	4
30–39	2	6	9	1	3	5
40–49	2	7	11	2	4	5
50–59	4	9	15	2	5	7
60–69	6	10	15	2	4	7

An important randomized double-blind trial (Cappucio) recently confirmed these findings with a reduction of 10/5 mmHg in older patients with a 100 mmol/L reduction in daily sodium intake.

Reducing salt intake in Western populations is difficult because manufacturers add 75 per cent of dietary salt. A reduction of 3 g/day (50 mmol/L or half a teaspoon) is, however, feasible and in people over 50 years old, the corresponding drop in SBP of 5 mmHg equates to reductions in age-specific mortality for stroke and CHD of 22 per cent and 16 per cent, respectively. Much of salt usage is habitual and health professionals should dispel the erroneous perception that salt enhances the flavour of food and urge patients to make low salt choices, reducing their intake.

Increasing potassium intake by 40 mmol/day is associated with a 2–6 mmHg fall in systolic blood pressure. Several prospective population studies have reported reduced stroke incidence and mortality with increased intake of potassium-rich foods such as fruit and vegetables, cereals, milk and nuts. In one study, a 40 per cent reduction in stroke mortality was associated with a 10 mmol/day increase in dietary potassium.

In Finland, where intensive cardiovascular programmes have raised life expectancy by 7 years over the last two decades, alteration in dietary electrolytes is identified as probably the biggest factor responsible. A modified table salt, 'Pansuola', has been introduced with the composition: 57 per cent NaCl, 28 per cent KCl, 12 per cent $MgSO_4$, 2 per cent L-lysine, KI and anti-caking agent. Using Pansuola, sodium intake is reduced by 30–50 per cent with improvement in the sodium/potassium ratio. The taste and properties of Pansuola are acceptable and food manufacturers elsewhere are beginning to incorporate it into some products.

OTHER DIETARY FACTORS

COFFEE

Strong relationships between heavy coffee drinking (more than 5 cups/day) and CHD have been described in Scandinavian countries and parts of North America. The interpretation of these findings is difficult, as heavy coffee drinkers are often heavy smokers, but La Croix showed that amongst American doctors (largely non-smokers) there was a two- to threefold increased risk of CHD in heavy consumers. In Norway, total cholesterol differences of up to 0.79 mmol/L in men and 0.72 mmol/L in women were found between the highest and lowest consumers. In Italy, where coffee is filtered rather than boiled, the differences were more modest, at 0.25 mmol/L.

It is proposed that the preparation of coffee by boiling releases substances (the diterpenes cafestol and kahweol have been identified) that probably stimulate LDL cholesterol synthesis. Experiments where coffee oil has been added surreptitiously to the diet have increased LDL cholesterol by 29 per cent. Filtering coffee, using decaffeinated coffee or granules, has much less adverse effects.

GARLIC

The medicinal properties of garlic (*Allium sativum*) have been recognized since Egyptian times and garlic is often to be found in Mediterranean cuisine. Preparations of garlic enjoy huge over-the-counter sales in Germany and it has been promoted as 'the world's most ancient, versatile and enjoyable medicine'. The active ingredients are organo-sulphur compounds (hence the smell) and crushing a clove releases enzymes, which form allicin from odourless alliin. Other metabolites may be important and both they and allicin are refined with considerable variation into several commercial products.

Claims are made that garlic will reduce cholesterol, LDL cholesterol, triglycerides, blood pressure, fibrinogen and platelet aggregation and increase HDL cholesterol and vessel flow. Many studies are poorly conducted and a recent meta-analysis that showed an overall reduction of 0.5 mmol/L in serum cholesterol may have suffered from publication bias. In 1989, Kleijnen suggested that whilst 7–28 cloves/day (!) may help, the data for commercial preparations were less convincing. In 1990 a double-blind controlled trial was conducted in Germany, which showed reductions of 11.7 per cent and 17 per cent in total cholesterol and triglycerides, respectively. It is significant that 21 per cent of the participants reported the observation of odour. By contrast, a well-conducted trial from British general practice (Neil, 1996) found no significant differences in lipid concentrations after 6 months between treatment and control groups.

The mechanisms whereby garlic exerts its cardiovascular benefit are unknown but it is interesting to note that extracts of garlic other than allicin have been found to inhibit HMG-CoA reductase.

NUTS

Some years ago, clinical studies showed that diets supplemented with walnuts and almonds reduced total and LDL cholesterol. Despite this evidence, nuts 'belonged to the provinces of cranky vegetarian sub-culture' until a reappraisal from the Nurses' Health Study in 1998. One nurse in 20, from the 84 409 nurses followed for 14 years, ate five or more helpings of nuts a week. In this group, CHD risk was reduced by 35 per cent compared with the third of nurses who hardly ever ate them. The effect is large and adjustments for other, potentially confounding, healthy behaviours did not appreciably alter the result.

The authors speculate that in addition to the lipid-lowering effect, other mechanisms might invoke vitamin E, linolenic acid (high in walnuts) and the fibre and mineral content, but essentially the answer is not known.

SOYA

A meta-analysis of 38 clinical trials showed that daily consumption of 25 g soya protein results in a mean fall in total cholesterol of 9.3 per cent, in LDL cholesterol of 12.9 per cent and in triglycerides of 10.5 per cent. The increase in HDL cholesterol of 2.4 per cent was non-significant. The effect was greater where baseline cholesterol levels were higher. Whilst a substitution effect for animal protein and the effect of its high PUFA content account for a large part of its action, constituent isoflavones are also likely to be involved. Soy is rich in phytoestrogen isoflavones, which have weak oestrogenic activity. In 1999, the FDA in the USA approved the claim for reducing heart disease using 25 g/day of soy protein.

PLANT STEROLS

Margarine has been used as a substitute for butter since the Napoleonic War. Subsequent compositional development has not only improved taste and texture but also expanded the potential of additional health benefits. In the Second World War, the fat-soluble vitamins A and D were added to margarines and as a response to Ancel Key's seminal work in the 1950s, the first margarines high in PUFA and low in SFA were produced. More recently, the *trans* fatty acid content of margarines has been reduced and vitamin E levels increased. Replacing butter with margarine high in PUFA lowers total serum and LDL cholesterol by about 0.3 mmol/L and margarines high in PUFA and MUFA are widely recommended as part of the cholesterol-lowering diet. Additional reductions in serum cholesterol are now achievable with the incorporation of naturally occurring plant sterols into the newest products.

Sterols are produced in both animals and plants and are essential components of all cell membranes. They share a similar carbon skeleton, the sterol ring, with an alcohol group and differ only in their side chains (Figure 7.6). Cholesterol is, of course, the best-known sterol, but is exclusive to animals. Over 40 plant sterols (or phytosterols) have been identified with beta-sitosterol, campesterol and stigmasterol the most common. Plant stanols are formed when the delta-5 double bond of the sterol ring of plant sterols is hydrogenated and trace amounts are present in the diet. The terminology is confusing as 'plant sterols' can both generically include unsaturated sterols and saturated stanols together or just refer specifically to the unsaturated compounds.

Under normal circumstances humans ingest 300–400 mg of dietary cholesterol per day and between 30 and 50 per cent is fully absorbed. Biliary cholesterol usually exceeds dietary cholesterol and approximately 1000 mg/day is secreted into the bowel, of which about 60 per cent is reabsorbed. Plant sterols are mostly ingested from edible vegetable oils (sunflower, soya, rape, sesame and maize) but are also present in legumes. Bread and cereals do not contain high amounts but account for about 17 per cent of plant sterol intake. The average intake in the UK is just under 200 mg/day, whilst in Finland and Japan it averages 400 mg/day. Intakes of 600–800 mg/day are seen in vegetarians. The specificity of intestinal transport mechanisms, which favour cholesterol absorption, means that typically only 4–5 per cent of beta-sitosterol, 15 per cent of campesterol and less than 1 per cent of dietary stanols are absorbed.

It is likely that plant sterols and stanols act by reducing cholesterol absorption from the gut by competing with cholesterol for solubilization within mixed micelles, but there may also be specific actions at the level of the enterocyte. Reducing cholesterol absorption (by about 50 per cent) invokes a compensatory mechanism to increase cholesterol synthesis in the liver but this is not enough to compensate the loss of cholesterol in the stool, LDL cholesterol receptors are up-regulated and net serum cholesterol is reduced. The effect of plant sterols is specifically to reduce total and LDL cholesterol. HDL cholesterol and triglyceride levels are unaltered and, thus, the total cholesterol to HDL cholesterol ratio becomes more favourable.

The knowledge that plant sterols can reduce cholesterol levels is not new. The first study evaluating plant sterols as cholesterol-lowering agents was published in 1953 and by 1976, more than 100 papers confirmed the results. In these early studies, between 10 g and 40 g of sitosterol were consumed, usually in solid, crystalline form and such amounts were found to lower serum cholesterol levels by 10–20 per cent. The preparations were well tolerated by patients treated for up to 5 years or longer. Unfortunately, enthusiasm waned as the erroneous perception grew that high doses of plant sterols were required to achieve a cholesterol-lowering effect. It was not until 1977 that dose-ranging experiments established that a sitosterol dose of 2–3 g/day appeared to maximize interference with cholesterol absorption and in 1986, similar results were achieved with low-dose sitostanol. A further breakthrough came in 1989 when Wester discovered that plant sterols could be incorporated into margarine by their prior esterification with long chain fatty acids. This led Miettinen and Puska, in 1993, to embark on a year-long landmark study evaluating the cholesterol-lowering efficacy of plant sterol-enriched margarine in 153 patients with mild hypercholesterolaemia. One hundred and two subjects replaced 24 g of daily fat intake with a rapeseed oil margarine fortified with sitostanol, sufficient to cover a slice of bread with each of three meals, resulting in an intake of sitostanol of either 1.8 or 2.6 g/day. The higher dose resulted in reductions of total

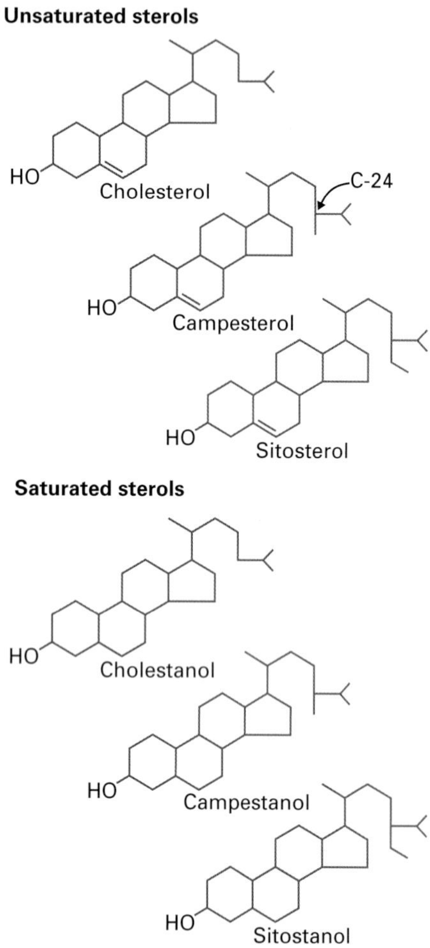

Unsaturated sterols

Saturated sterols

FIGURE 7.6 • The structure of sterols including cholesterol and common plant sterols (top) and stanols, i.e. saturated sterols (bottom).

cholesterol and LDL cholesterol of 10.2 per cent (control 0.1 per cent) and 14.1 per cent (control 1.1 per cent), respectively, at 12 months (Miettinen *et al.*, 1995). The margarine used in this trial was marketed in Finland in 1995 under the brand name Benecol and is now widely available not only as a spread but also as cream cheese, salad dressing, snack bars and yogurt. The sitostanol in Benecol is produced from tall oil, a byproduct derived when wood from tall trees such as pines is pulped to make paper. A second spread, fortified with unsaturated plant sterols, from soya bean, rapeseed and sunflower seed oils has been marketed in the USA as Take Control and in Europe as Flora pro.activ, Becel pro.activ and Fruit d'Or pro.activ.

Plant sterol margarines appear to be effective both in normocholesterolaemic and hypercholesterolaemic subjects. One non-randomized study achieved notoriety when disappointing LDL cholesterol reductions were achieved in patients already on a cholesterol-lowering diet. This may have been a chance finding, but probably was due to the administration of plant sterols in capsule form, thereby limiting effectiveness. Subsequent research in patients on cholesterol-lowering diets has confirmed the findings of earlier studies where the intake of dietary fat was higher.

In 1998, Weststrate and Meijer compared the efficacy of the Flora formulation with equivalent test margarines derived from tall oil, ricebran oil and sheanut oil against standard high-PUFA margarine without plant sterols. The five treatments were randomized over 3.5-week periods in 95 subjects. The effects were observable after only 2.5 weeks and the results are shown in Figure 7.7. Two other comparative trials suggest that there is little difference in the efficacy of stanols or sterols to lower cholesterol.

Fat-soluble vitamins are also absorbed via mixed micelles but levels of vitamins A, D, E and K are unaffected. Levels of alpha and beta-carotene and lycopene are slightly decreased but this is of questionable importance. Benecol has been used in Finland since 1995 without evidence of hazard.

Familial phytosterolaemia is a very rare autosomal recessive disorder with only approximately 50 cases of the homozygous condition reported world wide. In this condition,

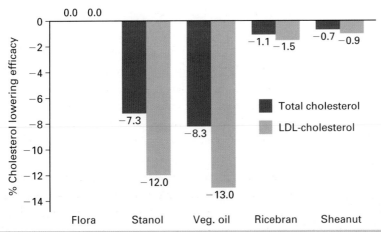

FIGURE 7.7 • A comparison of the efficacy of margarines with and without plant sterols. Adapted from Westrate and Meijer (1998).

increased absorption of sitosterol and campesterol leads to premature atherosclerosis. In heterozygotes, sitosterol absorption is also increased but the body pool remains normal as the ability to excrete the excess remains intact.

The effects of plant sterols and statins appear additive. In theory, the combination of reducing cholesterol absorption and synthesis would predict this and in several studies, co-administration of sitostanol margarine with a statin increased the LDL cholesterol reduction achieved by the statin by about 10 per cent. New data confirm the same results with unsaturated sterol spread. Further benefits would also be predicted when plant sterol spreads are used with other lipid-lowering agents and a French study shows additional LDL cholesterol reduction in patients taking fibrates with Flora pro.activ. Plant sterols have been tested in high-risk individuals and benefits are seen in type 2 diabetics and patients with familial hypercholesterolaemia.

Occasionally patients are encountered who do not respond well to statins. Analysis of the 4S trial suggests that those who benefited most from simvastatin had a high absorption and low rate of synthesis of cholesterol at baseline. Response is poorest in those with the Apo E4 allele and it is tempting to suggest that plant sterols would be useful in this situation.

The cost of plant sterol margarines is borne by the patient. Average table spread consumption ranges from 15 to 25 g/day and the formulations of both Benecol and Flora pro.activ are designed to provide sufficient plant sterol intake within this range. The cost is significant and unlikely to reduce as, first, the industrial refining process requires about 2500 parts of raw material to extract one part of plant sterol and, second, the amount of raw materials available is ultimately limited.

With the ability to achieve 10 per cent reductions in cholesterol, using mechanisms discrete from other agents, plant stanol and sterol spreads represent an important innovation in CHD prevention.

PATTERNS OF EATING

The Oxford Vegetarian Study is a prospective study of 6000 subjects who do not eat meat and 5000 meat-eating controls. The meat eaters have serum cholesterol levels near the UK average (5.9 mmol/L) with lower levels for fish eaters (5.6 mmol/L) and vegetarians (5.3 mmol/L) and lowest of all for vegans (5.0 mmol/L). Several studies from Britain and California show that CHD mortality is reduced in vegetarians by about 30 per cent.

There is some evidence that the way in which we eat may influence cholesterol levels. 'Nibbling' or 'grazing' is associated with a reduction of 8.5 per cent when compared with 'gorging'.

DIET STRATEGIES

I want to buy some real farmhouse butter, some real farmhouse eggs and some clotted cream – and I am not going to listen to those dietary faddists who say don't eat it. (Margaret Thatcher, *The Independent*, 1987).

TABLE **7.11** • Population goals for nutrients and foods

Nutrient or food	Population intake limit
Saturated (and *trans* fatty acids) (% energy)	<10
Polyunsaturated fatty acids (% energy)	3–7
Dietary fibre (g/day)	27–40
Fruits and vegetables (g/day)	>400
Legumes, nuts, seeds (g/day)	>30
Cholesterol (mg/day)	<300
Fish (g/day)	>20
Salt (g/day)	<6

From WHO Study Group (1990) *Diet, Nutrition and the Prevention of Chronic Diseases.* World Health Organization, Geneva.

There is much discussion about the optimal diet for CHD prevention. The Mediterranean diet is low in saturated fat and high in unsaturated fat, whereas the traditional Japanese diet is low in saturated fat but rich in complex carbohydrates. The Mediterranean diet will provide better lipoprotein levels, yet both diets are associated with the best life expectancies in the world.

Population goals for nutrients and foods to achieve a healthy diet have been proposed by the WHO (Table 7.11).

Pragmatic advice would seem to be to use a diet low in saturated fats, substituting them in part by mono- and polyunsaturated fatty acids, as well as with complex carbohydrates. With small differences, there is broad agreement between consensus bodies about the composition of the cholesterol-lowering diet which can be summarized as:

- Total fat: <30 per cent of energy requirement;
- Saturated fat: <7–10 per cent;
- Polyunsaturated fat: 7–10 per cent (including sources of omega-3 PUFA);
- Monounsaturated fat: 10–15 per cent;
- Cholesterol: <300 mg/day;
- Complex carbohydrates: 55 per cent (especially vegetables, grains and legumes);
- Protein: 15 per cent;
- Total calories: reduce when weight loss needed.

Issuing dietary strategies in percentage terms leads to a problem in interpretation for health professionals, very few of whom are well versed in aspects of nutrition. Not many individuals can identify what percentage of their day's energy has been derived from saturated fat. There is a need for more dietitians and clinical nutritionists to provide practical advice and education not only for patients and health professionals, but also in the workplace, schools and ethnic communities. Table 7.12 illustrates food choices in a way that is more interpretable by patients and their advisors.

TABLE **7.12** • Food choices for a healthy diet

	Best choice	In moderation	Best avoided
Cereals and starchy foods	Bread, chapatis, breakfast cereals, oats, porridge, rice, pasta, popcorn (without butter) and all other cereals	Naan bread	Puppodums (fried), waffles, croissant, Danish pastry, fried rice, pot noodles
Potatoes	Boiled, mashed, jacket, instant (without fat)	Oven chips, roast potatoes cooked in best choice of oil, fat-free crisps	Chips, potato croquettes, all other crisps
Vegetables and fruits	A wide variety of vegetables, fruit, salads, pulses – raw, baked, boiled, steamed and include all fresh, frozen, dried, canned	Stir-fried vegetables in best choice of oils. Coleslaw in home-made dressing	Coleslaw, vegetables in batter
Fish	White fish: cod, haddock, plaice, lemon sole, whiting. Oily fish (a good source of omega-3 fatty acids): mackerel, herring, salmon, tuna, trout. Canned fish in water or tomato sauce, tuna, pilchards, sardines. Shellfish: oyster, mussels, whelks, winkles, scallops, squid	Canned fish in oil (drain off excess oil); fish in breadcrumbs. Shellfish: shrimps, prawns, lobster, crab	Fried fish in batter, scampi, whitebait, roe, fish paté, taramosalata
Meat	Well trimmed grilled steak, chicken and turkey (with skin removed), venison, rabbit, veal	Lean cuts of lamb, beef, pork. Lean minced beef. Grilled lean burgers. Very lean ham, gammon and well-trimmed bacon. Liver and kidney. Low-fat sausages	Fatty meats, crackling and skin. Duck, sausages, sausagemeat, luncheon meat, corned beef, paté, scotch eggs, meat pies and pastries
Vegetarian choices	Quron, tofu, soya protein meat substitute, pulses (beans, peas and lentils), chestnuts	All fresh nuts (see eggs and dairy section)	Check fat content of vegetarian ready-prepared dishes
Eggs and dairy	Egg white, skimmed milk, very low fat cheese (cottage, low-fat yogurt, fat-free fromage frais)	Semi-skimmed, soya, goat, sheep milk and their products. Greek yogurt, fromage frais, crème fraiche, evaporated milk. Cheese: reduced-fat cheddar, Edam, Brie, Camembert, Feta, Mozzarella, Ricotta, cheese spread	Whole eggs (no more than 2 a week). Whole milk, condensed milk, cream. Cheese: Cheddar, Gouda, Gruyere, Roquefort, Stilton, cream cheese

(continued)

TABLE **7.12** • *(continued)*

	Best choice	In moderation	Best avoided
Oils	Olive oil, rapeseed (canola) oil	Sunflower oil, corn oil, safflower oil, groundnut oil and sesame seed oil	Lard, suet, ghee and vegetable oils, particularly palm and coconut oil
Spreads	Plant sterol or stanol spreads, low-fat spreads	Olive, rapeseed (canola), sunflower and soya oil spreads	Butter, hard margarines
Meals	Pasta with vegetable sauce, paella, kedgeree, kebabs skewered with best choice ingredients, home-made soups	Home-made pizza, cottage pie, chilli, fish pie, casseroles	Fish and chips, lasagne, pasta in cream sauce, pies, quiches, samosas, cream soups
Cakes and biscuits	Home-made using best choice ingredients. Crispbreads, crumpets, rice cakes, matzos, breadsticks	Currant buns, scones, tea bread, malt loaf, fatless sponge. Biscuits: rich tea, ginger nuts, garibaldi, cream crackers	Cakes: bought, rich, sponge, fresh cream. Doughnuts, pastries, chocolate biscuits
Puddings	Home-made using best choice ingredients. Baked or stewed fruit, meringue, low-fat rice pudding, jelly, sorbet, summer pudding	Frozen yogurt, ice cream, milk puddings, crumbles	Cheesecake, pastry, suet puddings
Flavourings, sauces, jams and sweets	Pepper, herbs, spices, lemon juice, vinegar, garlic, tomato purée, mustard. Home-made salad dressings and sauces made with best choice ingredients. Jam, marmalade, honey	Tomato ketchup, brown sauce, Worcester sauce, pickles, Bovril, Marmite, stock cubes, gravy granules, reduced calorie salad cream and mayonnaise. Houmous, peanut butter. Mints and boiled sweets	Salt, salad cream, mayonnaise, cream sauces, cook-in sauces, chocolate spread, chocolates, toffees, fudge

Source: www.heartuk.org.uk

In November 2000, the American Heart Association published revised dietary guidelines, which emphasize a more global approach to the dietary prevention of cardiovascular disease than previous advice. The step 1 designation had been the population-orientated recommendation and the step 2 approach for those at higher risk (Table 7.13).

The new guidelines:

▓ are orientated to foods and dietary patterns with broad health benefits:
   (a) fruit and vegetables five times a day
   (b) increased grain products (especially whole grains) six times a day
   (c) fat-free and low-fat dairy products

TABLE **7.13** • NCEP two-step dietary approach

Dietary factor	Step 1	Step 2
Total fat	<30%	<30%
SFA	<10%	<7%
PUFA	10–15%	10–15%
MUFA	<10%	<10%
P/S ratio	1.0	1.4
Cholesterol	300 mg/day	200 mg/day

(d) fish twice a week
(e) legumes, poultry and lean meat
■ place greater emphasis on weight loss and obesity control:
  (a) match intake of energy to needs to prevent obesity and maintain a healthy body weight
  (b) limit intake of foods with high caloric value (especially sugars)
  (c) achieve a level of appropriate physical activity for weight maintenance or loss
■ maintain desirable blood cholesterol, lipoprotein profile and blood pressure
  (a) limit intake of saturated fatty acids (<10 per cent) and cholesterol (<300 mg/day)
  (b) minimize *trans* fats
  (c) substitute with grains, unsaturated fatty acids (especially from vegetables, fish, legumes and nuts)
  (d) limit salt to <6 g/day
  (e) limit alcohol to two drinks per day for men, one for women
  (f) maintain healthy body weight
  (g) emphasize fruit and vegetables and low-fat products
■ target higher risk subgroups with individual approaches:
  (a) those with elevated LDL cholesterol, pre-existing cardiovascular disease, diabetes mellitus, heart failure or renal problems.

DIETS WITH EXTREMES OF MACRONUTRIENT INTAKE

The 'diet industry' is global and vast. Americans spend US$33 billion per year on diet foods and 'The Atkins Diet' ranks in the top 50 best-selling books of all time. Atkins proposed a **high protein** (>20 per cent), reduced carbohydrate diet but there is no scientific evidence for benefit in terms of body weight, metabolic changes or improved health. Protein sources, such as meat, are expensive and potentially higher in fat, saturated fat and cholesterol. In addition, when carbohydrates are reduced, the palatability of the diet suffers and compliance problems emerge.

Very low fat diets (<15 per cent) may lead to weight loss and improved lipid profiles under close supervision but, again, there is no clear evidence of superiority compared to less aggressive regimens. Weight loss is not always maintained and the intake of essential fatty acids may be inadequate. Very low fat foods may be calorie dense and, finally, in individuals with the insulin resistance pattern, levels of triglyceride may rise and HDL cholesterol may fall.

In diets **high in unsaturated fat**, the energy derived from fat may exceed 30 per cent. Total and LDL cholesterol are reduced by replacement of saturated fat by unsaturated fat or carbohydrate during weight maintenance conditions. This diet (typified by the Mediterranean diet) may also improve insulin sensitivity and may be useful for those with insulin resistance, offsetting the rise in triglyceride and reduction in HDL cholesterol, commonly seen in these individuals.

IS DIET WORTHWHILE?

The effect of dietary factors on serum lipids is summarized in Table 7.14.

Dietary studies are often criticized because community studies, with free-living subjects, are potentially unreliable and experimental 'metabolic ward' studies, which show cholesterol reductions of 10–15 per cent, do not reflect real world experience and are often too small. In 1991, Ramsay *et al.* reopened the debate on the efficacy of cholesterol lowering by diet. Ramsay's group divided 16 published trials of dietary intervention into NCEP step 1 and more rigorous diet groups. The NCEP had recommended a two-step dietary approach: step 1 for the general public and for most people under treatment and step 2 for more severe cases of hypercholesterolaemia (Table 7.13).

In Ramsay's analysis, the step 1 trials showed a fall in serum cholesterol ranging from 0 to 4 per cent, whereas the more rigorous diet group showed up to 15.5 per cent reduction. The analysis achieved notorious publicity ('Hole in the Heart of the Cholesterol Cult' – *The Times*) but has been criticized on several counts:

■ The diets in the more rigorous group are not significantly different
  from those in the step 1 group. For example, in the Oslo Study (page 243),

TABLE **7.14** • Effect of dietary factors on serum lipids

Dietary component	Total cholesterol	LDL	HDL	TG
Saturated fats	↑↑	↑↑	↑	↑↑
Omega-3 polyunsaturates	↓	↓	↑→	↓↓
Omega-6 polyunsaturates	↓↓	↓↓	↓	
Monounsaturated	↓	↓	↑→	↓
Dietary cholesterol	↑	↑	↑	
Soluble fibre	↓	↓		
Alcohol			↑	↑↑
Excess calories	↑↑	↑↑	↓	↑↑
Plant sterols	↓↓	↓↓	→	→

which was included in the second group, total fat was 28 per cent, P/S ratio 1.01 and cholesterol 289 mg/day. The Oslo trial was well conducted on free-living men over a period of 5 years and showed serum cholesterol reduction of 13 per cent and a reduction of MI and sudden death of 47 per cent.

- The population effect in the control groups of major studies such as MRFIT (page 39) was discounted.
- Compliance with some of the diets of the step 1 group was suboptimal.
- The common experience of most clinicians is that many patients do in fact show significant reductions in serum cholesterol with diet alone.

Denke's more selective review in 1995 claimed that dietary counselling could achieve reductions in cholesterol concentration of 10 per cent or more but Tang *et al.*'s (1998) meta-analysis of 19 randomized controlled trials again showed modest effects in free-living subjects. Those on a diet of step 1 intensity achieved a reduction of cholesterol concentration of only about 3 per cent, with those on more intensive regimens only managing 6 per cent. Although a sustained reduction in blood cholesterol of 1 per cent is associated with a reduction of 2–3 per cent in the incidence of CHD, the results are disappointing. These findings are in line with Truswell's review, in 1994, of 17 dietary intervention studies, which showed that the odds ratio of intervention versus control groups was 0.94 for total deaths and 0.87 for coronary events.

Dietary trials in free-living individuals are difficult to conduct. The alteration of one dietary component frequently upsets another, compliance is a problem and the trials are often impossible to blind. The meta-analyses disguise a variation of response and this is typified in a study of step 2 diets conducted by Schaefer in normocholesterolaemic and hypercholesterolaemic subjects. He found total cholesterol reductions of 20 per cent and 16 per cent, respectively, and LDL cholesterol reductions of 21 per cent and 18 per cent. There was a wide range of diet responsiveness within the study group and LDL cholesterol actually ranged from +5 per cent to −40 per cent.

Diets focusing solely on saturated fat reduction and reducing dietary cholesterol ignore the range and potential of available dietary and lifestyle interventions. Singh and colleagues published some evidence in favour of a more cardioprotective diet in 1997. Four hundred and six post-MI patients were randomized to a low (25 per cent) fat diet or to a healthy diet rich in fruit, vegetables, nuts and grains. Total cholesterol was reduced by 5.4 per cent, LDL cholesterol by 5.6 per cent and patients lost 3 kg weight in the standard group but in the healthy diet group, values were 12.7 per cent, 12.3 per cent and 7 kg, respectively. In addition, the healthy diet group had a 42 per cent reduction in cardiac mortality and a 45 per cent reduction in all-cause mortality. Trials like this and the Lyon Diet Heart Study are, however, small and should be repeated on a larger scale.

Dietary change, even with full compliance, is clearly less effective for some. There is increasing evidence that the effect of lipid-lowering medication is enhanced by diet and this is important for groups at high risk such as those with genetic hyperlipidaemia or pre-existing vascular disease.

PRACTICAL ADVICE

Rather than handing out diet sheets, which by their long lists of negatives can be intimidating, health professionals should be able to impart a series of simple dietary messages to patients. The advice, though, is practical for all of us!

Here are 10 simple dietary measures to avoid CHD:

- Optimize body weight.
- Eat less saturated fat.
- Substitute with poly- and monounsaturated fat.
- Choose lean meat, poultry, legumes, nuts, soya and low-fat dairy foods.
- Eat fish twice a week (especially oily fish).
- Eat more fruit and vegetables (at least five portions per day).
- Eat more starchy carbohydrate foods like potatoes, bread, cereals, rice and pasta.
- Eat less salt.
- Maintain sensible alcohol limits.
- Enjoy your diet!

Patients should be encouraged to look at their sources of fat and scrutinize food labels. Unfortunately, food labelling is often misleading, fat content being described as grams of fat/100 g. A pie, for example, may contain 25 per cent fat by weight but 75 per cent of the energy of the pie may be supplied from fat once the water content is removed.

Alternative cooking methods such as grilling, boiling, baking, steaming, poaching, microwaving and casseroling, using the barbecue or the stir-fry, can reduce the fat content of our diet.

Most people eat on average at least three meals per week out of the home and this can upset the best of plans. Even 'foreign' menus have become westernized and it may be better to have fish and chips fried in vegetable oil rather than doner kebabs or Indian take-aways.

A patient's diet should also be discussed in the context of the rest of the family, shopping facilities and financial constraints.

No diet that is dull, uninteresting or unpalatable will secure compliance and cholesterol-lowering diets have this reputation. The variety of flavour and appearance in the diet of many Mediterranean countries, however, proclaims the reverse and with proper advice and imagination we can all receive the cardiovascular benefit of a healthier diet.

POPULATIONS, INDIVIDUALS, GOVERNMENTS AND THE FOOD INDUSTRY

The underlying premise of the population strategy (see page 93) is that it seeks to change features of behaviour or the environment that are responsible for the overall rate of CHD. In essence this means informing and motivating the population to modify dietary, smoking and exercise habits.

Central government should stimulate public education through health professionals, educationalists and the media. Local government can influence schools, industry, shops, restaurants and the provision of exercise facilities. Sadly, changes are more often dictated by public demand, although there is evidence to suggest that a coordinated approach can be effective (e.g. the Minnesota Heart Health Project and the North Karelia project in Finland).

If, for example, British dietary reference values were to be adopted in the UK, mean serum cholesterol levels in 25–60 year olds would reduce by approximately 12 per cent from about 6.0 to 5.2 mmol/L. Compliance with the more restrictive WHO dietary recommendations would lead to a greater fall (of 17 per cent) and a major distribution shift in the prevalence of hypercholesterolaemia. Moreover, as cholesterol-lowering diets tend also to be weight optimizing, the fall in numbers with obesity would also further shift the cholesterol curve.

The right of an individual 'to die as I choose' often baulks the best efforts of health professionals to induce lifestyle change. Too often this is rooted in ignorance and ill-informed traditional belief. The counters to this include not only information, education and motivation, but also government-directed democratically developed social policy. Individual restrictions for the good of others already exist – for example, the use of seat belts, drink/driving regulations, restrictions in the sale of tobacco and alcohol and advertising limitations. The effect of increasing tobacco taxation is linked to a decline in smoking, but much more could be done to reduce the social acceptability of smoking.

The fact that food production in much of Europe is still linked to the nutritional priorities of the 1950s has led to massive agricultural surpluses, particularly surplus animal products and especially from the dairy industry (Table 7.15). This has led to the introduction of quotas and subsidies, which have not only maintained production values, but also flooded poorer countries (e.g. eastern Europe) with excess cheap saturated fat.

Until recently, meat carcasses were appraised for quality on their 'shape', 'finish' and 'marbling', all reflective of increased fat content and luxury status. There is now increased demand for lower-fat meats and this is most dramatically met in pig farming, where lean pork now contains less fat than chicken. Intensive feeding practices by poultry farmers have raised fat content compared with free-range varieties. Unfortunately, dairy cows, whose breeding attracts subsidized payments, tend to produce high-fat meat. Similarly, castrated bulls produce high-fat meat unless treated with anabolic steroids. Excess fatty meat that cannot be sold direct is then incorporated into meat products, sausages, meat pies, salamis,

TABLE **7.15** • Fat consumption in the UK (OPCS, 1990)

Fat source	Percentage of total fat consumption
Butter and margarines	16
Meat	14
Milk	9
Vegetables (including chips and crisps)	11
Cheese	6
Meat products	10
Cakes, biscuits, puddings	19
Other fats (e.g. cooking oil, etc.)	15

etc., which, being cheaper, are more attractive to the economically deprived.

In the UK, 70 per cent of products are now packaged or manufactured and are often high in hidden salt and sugar, providing an invisible intake for the consumer. Salt content is increased to allow for greater water content, thereby increasing bulk and ultimately profit.

To offset these hidden problems in nutrition, there is obviously a need for compulsory standardized food labelling, using language that is comprehensible to ordinary people. For example, bread is probably our chief source of salt currently with content as high as 1.1 g sodium/100 g. Consumers might purchase lower-salt brands if they were aware that this amount comfortably exceeds the concentration in seawater (0.9 g sodium/100 g). Low-fat cookies may indeed contain reduced fat, but invariably there is little difference in calorie content. Consumers, thinking they have chosen the

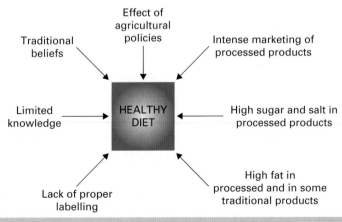

FIGURE **7.8** • Factors affecting a healthy diet.

healthy option are tempted to consume more cookies and thereby detrimentally, increase overall calorie intake.

In summary, the consumer is faced with a number of dilemmas when aiming to choose the components of a healthy diet (Figure 7.8).

There are clear roles for governments:

■ to establish an independent food protection agency to protect the public from misleading information and institute better food labelling;
■ to review agricultural strategies;
■ to establish services to implement and publicize health recommendations, particularly nutrition education, smoking policies and the facilitation of exercise.

REFERENCES AND FURTHER READING

American Heart Association (2000) AHA dietary guidelines: revision 2000. *Circulation* **102**, 2284–99.

Boaz, M., Smetana, S., Matas, Z. *et al.* (2000) Secondary prevention with antioxidants of cardiovascular disease in endstage renal disease (SPACE): randomized placebo-controlled trial. *Lancet* **356**, 1213–18.

Brown, L., Rosner, B., Willett, W. *et al.* (1999) Cholesterol-lowering effects of dietary fiber: a meta-analysis. *Am J Clin Nutr* **69**, 30–42.

Burr, M.L., Fehily, A.M., Gilbert, J.F. *et al.* (1989) Effects of changes in fat, fish and fibre intakes on death and myocardial reinfarction: diet and reinfarction trial (DART). *Lancet* **2**, 757–61.

Dattilo, A.M. and Kris-Etherton, P.M. (1992) Effects of weight reduction on blood lipids and lipoproteins: a meta-analysis. *Am J Clin Nutr* **56**, 320–8.

de Lorgeril, M., Salen, P., Martin, J.L. *et al.* (1999) Mediterranean diet, traditional risk factors and the rate of cardiovascular complications after myocardial infarction: the final report of the Lyon Diet Heart Study. *Circulation* **99**, 779–85.

Erdman, J.W. (2000) Soy protein and cardiovascular disease. *Circulation* **102**, 2555–9.

GISSI-Prevenzione Investigators (1999) Dietary supplementation with n-3 polyunsaturated fatty acids and vitamin E after myocardial infarction: results of the GISSI-Prevenzione Trial. *Lancet* **354**, 447–55.

Hooper, L., Summerbell, C.D., Higgins, J.P.T. *et al.* (2001) Dietary fat intake and prevention of cardiovascular disease: systematic review. *Br Med J* **322**, 757–63.

Hu, F.B. and Stampfer, M. (1999) Nut consumption and risk of coronary heart disease: a review of epidemiological evidence. *Curr Atherosclerosis Rep* **1**, 205–10.

Khaw, K.T., Bingham, S., Welch, A. *et al.* (2001) Relation between plasma ascorbic acid and mortality in men and women in EPIC-Norfolk prospective study: a prospective population study. *Lancet* **357**, 657–63.

Law, M. (2000) Salt, blood pressure and cardiovascular disease. *J Cardiovasc Risk* **7**, 5–8.

Miettinen, T.A., Puska, P., Gylling, H. *et al.* (1995) Reduction of serum cholesterol with sitostanol-ester margarine in a mildly hypercholesterolemic population. *N Engl J Med* **333**, 1308–12.

Ramsay, L.E., Yeo, W.W. and Jackson, P.R. (1991) Dietary reduction of serum cholesterol concentration: time to think again. *Br Med J* **303**, 953–7.

Robertson, R. and Smaha, L. (2001) Can a Mediterranean-style diet reduce heart disease? *Circulation* **103**, 1821–2.

Singh, R.B., Niaz, M.A., Sharma, J.P. *et al.* (1997) Randomized, double-blind, placebo-controlled trial of fish oil and mustard oil in patients with suspected acute myocardial infarction: the Indian experiment of infarct survival–4. *Cardiovasc Drugs Ther* **11**, 485–91.

Sjöström, L., Rissanen, A., Andersen, T. *et al.* (1998) Randomised placebo-controlled trial of orlistat for weight loss and prevention of weight regain in obese patients. *Lancet* **352**, 167–73.

Tang, J.L., Armitage, J.M., Lancaster, T. *et al.* (1998) Systematic review of dietary intervention trials to lower blood cholesterol in free-living subjects. *Br Med J* **316**, 1213–20.

Weststrate, J.A. and Meijer, G.W. (1998) Plant sterol-enriched margarines and reduction of plasma total and LDL cholesterol concentrations in normocholesterolaemic and mildly hypercholesterolaemic populations. *Eur J Clin Nutr* **52**, 334–43.

Williamson, D.F., Pamuk, E., Thun, M. *et al.* (1995) Prospective study of intentional weight loss and mortality in never-smoking overweight US white women aged 40–64 years. *Am J Epidemiol* **141**, 1128–41.

LIPID-LOWERING DRUGS

In recent years, major new therapeutic agents have been added to available lipid-lowering drugs such that goals of therapy can be achieved in the majority of patients. In most cases this will be possible with monotherapy; others, particularly the more severe monogenic disorders, will require combination therapy.

In this section the available classes of lipid-lowering drugs are discussed in detail. Where significant differences are apparent between individual drugs of a particular class, these are highlighted. It is convenient to consider the various drug classes as those that primarily lower cholesterol concentrations, those that primarily lower triglyceride concentrations and those that lower both cholesterol and triglycerides.

CHOLESTEROL-LOWERING DRUGS

BILE ACID SEQUESTRANTS

These drugs have been available for many years (cholestyramine was introduced in 1967) and considerable clinical experience has accumulated from extensive well-conducted clinical trials, including endpoint studies. They have a major advantage in that they are not absorbed and therefore do not have the potential to produce toxic side-effects. Major disadvantages are that some patients find them tiresome and inconvenient to take and the frequency of gastrointestinal side-effects. The available compounds are cholestyramine and colestipol. As there are no clinically important differences between the two agents, they are considered together.

Mechanism of action

Cholestyramine is a copolymer of styrene and divinyl benzene; colestipol is a copolymer of diethylpentamine and epichlorohydrin. Unabsorbed after oral administration, they bind bile acids in the intestinal lumen – interrupting the enterohepatic circulation

No drugs   Bile acid depletion

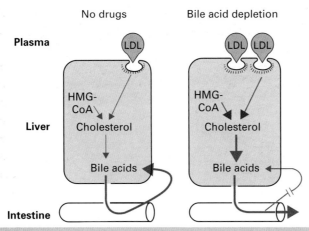

FIGURE 8.1 • Mechanisms of resins.

(Figure 8.1). As a result, the faecal loss of bile acids and cholesterol is increased, which leads to compensatory changes in hepatic metabolism. The conversion of cholesterol to bile acids is stimulated through activation of the enzyme 7α-hydroxylase, which catalyses the rate-determining step in bile acid synthesis. As hepatic cholesterol content is reduced through this process, there is up-regulation of LDL receptor activity, enhanced hepatic extraction of LDL from the circulation and decreased plasma LDL cholesterol concentrations. Part of the ability of resins to up-regulate LDL receptor activity is offset, because hepatic cholesterol synthesis is also stimulated through increased activity of HMG-CoA reductase, which catalyses the rate-determining step in cholesterol metabolism.

Pharmacology and clinical efficacy

The major effect is to reduce LDL cholesterol. The effect is maximal at about 2 weeks. After discontinuation, LDL levels return to baseline after 3–4 weeks. A small increase in HDL cholesterol is usually observed, though the mechanism of this effect is not understood. During the first few weeks of therapy, there is often a transient increase in VLDL triglyceride (5–20 per cent), which generally reverts to baseline levels after 2–3 months. This effect is more pronounced in individuals with pre-existing hypertriglyceridaemia.

At moderate doses (cholestyramine 16 g/day; colestipol 20 g/day), LDL cholesterol reductions of 15–30 per cent can be expected in hypercholesterolaemic individuals already on dietary measures. Reported increases in triglyceride concentrations range between 5 and 15 per cent. Several studies have been performed in heterozygous FH and similar results on LDL cholesterol have been observed. With good compliance, the effects on LDL cholesterol are maintained in the long term. In FH patients, regression of tendon xanthomata has been observed.

Cholestyramine was used in an important early primary prevention trial – the Lipid Research Clinics Coronary Primary Prevention Trial (LRCCPPT). In this randomized, double-blind study involving 3806 hypercholesterolaemic (>6.8 mmol/L) men, LDL reduction with cholestyramine over an average 7.4 years of follow-up was associated with a significant reduction in definite CHD death and/or non-fatal myocardial infarction. Subsequently, both cholestyramine and colestipol have been used, either alone or in combination with other lipid-lowering agents in angiographic trials, with beneficial effects (see page 256).

Adverse effects

Cholestyramine and colestipol are administered as powders. The powder is either scooped from a tin with a measured spoon or provided in sachets (cholestyramine 4 g; colestipol 5 g). The powders are mixed well with water or juice and are taken before a meal. The powder can also be sprinkled on food. These procedures are clearly a nuisance in comparison with simple tablet taking and patients often complain about the resins' gritty texture.

The adverse effects are more annoying than serious but do make a considerable impact on compliance. The main complaints are of constipation, a bloated feeling, flatulence, heartburn and nausea in up to a quarter of patients.

The resins can interfere with the absorption of other drugs. It is important that resins are taken either 1 hour before or 4 hours after other medications. In very high doses, malabsorption of fat may occur with decreased absorption of fat-soluble vitamins, and hypoprothrombinaemia has been described. Vitamin supplements may be required with prolonged high dosage. The gastrointestinal side-effects of resins tend to ameliorate with prolonged use. Patient disenchantment at the initiation of treatment can be partly overcome by low dosage (half a sachet daily) with a gradual increase over 4–6 weeks. Some patients mix the whole of their daily dose the day before and refrigerate it overnight, as they find the texture becomes more acceptable.

Various alternative preparations have been made available in some countries to try to improve compliance, e.g. tablet forms and chewy fruit-flavoured bars. However, in our experience these preparations do not offer any striking advantages.

Indications

The resins are indicated for the treatment of isolated primary hypercholesterolaemia but in practice they are used mainly in the rare patient who is statin intolerant. In mixed lipaemia they can be combined with a fibrate or nicotinic acid. In severe hypercholesterolaemia they can be combined with an HMG-CoA reductase inhibitor. It is our current practice to use low-dose therapy (2 sachets/day) for mild to moderate hypercholesterolaemia in individuals who have concerns about systemically active drugs. The resins are useful in children and in women of child-bearing potential.

TRIGLYCERIDE-LOWERING DRUGS

OMEGA-3 FISH OILS

Fish oils rich in the omega-3 fatty acids, eicosapentaenoic acid (EPA) and docosahexaenoic acid (DHA), have a limited but useful place in the therapy of lipid disorders. Interest in fish oils stemmed from epidemiological studies that contrasted the plasma lipid levels of Greenland Inuits and Danes. Despite the high-fat diet of the Inuits, their plasma triglyceride levels were lower. If non-Inuits were fed the Inuit diet, with a large percentage of calories derived from oily fish, reductions in plasma triglycerides were observed.

Mechanism of action

Fish oils reduce plasma triglyceride by reducing hepatic VLDL triglyceride synthesis. At very high doses VLDL apoprotein B secretion is also reduced, with reductions of plasma cholesterol. At lower doses, although triglyceride levels are reduced, LDL cholesterol may increase – possibly through enhanced conversion of VLDL to LDL. HDL cholesterol remains largely unchanged.

Pharmacology and clinical efficacy

In some countries, including the UK, fish oil preparations are licensed for use in the treatment of severe hypertriglyceridaemia. Maxepa (gelatin capsules or liquid) contain 18 per cent by weight of EPA and 12 per cent by weight of DHA. Omacor is a highly purified oil containing approximately 92 per cent omega-3 fatty acids, 47 per cent EPA, 37 per cent DHA and 8 per cent other omega-3 fatty acids.

The recommended dosage is 10 capsules a day in divided doses or 5 mL twice daily of the liquid form for Maxepa. As Omacor contains a higher percentage of omega-3 fatty acids the equivalent dose is 4 capsules daily. At these doses triglyceride concentrations will be reduced by 50–60 per cent in severely hypertriglyceridaemic patients. LDL cholesterol concentrations, which are low in these patients, tend to rise.

Fish oil administration in doses needed to reduce hypertriglyceridaemia has not been subjected to a long-term, randomized, controlled clinical trial with hard CHD endpoints. However, dietary measures to increase the consumption of fatty fish were associated with a significant reduction in CHD death in post-myocardial infarction patients in the DART study (see page 182). The largest trial to date was reported by the GISSI-Prevenzione Investigators (1999); the trial involved 11 300 patients who were myocardial infarction survivors; 1 g/day omega-3 fatty acid (as Omacor) administration over 3.5 years was associated with a 30 per cent reduction in cardiovascular death, a 45 per cent reduction in sudden death and a 20 per cent reduction in total mortality when compared with placebo.

Adverse effects

Although a 'natural' product, it cannot be assumed that the long-term consumption of fish oils at pharmacological doses will be harmless. Nevertheless, the intake of omega-3 fatty acids by some population groups throughout the world probably approaches the equivalent of Maxepa 10 g/day or Omacor 4 capsules/day with no apparent untoward effects. The most common side-effects are nausea and eructation.

Indications

Omega-3 fish oils are useful for the treatment of severe hypertriglyceridaemia and the authors often use it in combination with a fibrate drug. In patients with mixed hyper-lipidaemia with more modest elevations of triglyceride concentration, some patients respond well to a combination of fish oil with an HMG-CoA reductase inhibitor.

We have used fish oils successfully in women with familial hypertriglyceridaemia at risk of pancreatitis during pregnancy.

More research is needed on the optimal dosing for fish oil supplementation and the differential effects of purified EPA versus DHA (Mori and Beilin, 2001). The potential of omega-3 fatty acids to influence other important processes in atherogenesis and thrombosis (e.g. platelet function and vascular tone) is exciting.

DRUGS THAT LOWER CHOLESTEROL AND TRIGLYCERIDE ▬▬▬

NICOTINIC ACID (NIACIN)

Altschul and colleagues in the 1950s first demonstrated that nicotinic acid could reduce plasma lipids. This effect is independent of its action as a vitamin and is only observed at high dose. Importantly its amide derivative, nicotinamide (vitamin B_3) is ineffective.

There is no doubt that in terms of its broad spectrum of effect in modulating plasma lipid and lipoprotein concentrations, nicotinic acid could be considered to be the ideal drug. Sadly its wider use is markedly restricted because of poor patient acceptability and metabolic side-effects.

Mechanism of action

Kinetic studies have shown that the major effect is to reduce hepatic output of VLDL with consequent reductions in IDL and LDL. The increase in HDL (often pronounced) seen with nicotinic acid is most marked in hypertriglyceridaemic individuals and is due to decreased clearance of the lipoprotein. It is known that HDL clearance is enhanced in hypertriglyceridaemia and the reduction in plasma triglycerides by nicotinic acid appears to correct this.

Whilst the reduction in VLDL output is clear, the cellular mechanisms underlying this effect remain to be explained. It is not only VLDL triglyceride that is reduced, its protein components – apoproteins B, C and E – are all reduced.

Nicotinic acid inhibits hormone-sensitive lipase in adipose tissue with consequent reduction of free fatty acid flux to the liver. As this is a major determinant of VLDL out-put, it is attractive to hypothesize that this is the major explanation for nicotinic acid's effect. However, this effect is relatively short term. Two to three hours after dosing, free fatty acid concentrations are back to baseline and continue to rise with a significant overshoot, whilst triglyceride concentrations may remain reduced for 12–24 hours.

Nicotinic acid is unique amongst current lipid-modifying drugs, in that it reduces lipoprotein(a), but the mechanism of this effect is unknown.

Pharmacology and clinical efficacy

For effective reduction of plasma cholesterol and triglyceride, doses of nicotinic acid in the region of 2–8 g/day are required. At this dosage, reductions of total cholesterol of up to 30 per cent are to be expected, and LDL cholesterol concentrations fall by a similar amount. Reductions in plasma triglyceride vary depending on baseline levels. If triglyceride concentrations are in the normal range, then small decreases ($\cong$20 per cent) are usual, but in hypertriglyceridaemic patients, reductions of up to 60 per cent are not uncommon. It is of interest that increases in HDL cholesterol may be observed with lower doses (1 g/day). Nicotinic acid is particularly effective in increasing HDL cholesterol concentrations in hypertriglyceridaemic patients; increases of up to 30 per cent are not uncommon and occasionally increases of 50 per cent are observed.

Nicotinic acid is highly effective in patients with dysbetalipoproteinaemia and reductions in remnant particles of 50–60 per cent are to be expected.

In patients with elevated LDL and/or VLDL, nicotinic acid at a dose of 4 g/day reduces lipoprotein(a) concentrations; the most marked effect (a reduction of 38 per cent) has been observed in hypertriglyceridaemic patients.

Nicotinic has been used alone or in combination as the therapeutic agent in two secondary prevention trials and several angiographic progression/regression trials. In the Coronary Drug Project, nicotinic acid (3 g/day) was one of the five treatment arms, with 1119 men (aged 30–64 years) randomized to receive the drug. A placebo group consisted of 2789 men. In the nicotinic acid treated group, sustained reductions in total cholesterol of 10 per cent and in triglycerides of 26 per cent were achieved. After 5 years a significant reduction was observed in definite non-fatal myocardial infarction, but there was no difference in cardiovascular death or overall mortality. When the vital status of the study participants was ascertained 9 years after the completion of the study, mortality in the group treated with nicotinic acid was 11 per cent lower than in the placebo group.

In the Stockholm Ischaemic Heart Disease Study, nicotinic acid was used in combination with clofibrate. At 5 years there was a 26 per cent reduction in total mortality and a 36 per cent reduction in ischaemic heart disease mortality (Carlson and Rosenhamer, 1988).

Nicotinic acid was used in combination with other drugs in several angiographic trials, including the Cholesterol Lowering Atherosclerosis Study (CLAS) and Familial Atherosclerosis Treatment Study (FATS), with positive results, as detailed on page 256. Recently, a combination of simvastatin plus nicotinic acid has been shown to produce clinical and angiographically measurable benefits in CHD patients and low HDL cholesterol levels (Brown et al., 2001).

Adverse effects

Adverse effects associated with nicotinic acid are many and various. Undoubtedly, this is a drug that requires a clinician experienced in its use. Furthermore, very detailed clinical and biochemical monitoring is required.

Most patients will experience cutaneous flushing associated with a prickly feeling in the skin, which can be frightening if the patient is not forewarned. This was a frequent finding a few years ago when the virtues of nicotinic acid were extolled in a book written for the lay public. Unsuspecting individuals having purchased large tablets (0.5 g) of nicotinic acid from health food stores were startled and alarmed by faces the colour of a ripe strawberry. Tachyphylaxis to the flushing occurs rapidly and aspirin is useful in alleviating this symptom (as it is in prostaglandin-mediated flushing). Other skin reactions include pruritus, rash, dry skin and (rarely) acanthosis nigricans.

Gastrointestinal side-effects including abdominal pain (peptic ulceration may be reactivated) and nausea are quite common. More serious but rarer adverse effects include cardiac arrhythmias. In the Coronary Drug Project, atrial fibrillation occurred in 4.7 per cent of the nicotinic acid group compared with 2.9 per cent in the placebo group (Coronary Drug Project Research Group, 1975).

Cystic maculopathy leading to loss of visual acuity was observed in 0.7 per cent of patients taking nicotinic acid at high dose (3–6 g/day). This disorder regresses after the drug is discontinued. Rarely myopathy can occur, with increased creatinine phosphokinase (CPK) levels.

Metabolic abnormalities are quite commonly associated with nicotinic acid therapy. Elevated uric acid levels can occur but precipitation of an attack of gout is rare. Glucose tolerance is decreased and this is particularly important if nicotinic acid is used in Type 2 diabetic patients. Elevated liver enzymes occur in up to 5 per cent of patients and hepatic failure has been reported.

Indications

Nicotinic acid is widely used in the USA, where its relative cheapness is an advantage. In other countries (including the UK) it is rarely used because of the adverse effects described above. Attempts have been made to produce nicotinic acid derivatives to improve acceptability. Acipimox, for instance, received a licence in the UK. However, at the recommended doses this compound was considerably less effective than nicotinic acid.

Lack of availability of large-strength tablets also hinders the use of nicotinic acid in some countries. Some specialist clinics have arranged with their hospital pharmacy to import larger-strength tablets or to manufacture their own.

Nicotinic acid is indicated in all types of lipid disorder, either alone or in combination with other drugs. For the reasons indicated above, it is relatively contraindicated in diabetes and patients at risk of cardiac arrhythmia.

FIBRIC ACID DERIVATIVES

First reports of these compounds appeared in the early 1960s. A series of phenoxyisobutyric acids led to reduction in both cholesterol and triglyceride in experimental animals. Of these compounds, clofibrate (chlorophenoxyisobutyrate) was developed for clinical use. Since then clofibrate has had a chequered career and is now largely redundant. However, several other fibrates have been developed that are generally more effective with fewer adverse effects on the lithogenicity of bile and gallstone formation – this was clofibrate's major problem.

Although these compounds have been available for study for over 30 years, their mechanism of action at a molecular level is only just beginning to be identified.

The fibrates are perhaps the most heterogeneous class of lipid-modifying drugs and clinicians experienced in their use often try a second member of the class if the first-choice agent fails to achieve the desired effect in a particular patient.

It is disappointing that there are not more large, controlled clinical trials with hard CHD endpoints, which have employed fibrates.

Mechanism of action

The major action of fibrate drugs is to reduce plasma triglycerides; hepatic triglyceride synthesis is reduced and peripheral clearance is enhanced. The effects on the liver are thought to be secondary to increased cellular fatty acid catabolism resulting in inhibition of hepatic VLDL triglyceride synthesis and secretion. The enhanced triglyceride clearance is due to an increase in activity of the enzyme lipoprotein lipase through induction of the gene for lipoprotein lipase and repression of the gene for apoprotein C-III, an important inhibitor of the enzyme.

Kinetic studies of lipoprotein turnover point to an effect of fibrate drugs on LDL clearance, probably through effects on LDL structure. By decreasing VLDL triglyceride and consequently VLDL size, fibrates enhance the production of rapidly catabolized LDL. LDL produced from smaller VLDL particles are larger and less dense and are better ligands for the LDL receptor. When fibrates are used to treat isolated hypertriglyceridaemia, LDL concentrations can increase, albeit from previous low levels. However, this increase in LDL mass is accompanied by a change in LDL distribution to larger, more buoyant particles.

HDL cholesterol concentrations tend to rise with fibrate therapy. This increase appears to be due to increased synthetic rates of apoproteins A-I and A-II, the major protein constituents of HDL. Fibrates induce the transcription rates of the A-I and A-II genes through binding of activated PPARα to promotor regions of the genes. HDL concentrations may also be increased secondary to the reduction in triglycerides, which would tend to reduce the action of cholesterol ester transfer protein.

Despite the fact that it is over 30 years since the fibrate drugs were discovered, it is only recently that details of their mechanism of action at a cellular level have been discovered. Fibrates are activators for PPARα (peroxisome proliferator-activated receptor alpha) (Duez et al., 2001). PPARs, members of the nuclear hormone receptor family (includes oestrogen receptor and thyroid hormone receptor) are transcription factors that regulate gene expression in response to certain ligands (Figure 8.2). When activated by their various ligands, PPARα heterodimerizes with RXR (retinoid X receptor) and activates the transcription of genes by binding to PPAR response elements in the regulatory region of target genes. PPARs can also repress gene expression by interfering with other signalling pathways such as NF-κB. The first PPAR to be identified was PPARα and its role in modulating important genes in lipid metabolism has become clear.

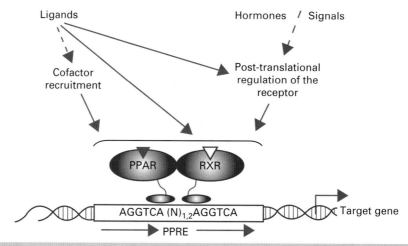

FIGURE **8.2** • PPARs and transcriptional regulation via PPAR response element. Source: Staels (2001).

Natural ligands for PPARα include fatty acids such as certain eicosanoids derived from arachidonic acid such as leukotriene B4 linoleic acid. The receptor is expressed mainly in the liver, heart, kidneys and muscle – tissues exhibiting a high rate of β-oxidation. Genes known to be controlled by PPARα include acyl-CoA synthetase, HMG-CoA synthetase, Apo A-I and Apo C-III.

PPARα receptors are also expressed in vascular smooth muscle cells, endothelial cells and monocyte/macrophages (Marx *et al.*, 2001), where they alter the expression of inflammatory mediators involved in atherogenesis, e.g. interleukin-1-induced interleukin-6 production and cytokine-induced expression of vascular cell adhesion molecule 1 (VCAM-1). These effects are likely to be important when considering the effects of PPARα agonists on the progression of atherosclerosis.

Pharmacology and clinical efficacy

The availability of different fibrates varies from country to country. In the UK there are five licensed for clinical use: the original drug clofibrate together with gemfibrozil, bezafibrate, ciprofibrate and fenofibrate. In the USA, on the other hand, fibrate availability is limited to clofibrate, gemfibrozil and fenofibrate.

Clofibrate, rapidly absorbed after oral administration, is hydrolysed to clofibric acid (*p*-chlorophenoxyisobutyrate), the active compound, peak plasma concentrations occurring at 6 hours. The drug is highly (95–98 per cent) protein bound and the elimination half-life ranges between 12 and 25 hours and rises to 29–88 hours in patients with renal dysfunction. Approximately 60 per cent is converted to the glucuronide and it is mainly excreted in the urine.

Gemfibrozil, although considered a fibric acid derivative, is structurally dissimilar to the other members of the class as it lacks the parachloride group. It is well absorbed with peak plasma concentration at 1–2 hours. The elimination half-life is approximately

112 hours. Gemfibrozil is highly metabolized, the major metabolite being a benzoic acid derivative. Seventy per cent of the drug is excreted in the urine – less than 2 per cent unchanged. The drug does not appear to accumulate in patients with abnormal renal function. As with clofibrate, gemfibrozil is highly (95 per cent) protein bound.

Bezafibrate, first introduced in 1978, is a second-generation clofibrate derivative. It is rapidly and completely absorbed with maximum plasma concentration at about 2 hours. Approximately 50 per cent of the drug is excreted unchanged, with 22 per cent as a glucuronide metabolite and 22 per cent as unidentified metabolites. After 24 hours, about 9 per cent of the drug is excreted in the urine – the elimination half-life being 2.1 hours. Bezafibrate is highly ($\cong$94–96 per cent) protein bound.

Ciprofibrate is characterized by a long elimination half-life (80 hours), which enables once-daily dosing. Similar to other fibrates, it is rapidly and almost fully absorbed and the maximum plasma concentration occurs at 1 hour. There are three as yet unidentified metabolites but these constitute only a tiny proportion of the excreted dose. Seventy-three per cent of an oral dose is excreted in the urine as conjugated metabolites. The drug is highly (99 per cent) protein bound.

Fenofibrate, first introduced in 1973, is rapidly and completely absorbed when taken with food. It is renally excreted and accumulates in patients with renal impairment. Fenofibrate is highly (99 per cent) protein bound.

There are other fibric acid derivatives available for clinical use such as simfibrate, theofibrate and nicofibrate, and several others. As they are licensed only in a minority of countries (on average one or two), they are not considered further here. Etofibrate, which is licensed in Spain, Germany and Switzerland, is the ethylene glycol diester of clofibric acid and nicotinic acid. After administration, the drug is hydrolysed and the two active components are released. To date it does not appear to have any advantages over the usual fibrates.

The effect of fibrate therapy on plasma lipid and lipoprotein concentrations depends on the particular lipid phenotype and the particular fibrate chosen. As discussed above, there is considerable heterogeneity within the class, particularly with regard to effects on LDL cholesterol.

The major effects are on triglycerides and HDL cholesterol, as might be predicted from what is understood about their mode of action. The degree of triglyceride reduction is generally similar amongst the newer fibrates and depends on the baseline plasma triglyceride concentration. With high baseline levels, reductions of 60 per cent would be expected.

Effects on LDL cholesterol of the various fibrates have been reviewed and on average gemfibrozil would be expected to produce a 10 per cent reduction, bezafibrate a 15 per cent reduction and fenofibrate and ciprofibrate a 25 per cent reduction. As a general rule, LDL cholesterol reductions are greater in patients with pure hypercholesterolaemia than in those with mixed hyperlipidaemia. The paradoxical increase in LDL cholesterol in patients with hypertriglyceridaemia has already been discussed.

In addition to effects on plasma lipid levels, various other potentially beneficial effects have been described with fibrate drugs. Fibrinogen, an important independent risk factor for CHD, is reduced by therapy with clofibrate particularly, but also with bezafibrate, fenofibrate and ciprofibrate. Interestingly, gemfibrozil does not appear to share this property. Other effects have been described on platelet function and other coagulation parameters but more studies are needed to clarify the situation. Gemfibrozil has been shown to decrease factor VII–phospholipid complex and plasminogen activator inhibitor 1 (PAI-1) activity, with consequent improved fibrinolytic capacity.

A frequent concomitant finding in hypertriglyceridaemic patients is hyperuricaemia and clinical gout. Fenofibrate therapy is associated with a sustained reduction in serum urate levels and this appears to be due to increased renal urate excretion.

Several major large, randomized, controlled clinical trials have assessed the effect of fibrate therapy on CHD events. In the Coronary Drug Project, 1103 middle-aged men with previous myocardial infarction received clofibrate for 5 years. Clofibrate therapy was associated with a modest 6 per cent reduction in plasma cholesterol and a 16 per cent reduction in plasma triglyceride. There was a reduction in fatal and non-fatal CHD in the clofibrate group compared with a placebo group ($n = 2789$) but this difference did not reach statistical significance. No difference in overall mortality was observed between the two groups.

In the large WHO Cooperative primary prevention trial (see page 245), clofibrate (1.6 g/day) was given to approximately 5000 men whose cholesterol was in the upper third of the distribution. Individuals were followed for a mean of 5.3 years. Clofibrate therapy produced a modest 9 per cent reduction in plasma cholesterol but this was associated with an overall decrease in CHD events of 20 per cent, mainly due to a reduction in non-fatal myocardial infarction. However, deaths from non-cardiac causes were significantly higher in the treatment group. This finding, together with its limited efficacy and its undoubted predisposition to gallstone formation, has led to a decline in the use of clofibrate and the drug is now virtually redundant.

In the Helsinki Heart Study (see page 247), gemfibrozil (600 mg b.d.) or placebo was administered to over 4000 middle-aged men with primary hyperlipidaemia (non-HDL cholesterol greater than 5.2 mmol/L). Gemfibrozil therapy reduced LDL cholesterol by 11 per cent, plasma triglyceride by 35 per cent and increased HDL cholesterol by 11 per cent. The cumulative CHD endpoints (fatal and non-fatal myocardial infarction) at 5 years were 27.3/1000 in the treated group compared with 41.4/1000 in the placebo group, representing a significant 34 per cent reduction.

In this trial, non-cardiac deaths were not increased and there was no significant increase in the rate of cholecystectomy. The beneficial effects observed with gemfibrozil were related not only to the reduction in LDL but also to the increase in HDL cholesterol. In a subsequent analysis, a subgroup with an LDL/HDL cholesterol ratio greater than 5 together with a triglyceride concentration greater than 2.3 mmol/L was identified as showing most benefit, with a 71 per cent reduction in CHD events (Manninen et al., 1992).

More recently, information on the potential benefits of fibrate drugs has come from two secondary prevention trials. The Veterans Administration HDL Intervention Trial (VA-HIT) was designed to test the benefit of therapy to increase HDL cholesterol in CHD patients where the primary lipid abnormality was a low HDL cholesterol (Rubins *et al.*, 1999). Gemfibrozil therapy in 2531 men with established CHD (baseline HDL 0.8 mmol/L; baseline LDL cholesterol 2.9 mmol/L) was associated with a 6 per cent increase in HDL cholesterol and a 31 per cent reduction in plasma triglyceride with no change in LDL cholesterol. The primary outcome measure (combined incidence of non-fatal myocardial infarction or CHD death) was reduced by 22 per cent (275 events versus 219) in the gemfibrozil group, $P = 0.006$. For the combined outcome of CHD death, myocardial infarction and stroke, there was a 24 per cent reduction, $P < 0.001$).

In the Bezafibrate Infarction Prevention (BIP) study (BIP Study Group, 2000), 3090 patients with established CHD (2825 men) received either bezafibrate (400 mg/day) or placebo. Baseline lipid values were total cholesterol 5.49 mmol/L, LDL cholesterol 3.83 mmol/L, HDL cholesterol 0.9 mmol/L and plasma triglycerides 1.6 mmol/L. Bezafibrate treatment was associated with an 18 per cent increase in HDL cholesterol and a 21 per cent reduction in plasma triglyceride. After 6.2 years the cumulative probability of the primary endpoint (a combination of fatal and non-fatal myocardial infarction or sudden death) was reduced by 7.3 per cent with bezafibrate ($P = 0.24$). A *post hoc* analysis of patients with high triglycerides ($\geqslant 200$ mg/dL) demonstrated a 39.5 per cent reduction ($P = 0.02$) in the primary endpoint. These conflicting findings are discussed elsewhere.

Adverse effects

The fibrates are well tolerated in the majority of patients and adverse effects are infrequent. In some patients gastrointestinal symptoms (abdominal pain, diarrhoea and nausea) lead to discontinuation of therapy. Skin rash may occur very rarely. The most important side-effect, which fortunately is rare, is myositis with muscle pain and tenderness and an elevated CPK level.

Fibrates tend to accumulate in patients with renal impairment, with the potential for increased side-effects – particularly myositis and deteriorating renal function. It is our practice to avoid the use of these drugs in such patients. Because the fibrates are highly protein bound, they have the potential to potentiate the action of anticoagulants and careful monitoring is required.

There is no doubt that the founder drug, clofibrate, increases the lithogenicity of bile with resultant increased risk of gallstone formation. However, this problem is considerably less with later compounds. Cholecystectomy rate was not significantly increased in the Helsinki Heart Study and no excess gallstone risk has been reported with fenofibrate, which has the longest clinical experience after clofibrate. Biliary lipid studies in patients receiving ciprofibrate showed an increase in the cholesterol saturation in the short term but at 1 year there was no significant effect. It is sensible to avoid the use of fibrate drugs in patients with known biliary disease but the risk of gallstone development in those free of disease appears to be small. Occasionally elevations of liver enzymes are seen. However, alkaline phosphatase levels tend to be reduced consistently.

In rodents, all fibrates produce hepatomegaly and peroxisome proliferation. This is species specific and does not occur in humans. Furthermore, hepatocellular carcinoma has been observed in rats receiving high-dose fibrate therapy. Again, this effect appears to be species specific. Nevertheless, these findings, together with the increase in non-cardiac deaths observed in the WHO clofibrate trial, led to concerns on the long-term safety of the fibrate class. A recent meta-analysis of the fibrate trials has also cast doubt on safety, but the increase in non-cardiac mortality associated with fibrate therapy in the meta-analysis was entirely attributable to the data from the WHO study.

As discussed elsewhere in this book, increasing concentrations of total serum homocysteine are associated with cardiovascular risk (Boushey *et al.*, 1995). Moreover, recently it has been shown that treatment with a combination of folic acid, vitamin B12 and pyridoxine which reduced homocysteine levels from $11.1 \pm 2.4\,\mu\text{mol/L}$ ($P < 0.001$) was associated with reduced re-stenosis rate following coronary angioplasty (Schnyder *et al.*, 2001). Importantly in this regard, it has been reported that fibrates can affect serum homocysteine concentrations (Dierkes *et al.*, 1999; Westphal *et al.*, 2001). Bezafibrate and fenofibrate increase homocysteine whereas gemfibrozil does not. The mechanism of this effect is not fully understood but effects on renal function have been suggested and fenofibrate therapy in one study reduced vitamin B6. Given recent evidence of benefit of homocysteine-lowering therapy, supplementation with folate might be advisable in patients taking bezafibrate and fenofibrate.

Indications

Fibrates are useful in the treatment of moderate to severe hypertriglyceridaemia, in mixed hyperlipidaemia where the predominant abnormality is hypertriglyceridaemia and in type III dyslipidaemia. They are not first-line agents for isolated hypercholesterolaemia.

Fibrates may be used in combination with anion exchange resins in mixed hyperlipidaemia and with nicotinic acid in severe hypertriglyceridaemia. In patients considered at high risk of CHD and mixed hyperlipidaemia, a fibrate may be used with a statin. Careful safety monitoring is required, because of the increased risk of side-effects, and patients should be warned to stop the drugs in the event of muscle pains. It has become clear that the potential increase in serious muscle adverse events such as myositis and rhabdomyositis are more common when statins are combined with gemfibrozil. In the authors' view, gemfibrozil should not be used in combination with statins.

The considerable heterogeneity amongst the fibrate class has already been discussed. In our experience and based on published trials, it is reasonable to infer that bezafibrate, ciprofibrate and particularly fenofibrate are most effective in patients with isolated hypercholesterolaemia. In terms of triglyceride-lowering efficacy, there seems to be little to choose between the drugs in mixed lipaemia. Gemfibrozil is particularly effective in type III dyslipidaemia. In isolated moderate hypertriglyceridaemia, ciprofibrate and fenofibrate are highly effective, whilst in the type V phenotype, bezafibrate and gemfibrozil are most effective.

HYDROXYMETHYLGLUTARYL COENZYME A (HMG-CoA) REDUCTASE INHIBITORS (THE STATINS)

The HMG-CoA reductase inhibitors, generally referred to as the statins, are inhibitors of cholesterol synthesis. Unlike earlier compounds such as triparanol and AY-9944, which inhibited steps towards the end of the pathway, resulting in accumulation of sterol intermediates and resultant toxicity (cataracts, ichthyosis), the statins inhibit cholesterol synthesis at an early stage.

The first compound, compactin, was isolated from culture broths of the fungi *Penicillium citrinum* and *Penicillium brevecompactum*. This compound was not developed for clinical use and it was the structural analogues lovastatin and simvastatin, from *Aspergillus terreus*, and pravastatin (first identified as a urinary metabolite of compactin) that were eventually licensed. More recently, three synthetic analogues of the early fungal metabolites have been developed and brought to market in several countries: fluvastatin, atorvastatin and cerivastatin. Cerivastatin was withdrawn from worldwide clinical use in 2001 because of an increased frequency of myositis (see page 227). These compounds share a fluorophenyl group and a dihydroxyheptanoic side chain and atorvastatin has a poly-substituted pyrole nucleus (Figure 8.3).

Mechanism of action

Statins are specific, competitive inhibitors of the enzyme HMG-CoA reductase, which catalyses the rate-determining and first committed step in cholesterol synthesis – the conversion of HMG-CoA reductase to mevalonate. The pathway is inhibited *in vivo* by approximately 40 per cent as assessed by measurement of mevalonate concentrations.

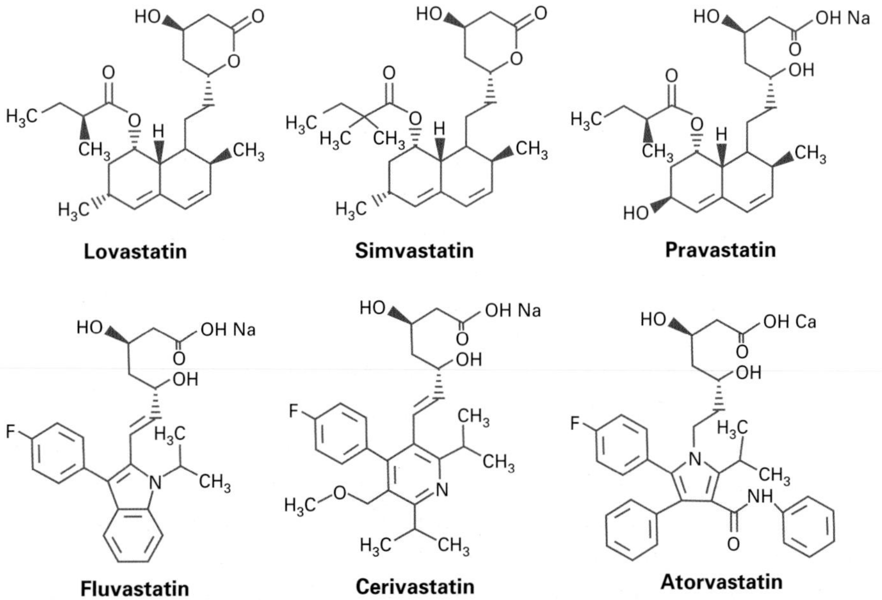

FIGURE 8.3 • HMG-CoA reductase inhibitors.

HMG-CoA reductase enzyme protein increases when its activity is blocked but this does not overcome the inhibition.

As a result of inhibition of cholesterol synthesis in the liver, hepatic LDL receptor activity increases to maintain equilibrium with increased uptake of LDL cholesterol and decreased plasma LDL cholesterol and Apo B concentrations (Figure 8.4). Proteolytic cleavage of cytoplasmic membrane-bound SREBP is promoted by reduced intracellular cholesterol concentration. Active SREBP, following translocation to the nucleus binds to gene promotors enhancing mRNA transcription of LDL receptors. In addition, LDL cholesterol synthesis is decreased in some patients. That the statins principally act through the LDL receptor has been confirmed *in vivo* by lipoprotein turnover studies and *ex vitro* measurement of LDL receptor activity in liver biopsy specimens. As might be expected, the statin drugs are much less effective in patients with homozygous familial hypercholesterolaemia. However, high-dose simvastatin and atorvastatin have been shown to reduce LDL cholesterol moderately but significantly in these patients. It is likely, therefore, that in addition to effects on the LDL receptor there is also a reduction in hepatic VLDL output and consequently LDL production. VLDL synthesis is a complex process involving coupling of lipid (triglyceride and cholesterol) to Apo B facilitated by microsomal transfer protein. Inhibition of HMG-CoA reductase may affect this process and therefore reduce VLDL synthesis and output. This effect also contributes to the moderate reduction in triglycerides.

Pharmacology and clinical efficacy

The statin drugs differ in the form in which they are administered: lovastatin and simvastatin are given as lactones, which are hydrolysed in the liver to the open acid form;

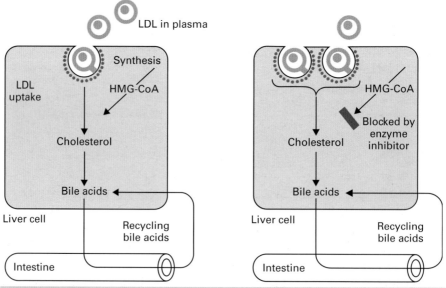

FIGURE 8.4 • Mechanism of action of HMG-CoA reductase inhibitors.

pravastatin, fluvastatin and atorvastatin, on the other hand, are administered in the open acid form. The structure of six statin molecules is shown in Figure 8.3. The open acid parts of the molecules bear a striking structural similarity to HMG-CoA, the substrate for HMG-CoA reductase.

The absorption of statin compounds varies between the members of the class. Simvastatin and fluvastatin are well absorbed (70–100 per cent) and lovastatin ($\cong$30 per cent) and pravastatin ($\cong$34 per cent) less so. The degree of protein binding also varies: simvastatin, lovastatin and fluvastatin are highly protein bound (>90 per cent) whilst pravastatin and its major metabolite show protein binding ranging between 46 and 57 per cent. The elimination half-time of the statins is generally short (<2 hours) and the major route of excretion is the liver. The elimination half-time of atorvastatin is longer (>12 hours). Atorvastatin, lovastatin and simvastatin are metabolized through cytochrome P450 3A4. Fluvastatin is metabolized through P450 2C9, whilst pravastatin is not metabolized via the cytochrome system. The major degradation product of pravastatin is the 3-hydroxy isomer.

Much has been made in the past of the differences between the various statins with regard to lactone versus open acid form and the degree of solubility in aqueous or lipid environment, i.e. hydrophilic versus hydrophobic. Because of its free hydroxyl group at position 6 of the decalin ring (Figure 8.3), pravastatin is a hydrophilic compound, whereas lovastatin and simvastatin are hydrophobic compounds as a result of the methyl group at this position. Fluvastatin is relatively hydrophilic. The differences in solubility characteristics may affect the degree to which the various drugs are taken up by non-hepatic tissues (hepatic uptake appears to be an active process), as hydrophobic compounds are better able to cross all membranes including the blood–brain barrier.

These differences, although undoubtedly present, do not appear to translate into significantly different clinical and biochemical adverse effects between the drugs. Through active uptake by the liver and major first-pass metabolism and the degree of protein binding, the exposure of extrahepatic tissues to these compounds is very low.

The statins are the most potent compounds for reducing plasma LDL cholesterol concentrations with LDL cholesterol reductions ranging from 30 to 60 per cent. Furthermore, there is little evidence of significant safety issues between the various statins apart from cerivastatin which was withdrawn because of a much greater risk of myopathy. Apo B concentrations tend to be reduced to a similar degree as LDL cholesterol. HDL cholesterol concentrations tend to increase but only to a small degree ($\cong$5 per cent), while triglycerides similarly show modest reductions (10–15 per cent).

Statins have been studied in a wide range of patients. They appear to be effective in patients with type III disease, with significant reductions in LDL and VLDL remnants. They have been studied in patients with secondary dyslipidaemia, including diabetes and nephrotic syndrome, and beneficial effects on plasma lipid and lipoprotein profiles have been observed. Initial studies with statins focused on effects on total and LDL cholesterol in patient populations with isolated hypercholesterolaemia. In these patients only modest effects on plasma triglycerides were observed. However, it has now become clear that in hypertriglyceridaemic patients more substantive effects of statins are seen.

Atorvastatin was the first statin to be studied in hypertriglyceridaemic patients. In a dose-ranging (5–80 mg/day) study in patients with hypertriglyceridaemia (>350 mg/dL; 3.95 mmol/L), reductions in plasma triglycerides of 26.5–45.8 per cent were observed with atorvastatin. Subsequently it has become clear from an analysis of pooled laboratory data that all statins lower plasma triglycerides in a dose-dependent manner if baseline triglycerides are raised (>250 mg/dL; 2.8 mmol/L) (Stein *et al.*, 1998). In this analysis, the reduction in plasma triglycerides was similar in proportion to the reduction observed in LDL cholesterol. Of interest, increases in HDL cholesterol were higher in this group of patients.

It is likely that the effects of statins in reducing plasma triglycerides are through increased removal of the remnant particles of the metabolism of triglyceride-rich lipoproteins through the Apo B_{100}/Apo E receptor. In addition, effects on hepatic production of VLDL are likely.

In severe hypercholesterolaemia, statins have been combined effectively with anion-exchange resins, resulting in reductions of LDL cholesterol of approximately 50 per cent. In severe mixed dyslipidaemia, statins have been combined with fibrates, with beneficial effects, but careful safety monitoring is required with this combination as the risk of side-effects, particularly myopathy, is increased (Sampson and Betteridge, 1999). As discussed elsewhere, statins should not be combined with gemfibrozil, which, through as yet unknown mechanisms, leads to increased plasma statin concentrations.

Statins have been used in long-term, randomized, controlled clinical trials to examine the impact of cholesterol lowering on atherosclerosis regression and on hard CHD endpoints. These trials have ended previous controversies in relation to overall benefit and to adverse events. Various statins – lovastatin, pravastatin and simvastatin – have been used in many atherosclerosis regression trials either alone or in combination with other drugs. These trials (described in detail in Chapter 9) have shown that coronary plaque progression can be delayed and in some cases plaque regression can occur.

The landmark 4S study (page 264) demonstrated a highly significant reduction in overall mortality with simvastatin in patients ($n = 4444$) with established CHD and cholesterol levels ranging between 5.8 and 8.0 mmol/L persisting after dietary measures. Subsequently this information on the benefits of simvastatin therapy in hypercholesterolaemic CHD patients was extended in the CARE study to CHD patients with average cholesterol levels – baseline total cholesterol concentrations below 6.2 mmol/L treated with pravastatin (see page 267). In the LIPID study, patients with established CHD (previous history of myocardial infarction or hospitalization for unstable angina), wide baseline cholesterol concentrations (4–7 mmol/L) and triglyceride concentrations up to 5 mmol/L showed benefit with pravastatin 40 mg/day (see page 268). Most recently, the HPS has provided massive data on the benefits of statin therapy (simvastatin 40 mg/day) not only in patients with established CHD (previous myocardial infarction or angina) but also in patients with carotid disease and peripheral vascular disease. In this study, benefit was demonstrable in patients with baseline LDL cholesterol concentrations <2.6 mmol/L, the current goal of therapy of the American NCEP guidelines. The HPS also provides copious information on the benefits in women, the elderly and those with diabetes (see page 275).

The first primary prevention trial using a statin was WOSCOPS (see page 248). This study showed that pravastatin therapy (40 mg/day) in middle-aged men with cholesterol concentrations of 6.5–8.0 mmol/L was associated with a highly significant reduction in the major study endpoint of combined non-fatal myocardial infarction and cardiac death. No excess of non-cardiac death was observed such that overall mortality was also reduced. AFCAPS/TexCAPS (page 251) extended the evidence base for statin therapy in the primary prevention of CHD to men and women with average total and LDL cholesterol but below average HDL cholesterol concentrations. In addition, the HPS provides further information on primary prevention in higher risk individuals across a wide range of cholesterol concentrations and a wide age range (page 275).

Adverse effects

Given the potency of the statins, it is remarkable that the safety profile is so good. Generally the drugs are well tolerated and adverse effects leading to discontinuation of drug are rare.

The nature of their mechanism of action raised the possibility of adverse effects through inhibition of synthesis of important biological compounds – ubiquinones and dolichols, formed from mevalonate. As can be seen in Figure 8.5, the biochemical pathways leading to ubiquinone and dolichol branch from farnesyl pyrophosphate prior to squalene synthetase. It is possible that inhibition of HMG-CoA reductase could reduce flux through these pathways. Dolichol is required for glycoprotein synthesis and ubiquinone is important in mitochondrial electron transport. There does not appear to be any significant reduction in the synthesis of these compounds. As previously discussed, mevalonate levels are reduced by only 40 per cent *in vivo* and the branch pathways appear to be preserved preferentially.

A further potential problem secondary to the action of statins is reduced hormone synthesis. Steroid hormones are produced from cholesterol and it is conceivable that

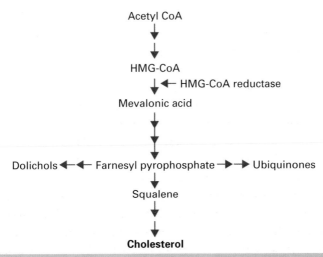

FIGURE 8.5 • Cholesterol synthetic pathway showing the branching points to ubiquinones and dolichols.

reduction in cholesterol synthesis could be associated with a fall in adrenal and gonadal steroids. However, clinically significant reductions of steroid hormones have not been observed with statin treatment.

A further possible adverse effect which could be related to inhibition of cholesterol synthesis is reduction of bile acid synthesis. This could lead to an increased risk of gallstones through an alteration in the lithogenic index of bile. Bile acid production is probably moderately decreased by statin therapy, as shown by cholesterol balance studies. However, biliary cholesterol is reduced to a greater extent than bile acid production such that the lithogenic index is actually reduced.

The most common side-effects of the statins are gastrointestinal disturbances but these tend to disappear if the drug is continued. Weakness, headache and aches and pains occasionally occur. Early studies in experimental animals given extremely high doses of some statin drugs had shown cataract formation. This has not been shown in human patients and ophthalmic assessment advised in early guidelines is no longer necessary.

The most serious adverse event with statin therapy is myopathy. This fortunately very rare complication is characterized by painful, tender muscles, often with flu-like symptoms. The CPK level is very high. Myopathy usually resolves when the drug is discontinued. In rare cases acute renal tubular necrosis has occurred following rhabdomyolysis. Patients should be warned to stop statin drugs if they develop severe muscle pains.

Myopathy is more likely to occur when statins and fibrates are combined. This is a particular problem with gemfibrozil. Drugs that interfere with excretion of the statins, such as cyclosporin, nicotinic acid, protease inhibitors and erythromycin, resulting in raised blood levels, also increase the risk of myopathy. Statins are also best discontinued in severe intercurrent illness to avoid the risk of myopathy, and should not be taken by individuals with liver dysfunction or alcoholics.

Apart from the drugs discussed above, the potential for interaction of statins with other compounds is low. Statins do not appear to influence the cytochrome P450 system. The high protein binding of most of the statins should be remembered in patients who require anticoagulants. With pravastatin, however, no changes in anticoagulant action of warfarin have been observed.

Guidelines for biochemical safety monitoring during statin therapy have changed with increasing clinical experience. When the drugs were first introduced, frequent measurement of liver function tests was advised. This is not now necessary and it is our practice to check liver function prior to initiation of therapy and thereafter when the lipid profile is measured. Analysis of the biochemical safety databases of the large prospective, randomized, controlled trials such as 4S, CARE and HPS have shown little difference in liver function abnormalities between placebo and active drug groups.

It is not our practice to measure CPK levels routinely. Levels of this enzyme vary, often quite markedly, in normal individuals after a visit to the gym, for example. However, if patients complain of muscle pain, then it is important to measure CPK levels. An important practice point, which is not generally known, is the higher levels of CPK in black patients.

The withdrawal of cerivastatin

The withdrawal of cerivastatin in the autumn of 2001 quite rightly has received considerable comment. Important lessons should be learned from it such that similar events are less likely in the future. It is clear that there is no room for complacency in terms of drug safety and individual drugs should be subject to risk-benefit assessments particularly when long-term therapy is required.

From the early years of statin therapy, it became clear that myotoxicity was the most important serious adverse event. Myositis with high creatinine kinase (CK) levels could, rarely, progress to acute rhabdomyolysis and renal failure. Fortunately this adverse event provided to be very rare indeed. In a recent meta-analysis of three major long-term, placebo-controlled trials with pravastatin involving about 20 000 patients, no case of rhabdomyolysis was identified. In the Scandinavian Simvastatin Survival Study (4S) trial using simvastatin, only six patients developed asymptomatic CK levels greater than ten times the upper limit of normal (ULN) compared with one patient on placebo. There was just one case of rhabdomyolysis, which reversed on stopping the drug. In the safety database of the massive HPS, there were nine cases (compared with five on placebo) of CK > 10 × ULN in the 10 269 patients on simvastatin. This confirms a previous meta-analysis of simvastatin safety data where muscle adverse events were 0.025 per cent (Gruer et al., 1999). In the AFCAPS/TexCAPS involving 6605 patients, the frequency of CK > 10 × ULN was similar in lovastatin and placebo groups (0.7 per cent). There were two cases of rhabdomyolysis in the placebo group and one in the lovastatin group but the patient was not taking the active drug at the time.

The mechanism of statin-induced myositis is ill-understood, although it has been suggested from in vitro studies that it relates to inhibition of HMG-CoA reductase and secondary depletion of metabolic intermediates such as geranylgeranylation of low molecular weight proteins or reduced ubiquinone (coenzyme Q). Whatever the cause of myositis, it became clear that the particular statin cerivastatin was associated with at least a 10-fold higher risk of serious rhabdomyolysis than other statins. Fifty-two deaths were recorded world wide associated with cerivastatin; of these 31 deaths occurred in the USA and 12 were associated with concomitant therapy with gemfibrozil. Furthermore, several of the cases involved use of the highest dose (800 μg), which had only been approved for a short time. It is clear that concurrent gemfibrozil therapy leads to increased plasma levels of statins and particularly cerivastatin through mechanisms as yet not fully documented but not through the cytochrome system. Clearly, it would be of enormous benefit if this mechanism could be identified. Nevertheless, cerivastatin across the dosage range and particularly at 800 μg proved to be a quantum more prone to cause rhabdomyolysis than the older, well-established statins and consequently was removed from the market.

This episode is a timely reminder of the importance of continued vigilance in terms of drug safety and the need to optimize the evaluation and monitoring of safety outcomes. As discussed elsewhere in this book, combination therapy of statin and fibrate is commonly used in specialist centres for the treatment of high-risk patients with mixed dyslipidaemia. Clearly gemfibrozil is best avoided in combination with a statin.

Indications

Simvastatin (10–80 mg daily), pravastatin (10–40 mg daily), fluvastatin (10–80 mg daily), atorvastatin (10–80 mg daily) and lovastatin (10–80 mg daily) are available in many countries world wide. Statins are first-line agents for the treatment of hypercholesterolaemic patients in whom dietary and lifestyle measures have failed to achieve goals of therapy. They are also first-line agents in mixed hyperlipidaemia when the major lipid abnormality is raised cholesterol. In severe hypercholesterolaemia, such as heterozygous familial hypercholesterolaemia, statins, if necessary, can be used in combination with resins.

Combination of statins with fibrates is justified only in severe mixed hyperlipidaemia in those patients considered to be at high risk of a coronary event. Increased safety monitoring is advised and intensive therapy of this nature is best left to the lipid expert. In the authors' opinion, gemfibrozil should not be used in combination with a statin. Similarly, in transplant patients receiving cyclosporin, careful monitoring is required in a specialized centre.

If statins are prescribed to premenopausal women of child-bearing potential, the patient should be counselled to discontinue therapy at least 6 weeks prior to planned conception.

Pleiotropic effects of statins

There has been considerable interest in effects of statins on important processes in atherogenesis which appear to be independent of cholesterol lowering: so-called pleiotropic effects. This area of both basic and clinical research was stimulated by an impression that the overall clinical benefits of statins observed in the major endpoint trials were greater than would be expected from effects on LDL cholesterol alone. This is a very interesting area and a brief discussion of pleiotropic effects is merited in this mainly clinical text. Readers are directed to extensive recent reviews for more detailed analysis and discussion (Davignon and Laaksonen, 1999; Takemoto and Liao, 2001; Gotto and Farmer, 2001). In the authors' opinion, these studies are likely to provide further insight into the mechanisms of action of statins and possibly identify new targets for therapeutic intervention. However, they should not detract from the major indication for statins, which is effective LDL cholesterol lowering in patients at increased risk of vascular disease.

Important pleiotropic effects of statins in relation to atherogenesis and the prevention of acute coronary events relate primarily to effects on:

- improving/restoring arterial endothelial function;
- stabilizing atherosclerotic plaques;
- decreasing oxidative stress and vascular inflammation.

These effects are, in the main, attributable to the major effect of statins, i.e. inhibition of HMG-CoA reductase with reduction of the formation of mevalonate (see Figure 8.4). Mevalonate is a precursor of important isoprenoid intermediates which serve to direct membrane localization and function of a variety of intracellular signalling molecules, particularly small GTP-binding proteins Rho, Ras and Rac. For instance, activation of Rho is associated with vasoconstriction, decreased nitric oxide and activation of pro-inflammatory pathways. The translocation of Rho to the cell membrane and consequently its activation depends on its post-translational modification by the isoprenoid intermediate of the cholesterol biosynthetic pathway geranylgeranylpyrophosphate (GGPP). By reducing the production of GGPP, statins decrease the activation of Rho and therefore ameliorate the effects of Rho on vasoconstriction, inflammation and nitric oxide. These LDL-independent effects are likely to be augmented by the LDL cholesterol lowering as oxidized LDL can activate Rho.

Endothelial dysfunction is generally considered to be an early manifestation of atherosclerosis and can be demonstrated in the absence of angiographic evidence of plaque. Abnormalities of synthesis, release and activity of nitric oxide (endothelium-derived relaxing factor) are central to endothelial dysfunction. Nitric oxide has been shown to inhibit important mechanisms of atherosclerosis; it is important in vasorelaxation, it has inhibitory effects on vascular smooth muscle cell proliferation, it inhibits platelet aggregation and leucocyte/endothelium interactions. Vasodilating properties of statins have been demonstrated using a variety of techniques in patients (e.g. endothelial-dependent flow-mediated dilatation measured by brachial artery ultrasound, plethysmography and positron emission tomography-assessed myocardial perfusion). Clearly, LDL cholesterol lowering is important in these effects as cholesterol lowering by other means (resin therapy and apharesis) improves endothelial function. However, pleiotropic effects are likely to contribute to improved endothelial function as in some experimental models effects of statins on endothelial function precede demonstrable effects on cholesterol levels. Direct effects of statins on endothelial nitric oxide synthase (eNOS) have been observed in several studies associated with stabilization of eNOS mRNA. Other actions of statins that may contribute to improving/preserving endothelial function include reduction of endothelin 1 (a potent endothelial-derived vasoconstrictor) synthesis and antioxidant effects. Nitric oxide is scavenged by reactive oxygen species (ROS) such as superoxide and hydroxyl radicals and statins reduce production of ROS. Statins also up-regulate tissue-type plasminogen activator and down-regulate PAI-1 through effects on geranylgeranylation of Rho.

Vascular smooth muscle cell (SMC) proliferation and migration are central features in atherosclerosis. Statins reduce SMC proliferation in a variety of experimental models. These inhibitory effects can be abolished by the addition of mevalonate. Proliferation requires the activity of second messengers such as Ras and Rho, which promote cell cycle progression and cellular proliferation. It is likely that statins, by reducing the availability of isoprene units, reduce the activation of these important second messengers.

It has become clear in recent years that inflammation is an important component of atherosclerosis; monocyte/macrophages and T lymphocytes are prominent cellular components of the lesion. Inflammatory cytokines produced by these cells can influence SMC proliferation, endothelial function, thrombosis and collagen degradation. Statins reduce inflammatory cell content of lesions in various experimental models probably through decreased cell recruitment by inhibition of adhesion molecules. In carotid endarterectomy specimens obtained from patients treated with a statin, the number of macrophages and T lymphocytes was reduced. The important beneficial effects of statins observed in organ transplant patients (decreased rejection episodes, improved survival) are likely to involve anti-inflammatory effects (such as decreased natural killer cell cytotoxicity) as well as anti-proliferative effects.

The acute phase protein CRP is produced in the liver in response to inflammatory cytokines such as interleukin-6. CRP is considered to be a risk factor for vascular disease and CRP levels are elevated in patients with CHD. Statins reduce CRP levels possibly by reducing interleukin-6 production from vascular tissue.

Of potential for great interest for the future is the possible impact of statins on carcinogenesis. Lovastatin can inhibit cell proliferation by inhibiting proteasome degradation of the cyclin-dependent kinase inhibitors p21 and p27. These molecules have tumour-suppressor effects. The effects of lovastatin can be overcome by mevalonate. Further evidence for the potential benefit of statins comes from *in vitro* effects on acute myeloid leukaemic and colon adenocarcinoma cell lines, malignant mesothelioma cell lines, and animal models of mammary tumours and malignant melanomas.

A further exciting development unrelated to atherogenesis is the unexpected finding that statins stimulate bone formation through morphogenic protein-2 transcription in experimental animals. These observations may herald new insights into the mechanisms and therapy of osteoporosis.

FUTURE DIRECTIONS FOR LIPID-LOWERING DRUGS

There will be patients who do not respond to current agents for a variety of reasons. It is possible that even lower targets for LDL cholesterol will be advocated in the future if ongoing trials prove positive. Furthermore, other parameters of atherogenic dyslipidaemia, particularly HDL cholesterol and reverse cholesterol transport and perhaps lipoprotein(a), triglyceride-rich lipoproteins and remnants will become targets for therapeutic intervention in certain patients in addition to aggressive LDL lowering.

Ongoing developments include newer agents in existing classes such as the statins and agents targeted to novel sites in lipid and lipoprotein metabolism. There are two new compounds of the statin class at an advanced stage of clinical development: rosuvastatin (previously known as ZD4522) and pitavastatin (previously known as NK104). These agents are potent LDL cholesterol-lowering agents. Rosuvastatin, (trade name Crestor) is closest to release for clinical use, and published data point to a highly effective compound.

Rosuvastatin is a single enantiomer administered as the calcium salt of the active hydroxy acid. It is a hydrophilic compound (similar to pravastatin), which has potential advantages in terms of tissue distribution and metabolism. In *in vitro* experiments it is the most potent inhibitor of the enzyme HMG-CoA reductase with a 50 per cent inhibitory concentration [IC_{50}] of 5.4 nM compared with 44.1 nM for pravastatin. Of interest in terms of the potential for drug interactions, rosuvastatin shows little or no metabolism by cytochrome P450 3A4 (McTaggart *et al.*, 2001). In a 12-week study in hypercholesterolaemic patients (LDL cholesterol $\geqslant$4.14 mmol/L and <6.5 mmol/L) rosuvastatin, 5 mg and 10 mg/day, reduced LDL cholesterol from baseline by 42 per cent and 49 per cent, respectively; HDL cholesterol rose by 6 per cent and 7 per cent, respectively, with corresponding increases in apoprotein A-I (Paoletti *et al.*, 2001). In a similar study performed in North America 10 mg/day of rosuvastatin reduced LDL cholesterol by 43 per cent with a 12 per cent increase in HDL cholesterol; 82 per cent of patients achieved NCEP ATP-III LDL cholesterol goals of therapy (Davidson *et al.*, 2002). Higher doses of rosuvastatin, 20 mg and 40 mg/day, reduced LDL cholesterol by 59 per cent and 63 per cent from baseline with corresponding reductions of apoprotein B of 49 per cent and 55 per cent. HDL increased by 9 per cent and 10 per cent. In the same study, 10 mg and 80 mg/day of atorvastatin decreased LDL cholesterol (Olsson *et al.*, 2000). In patients with type 2 diabetes, LDL cholesterol fell by 46 per cent and triglycerides by 29 per cent. HDL cholesterol increased by 10 per cent with 10 mg/day of rosuvastatin (Durrington *et al.*, 2001).

Pitavastatin is also a potent synthetic inhibitor of HMG-CoA reductase with a [IC_{50}] of 6.8 mmol/L and shows little or no metabolism by the cytochrome P450 pathway. In a 12-week study performed in Japan, 2 mg/day of pitavastatin reduced LDL cholesterol by 37.6 per cent from baseline compared with 18.4 per cent with 10 mg/day of pravastatin. A corresponding 33.8 per cent reduction in apoprotein B was observed. HDL cholesterol increased by 8.9 per cent with a 7.2 per cent increase in apoprotein A-I (Saito *et al.*, 2002). In patients with heterozygous familial hypercholesterolaemia LDL cholesterol was reduced by 41 per cent and 49 per cent by 2 mg and 4 mg/day of pitavastatin, respectively (Noji *et al.*, 2002).

Interruption of intestinal cholesterol absorption or bile acid absorption remains an attractive approach to lipid lowering. As discussed previously, currently available agents are bulky and poorly tolerated. The agent most advanced in clinical development is SCH 58235, now known as ezetimibe. Ezetimibe is a selective intestinal cholesterol absorption inhibitor, which, in milligram doses, blocks the absorption of dietary and biliary cholesterol. This compares to gram doses required with the anion-exchange resins. Furthermore, it does not interfere with the absorption of fat-soluble vitamins. Ezetimibe in a dose of 10 mg/day has been reported to reduce LDL cholesterol by 16–18 per cent. The potential for combination with statins (and indeed with fibrates in mixed lipaemia) is clearly appealing and preliminary results show an additional 18 per cent reduction over that seen with statin alone. Given that when statin doses are doubled an average 6 per cent further LDL lowering is observed, there is potential for a low-dose statin/ezetimibe combination to save three statin dose titrations.

Also in active development are inhibitors of the apical sodium-dependent bile acid transporter (ASBT), which is expressed at highest levels in the distal half of the ileum. An antagonist of ASBT such as S-8921, which is in early clinical studies, would be expected to increase bile acid excretion with consequent increased conversion of hepatic cholesterol to bile acids and up-regulation of LDL receptors.

Other drug targets in development include acyl coenzyme A:cholesterol acyltransferase (ACAT) inhibitors and inhibitors of cholesterol synthesis at the level of squalene synthase and squalene cyclase. Further towards the horizon are compounds that up-regulate ABC-1, LCAT, CETP, hepatic lipase, PPARs and SREBPs. Clearly the future is likely to continue to be full of interest and excitement.

RADICAL THERAPY FOR REFRACTORY HYPERLIPIDAEMIA ▪▪▪▪

Various forms of radical treatment have been used in patients with very severe hyper-cholesterolaemia, usually homozygous FH. These techniques are very much the province of the specialist centre.

ILEAL BYPASS

Prior to the advent of the statin drugs, the treatment of heterozygous FH was unsatisfactory, particularly in patients who were unable to take large doses of anion-exchange resins. This led to the introduction of partial ileal bypass by Buchwald (1964) in the USA. This operation involved sectioning the ileum and anastomosing it to the caecum so that the terminal third ($\cong 200$ cm) of the ileum was bypassed. As a result, the enterohepatic circulation was disrupted with consequent increased hepatic bile acid synthesis and up-regulation of the LDL receptor just as with resin therapy. This operation was highly successful in reducing cholesterol levels and improved long-term CHD outcome in the Programme on the Surgical Control of Hyperlipidaemias (POSCH) study (page 262). Although postoperative diarrhoea was an occasional problem with this operation, it lacked the serious side-effects of the jejunal ileal bypass used for obesity. As vitamin B12 is also absorbed from the terminal ileum, replacement vitamin B12 is required.

This operation is now largely redundant as most patients are tolerant of statin drug therapy. However, in the rare FH patient intolerant of all drugs, ileal bypass may still be indicated.

PORTACAVAL SHUNT

This operation has been used to treat homozygous FH, the rationale being to reduce hepatic lipoprotein production (Starzl et al., 1983). Unfortunately, the overall reduction in LDL cholesterol in two reported series was modest, ranging between 18 per cent and 34 per cent, and rarely was the total cholesterol reduced below 12 mmol/L. Xanthomata regressed in some patients but unfortunately most patients still succumbed to CHD. This operation is now redundant with the advent of liver transplantation and LDL apheresis.

LIVER TRANSPLANTATION

The first liver graft to a patient with homozygous FH was performed in 1984 in the USA (Starzl et al., 1984). This operation provides normal LDL receptors. The first patient was a 7-year-old girl who had already developed significant CHD requiring a heart transplant. Following this dual transplantation procedure, her plasma cholesterol fell from 25 mmol/L to 7 mmol/L. There was a further cholesterol reduction with the statin drug, indicating that the LDL receptors on the transplanted liver were functional. Since then other homozygous FH patients have received this treatment (Barbir et al., 1992). Liver transplantation remains a high-risk procedure and is reserved for FH homozygous patients who also require heart transplantation.

EXTRACORPOREAL LIPOPROTEIN REMOVAL

Various techniques have been developed for the regular removal of LDL from the circulation in patients with severe heterozygous or homozygous FH. These range from plasma exchange (Thompson *et al.*, 1975) to the more selective LDL apheresis, which employs the principle of affinity chromatography for the removal of Apo B-containing lipoproteins, leaving HDL to return to the patient (Richter *et al.*, 1993).

Using these techniques it is possible to produce substantial reductions in LDL cholesterol. For instance, twice-weekly sessions where 1–1.5 plasma volumes are passed through LDL apheresis columns results in a 40–50 per cent reduction in integrated mean LDL cholesterol concentrations.

Another technique that has been used in Europe is the HELP (Heparin Extracorporeal LDL Precipitation) system. LDL is precipitated from plasma by lowering the pH. The resulting precipitate is removed by filters; the plasma pH is readjusted and returned. This process also removes fibrinogen and lipoprotein(a) (Thiery and Seidel, 1993).

In the long term, these techniques have been shown to lead to xanthomata regression, improvement in coronary atherosclerotic plaques, reduction of vascular events and prolongation of life. HELP has been shown to be helpful in preventing and treating graft vessel disease in cardiac transplant recipients. However, these techniques are very expensive and can only be performed in specialist centres.

GENE THERAPY

Homozygous FH is a prime candidate disease for trials of gene therapy, as current treatment options are relatively unsuccessful and the prognosis is very poor. A protocol is in place for gene transfer in the USA, but current techniques are relatively crude, involving partial hepatectomy, the transfection of liver cells *ex vivo* with retrovirus carrying DNA for the LDL receptor and subsequent injection of the cells into the portal vein. The reduction in LDL in the first patient was relatively modest at 17 per cent (Grossman *et al.*, 1994). Clearly, gene transfer techniques are continually advancing and it is hoped that better results will be obtained in the future when novel vectors which are safe and efficient become available for clinical use.

REFERENCES

Altschul, R., Hoffer, A. and Stephen, J.D. (1955) Influence of nicotinic acid on serum cholesterol in man. *Arch Biochem Biophys* **54**, 558–9.

Barbir, M., Khaghani, A., Kehely, A. *et al.* (1992) Normal levels of lipoproteins including lipoprotein(a) after liver–heart transplantation in a patient with homozygous familial hypercholesterolaemia. *Q J Med* **85**, 807–12.

The BIP Study Group (2000) Secondary prevention by raising HDL-cholesterol and reducing triglycerides in patients with coronary artery disease. The Bezafibrate Infarction Prevention (BIP) Study. *Circulation* **102**, 21–7.

Brown, B.G., Zhao, X-Q, Chait, A., Fischer, L.D., Cheung, M.C., Morse, J.S. *et al.* (2001) Simvastatin and niacin, antioxidant vitamins or the combination for the prevention of coronary disease. *N Engl J Med* **345**, 1583–92.

Boushey, C.J., Beresford, S.A., Omenn, G.S. *et al.* (1995) A quantitative assessment of plasma homocysteine as a risk factor for vascular disease. Probable benefits of increasing folic acid intakes. *J Am Med Assoc* **274**, 1049–57.

Buchwald, H. (1964) Lowering cholesterol absorption and blood levels by ileal exclusion. *Circulation* **29**, 713–20.

Carlson, L.A. and Rosenhamer, G. (1988) Reduction of mortality in the Stockholm Ischaemic Heart Disease Secondary Prevention Study by combined treatment with clofibrate and nicotinic acid. *Acta Med Scand* **223**, 405–18.

Coronary Drug Project Research Group (1975) The Coronary Drug Project: clofibrate and niacin in coronary heart disease. *J Am Med Assoc* **231**, 360–81.

Davidson, M., Ma, P., Stein, E.A., *et al.* (2002) Comparison of effects of low-density lipoprotein cholesterol and high-density liproprotein cholesterol with rosuvastatin versus atorvastatin in patients with type IIa or IIb hypercholesterolaemia. *Am J Cardiol* **89**, 268–75.

Davignon, J. and Laaksonen, R. (1999) Low-density lipoprotein-independent effects of statins. *Curr Opin Lipidol* **12**, 543–59.

Dierkes, J., Westphal, S. and Luley, C. (1999) Serum homocysteine increases after therapy with fenofibrate or hezafibrate. *Lancet* **354**, 219–20.

Duez, H., Fruchart, J.-C. and Staels, B. (2001) PPARs in inflammation, atherosclerosis and thrombosis. *J Cardiovasc Risk* **8**, 187–94.

Durrington, P., Hamann, A., Tuomilehto, J., Smith, K. and Kallend, D. (2001) Rosuvastatin alone and in combination with fenofibrate in hyperlipidaemic patients with type 2 diabetes. *Diabetologia* **44**(Suppl 1), A165.

GISSI-Prevenzione Investigators (1999) Dietary supplementation with n-3 polyunsaturated fatty acids and vitamin E after myocardial infarction: results of the GISSI-Prevenzione Trial. *Lancet* **354**, 447–55.

Gotto, A.M. and Farmer, J.A. (2001) Pleiotropic effects of statins: do they matter? *Curr Opin Lipidol* **12**, 391–4.

Grossman, M., Raper, S.E., Kozarsky, K. *et al.* (1994) Successful *ex vivo* gene therapy directed to liver in a patient with familial hypercholesterolaemia. *Nat Genet* **6**, 335–41.

Manninen, V., Tenkanen, H., Koskinen, P. *et al.* (1992) Joint effects of triglycerides and LDL-cholesterol and HDL-cholesterol concentrations on coronary heart disease risk in the Helsinki Heart Study. Implications for treatment. *Circulation* **85**, 37–45.

Marx, N., Libby, P. and Plutzky, J. (2001) Peroxisome proliferator-activated receptors and their role in the vessel wall: possible mediators of cardiovascular risk? *J Cardiovasc Risk* **8**, 203–10.

McTaggart, F., Buckett, L., Davidson, R., *et al.* (2001) Preclinical and clinical pharmacology of resuvastatin, a new 3-hydroxy-3-methylglutaryl coenzyme A reductase inhibitor. *Am J Cardiol*, **87** (Suppl.), 28B–32B.

Mori, T.A. and Beilin, L.J. (2001) Long-chain omega-3 fatty acids, blood lipids and cardiovascular risk reduction. *Curr Opin Lipidol* **12**, 25–30.

Noji, Y., Higashikata, T., Inazu, A., *et al.* (2002) Long-term treatment with pitavastatin (NK-104), a new HMG CoA reductase inhibitor, of patients with heterozygous familial hypercholesterolaemia. *Atherosclerosis* **163**, 157–64.

Olsson, A.G., Pears, J.S., McKellar, J., Caplan, R.J. and Raza, A. (2000) Pharmacodynamics of a new HMG CoA reductase inhibitor ZD 4522 in patients with primary hypercholesterolaemi. *Atherosclerosis* **151**(1), 39.

Paloetti, R., Fahmy, M., Mahla, G., Mizan, J. and Southworth, H. (2001) Rosuvastatin demonstrates greater reduction of low-density lipoprotein cholesterol compared with pravastatin and simvastatin in hypercholesterolaemic patients: a randomized double-blind study. *J Cardiovasc Risk* **8**, 383–90.

Richter, W.O., Jacob, B.G., Ritter, M.M. *et al.* (1993) Three year treatment of familial heterozygous hypercholesterolaemia by extracorporeal low density lipoprotein immunoadsorption with polyclonal apolipoprotein B antibodies. *Metabolism* **42**, 888–94.

Rubins, H.B., Robbins, S.J., Collins, D. *et al.* (1999) Gemfibrozil for the secondary prevention of coronary heart disease in men with low levels of high-density lipoprotein cholesterol: Veterans Affairs High-Density Lipoprotein Cholesterol Intervention Trial Study Group. *N Engl J Med* **341**, 410–18.

Saito, Y., Yamada, N., Teramoto, T., *et al.* (2002) A randomized double-blind trial comparing the efficacy and safety of pitvastatin versus pravastatin in patients with primary hypercholesterolaemia. *Atherosclerosis* **162**, 373–9.

Sampson, M.J. and Betteridge, D.J. (1999) Hyperlipidaemia and combination drug therapy. In *Lipoproteins in Health and Disease* (eds D.J. Betteridge, D.R. Illingworth and J. Shepherd) Arnold, London, 1213–30.

Schnyder, G., Roffi, M., Pin, R. *et al.* (2001) Decreased rate of coronary restenosis after lowering of plasma homocysteine levels. *N Engl J Med* **345**, 1593–600.

Staels, B. (2000) The PPAR system and regulation of lipoprotein metabolism. In *Lipids and Vascular Disease: Current Issues* (ed. D.J. Betteridge). Martin Dunitz, London, 27–37.

Starzl, T.E., Chase, H.P., Ahrens, E.H. *et al.* (1983) Portacaval shunt in patients with familial hypercholesterolaemia. *Ann Surg* **198**, 273–83.

Starzl, T.E., Bilheimer, D.W. and Bahnson, H.T. *et al.* (1984) Heart–liver transplantation in a patient with familial hypercholesterolaemia. *Lancet* **1**, 1382–3.

Stein, E.A., Lane, M. and Laskarzewski, P. (1998) Comparison of statins I hypertriglyceridemia. *Am J Cardiol* **81**(4A), 66B–9B.

Takemoto, M. and Liao, J.K. (2001) Pleiotropic effects of 3-hydroxy-3-methylglutaryl coenzyme A reductase inhibitors. *Arterioscler Thromb Vasc Biol* **21**, 1712–19.

Thiery, Y. and Seidel, D. (1993) LDL apheresis: clinical experience and indications in the treatment of severe hypercholesterolaemia. *Transfus Sci* **14**, 249–59.

Thompson, G.R., Lowenthal, R. and Myant, N.B. (1975) Plasma exchange in the management of homozygous familial hypercholesterolaemia. *Lancet* **1**, 1208–11.

Westphal, S., Dierkes, J. and Luley, C. (2001) Effect of fenofibrate and gemfibrozil on plasma homocysteine. *Lancet* **358**, 39–40.

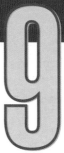

CHAPTER 9

LIPID-LOWERING TRIALS

Many trials of lipid lowering with various diet and drug therapies have been conducted during the last three decades but until 1994 no trial reported an unequivocal result. Over the years these trials have caused much controversy, not only in the medical press but also in the lay press. The controversy arose because of the failure of the early trials to demonstrate overall benefit.

THE CHOLESTEROL CONTROVERSY OF THE EARLY 1990s

In the majority of trials, the primary endpoint was a combination of non-fatal and fatal myocardial infarction. Most commentators accepted that these events were reduced, but the reduction in CHD deaths did not translate into an improvement in overall mortality because there was an apparent excess of non-CHD deaths. This led to the well-known statement, probably first made by the late Professor Mitchell (then Professor of Medicine at Nottingham University), that the only effect of reducing cholesterol is to change the diagnosis on the gravestone. Instead of dying of CHD, patients on cholesterol-lowering therapy would die of other causes, principally cancer, and, of particular interest because it attracted so much attention in the lay press, suicide or violent deaths.

The fact that the early trials did not have the statistical power to determine effects on overall mortality did not seem to deter the principal protagonists of the 'let's attack the cholesterol story' brigade. The effect on patients was often – as might be expected – very distressing, as various startling headlines appeared in the lay press. This situation was compounded by the fact (still a problem with all the major weekly medical journals) that controversial information becomes available to the lay press prior to receipt of the relevant journal by its subscribers. This led to immense problems during the height of the so-called cholesterol controversy in trying to deal with calls from concerned patients.

This problem is well illustrated by an article in the *British Medical Journal* (*BMJ*) in 1992 entitled 'For debate: should there be a moratorium on the use of cholesterol-lowering drugs?' (Smith and Pekkanen, 1992). A particularly outrageous headline based on this article appeared in *The Guardian* (February 14, 1992): 'Murders Linked to Low Fat Drugs!' Imagine reading that headline if you were a patient on drug therapy. The *BMJ* report was even predicted in *The Sunday Times* the week before publication. Under the headline 'Health Call', it was reported that:

> a moratorium on using cholesterol-lowering drugs is to be urged after evidence that they do not reduce – and may increase – death rates. A study in the *British Medical Journal* by researchers at the London School of Hygiene and Tropical Medicine confirms December's *Sunday Times* report that cutting cholesterol can be bad for you in certain circumstances.

In these circumstances it was difficult for physicians to reassure patients as the relevant *BMJ* issue had not by then reached its subscribers. When debate about important issues in medicine is conducted in this way it is often the headline message that is accepted by the profession as well as the patient.

The controversy arose because the cholesterol-lowering trials lacked the statistical power to provide a definitive analysis of overall mortality. In most trials there was no significant difference in non-CHD deaths (apart from the WHO collaborative trial of clofibrate, discussed later) but there were, literally, one or two more deaths in the drug treatment group from cancer or suicide or violent death – the most likely explanation being a chance effect.

In an attempt to address these possible adverse effects it became fashionable to adopt the technique of meta-analysis which emerged in the 1980s. The potential advantages and disadvantages of this technique are shown in Table 9.1. The application of the technique

TABLE **9.1** • Advantages and disadvantages of meta-analysis (Furberg and Furberg, 1994)

Advantages	Disadvantages
Increased patient numbers and therefore increased statistical power to detect treatment differences	Potential for bias from publication bias and choice of trials for inclusion/exclusion in the analysis
Identification of subgroups who do well (or badly)	*Post hoc* nature of the analysis
A robust test of whether the results can be generalized	'Similar' trials may have important differences, e.g. disease severity; therefore equivalent to combining apples, pears, etc.
Neutralization of extreme results (positive or negative) of individual trials	

Meta-analysis: a pooled analysis that employs formal statistical methods to combine outcome results from clinical trials of particular therapeutic interventions.

(which, by combining the results of similar trials, increases the statistical power for testing a treatment benefit or adverse effect) led to widely different conclusions with regard to the cholesterol story. Meta-analyses particularly highlighted the possibility of increased suicide and violent death in relation to cholesterol lowering (Muldoon *et al.*, 1990; Smith and Pekkanen, 1992). This disturbing claim was reiterated so many times that it was accepted as fact and hypotheses were published to explain the phenomenon. This was irksome to those of us working in the subject because researchers from the Food and Drug Association (FDA) had undertaken a detailed review of such deaths in the two largest trials where there appeared to be an issue and published their findings in 1990 (Wysowski and Gross, 1990).

In the Lipid Research Clinics (LRC) primary prevention trial using the anion exchange resin, cholestyramine (Lipid Research Clinics Programme, 1984), four individuals in the treatment group committed suicide, compared with two taking placebo. Of the four cases (three by gunshot wounds to the head and one by hanging) there was a history in three of tranquillizer use or psychiatric symptoms at entry into the study. Furthermore, three of the cases dropped out of the study. Only one suicide case showed good compliance with the study drug and had no previous history of psychiatric symptoms. In the study as a whole, there were no differences in the incidence of psychiatric symptoms or the use of antidepressants during the trial.

With regard to accidental deaths in the LRC study, there were six in the drug-treated group compared with two on placebo. Alcohol was detected at autopsy in three cases and was a possible factor in two others; also, the nature of some of the accidents suggested intoxication (a head-on collision while using a mobile phone and a single-car accident). Two of the accidents were probably unavoidable – a car driver was hit by a trailer which had broken loose from an oncoming truck and a motor cyclist was struck from behind by a hit-and-run driver. Compliance with the study drug in three of the cases was poor and four had a history of either tranquillizer use or psychiatric symptoms prior to the trial. In the six cases, the average cholesterol was 6.46 mmol/L.

The other trial that contributed to the suicide and violent death controversy was the Helsinki Heart Study (HHS) (Frick *et al.*, 1987) with the fibrate, gemfibrozil. In this study there were four suicides on gemfibrozil and two on placebo. Two cases in the treatment group were study drop-outs. Of the remainder, the mean cholesterol at the last study visit was 6.7 mmol/L. Based on population characteristics, 11 suicides should have been expected during the study and so the frequency of suicide observed was less than expected in both the drug and the placebo groups. There were four fatal accidents in the gemfibrozil group and four in the placebo group. Two of the accident cases were study drop-outs and alcohol was detected at post-mortem examination. In the treatment group, mean cholesterol at the last study visit was 7.2 mmol/L.

Remember the *Guardian* headline about murders? Indeed, there were two murders – one in the LRC study and one in the Helsinki study – but the trial participants were victims, not perpetrators of the crime. It would be interesting to consider the biochemical and cellular mechanisms induced by taking a lipid-lowering drug that are likely to lead to an increased risk of being a murder victim.

The conclusion of the meticulous analysis of Wysowski and Gross (1990) for the FDA on suicide and violent death was that:

> when drop-outs and known risk factors for the deaths such as alcohol intoxication and psychiatric histories are considered, little evidence remains to support the hypothesis that cholesterol-lowering drugs are causally associated with deaths due to homicides, suicides and accidents in these trials.

When the cholesterol-lowering trials were analysed (and up to 1993 there were nearly 50 controlled clinical trials involving approximately 85 000 participants), widely different conclusions were frequently obtained, often when similar data were examined. For instance, Holme (1990) found a strong correlation across the various trials between reductions in cholesterol level and mortality and pointed to the trend for mortality reduction when cholesterol was reduced by over 9 per cent. On the other hand, Ravnskov (1992) concluded that cholesterol lowering was unlikely to lower CHD, let alone overall mortality.

THE 'CHOLESTEROL PAPERS' OF 1994

Fortunately, there were attempts to put the record straight with regard to the cholesterol trials.

In an important contribution that comprised the third of the Cholesterol Papers (see Chapter 2) published in the *British Medical Journal*, Law *et al.* (1994a) examined the possible hazards of reducing serum cholesterol. Previous meta-analyses of selected cholesterol-lowering trials showed an apparent excess of non-CHD deaths, particularly suicides and violent death and possibly cancer. These small excesses, likely to be the play of chance, were nevertheless linked to epidemiological studies that demonstrated an upturn in overall mortality in the lowest part of the cholesterol distribution.

Law and colleagues analysed data from the ten largest cohort studies, two international studies and 28 randomized trials of cholesterol lowering – the mean outcome measure being excess cause-specific mortality with low or lowered cholesterol concentration. Non-CHD deaths were divided into other circulatory diseases, cancer, accidents and suicides, and other causes.

The question whether low cholesterol concentration predisposes to illness or whether low cholesterol is secondary to illness was addressed in an interesting way. The authors divided the available cohorts into those that recruited from employed populations and those that recruited from populations as a whole. The reasonable assumption is that those individuals in employment are on the whole likely to be healthier. No excess mortality was found associated with low cholesterol in cohorts of employed people. On the other hand, there was a significant excess mortality in the community cohorts. Law and colleagues interpreted these findings as evidence that preceding illness was likely to be the explanation for the low cholesterol/non-CHD death association seen in the community cohorts. The authors did find an excess of non-CHD deaths when they analysed the controlled trials but pointed to the difficulties of reaching meaningful conclusions, because of the small number of deaths in the studies, their relatively short duration and the fact that low cholesterol levels were not achieved.

In order further to assess possible hazards due to low cholesterol, they examined data from cohorts and international comparisons. They found no overall excess of cancer deaths in the randomized trials. This finding, together with observations from prospective studies showing that a low cholesterol/cancer association present at baseline and in the early years of follow-up disappeared with continued follow-up, suggests that the association is due to the well-described phenomenon that plasma cholesterol is reduced by cancers. The metabolic basis for this has been studied and increased LDL plasma clearance has been described in patients with malignancy, presumably to provide membrane cholesterol for the proliferating cells.

A difference between the employed and community cohorts was found for accidents and suicides, with a significant excess in the community cohorts in those with the lowest cholesterols (relative risk 1.48). Such an association was not found in the cohorts of employed people and in the international comparisons. The authors' conclusion was that the association could be explained by the plasma cholesterol reduction associated with the anorexia and weight loss of depression. As with the cancer association, the relationship of low cholesterol with suicide disappears after 5 years of follow-up. Importantly, no excess of accidents and suicides was seen overall in the randomized trials.

With regard to circulatory disorders other than CHD, Law and colleagues did conclude that the low cholesterol/haemorrhagic stroke association observed in cohort studies was likely to be causal in the presence of fairly high blood pressure. However, the increased mortality from haemorrhagic stroke is small when compared with the lower CHD mortality. For instance, in the large MRFIT database, mortality from haemorrhagic stroke in men with the lowest cholesterol concentration ($\leqslant 4.14$ mmol/L) was 0.3 per 10 000 man-years higher when compared with that in the next lowest concentration (4.14–15 mmol/L). However, CHD mortality was 3.3 per 10 000 man-years lower. Despite this conclusion, stroke overall in the three subsequent large statin trials (4S, WOSCOPS and CARE) was reduced.

Other-cause mortality (not cancer, accidents and suicides, and non-CHD circulatory disorders) was also investigated. There was a significant excess in the community studies (1.62) but again no excess was observed in the employed cohorts. Excess mortality was mainly related to chronic respiratory disorders and liver and bowel diseases. The authors concluded that the observed association was likely to be explained by the cholesterol-lowering effect of chronic disease. No excess of other-cause mortality was observed in the randomized trials or international comparisons.

There is no doubt that the monumental piece of work by Law and colleagues summarized above did much to reassure physicians about the safety of cholesterol lowering. Their final conclusion merits quoting in full (Law *et al.*, 1994a):

> The evidence is clear: the need is not to repeat research which has already
> been performed but to disseminate results, their interpretation and the

TABLE **9.2** • Meta-analysis of cholesterol-lowering trials (Law *et al.*, 1994a–c): percentage reduction of ischaemic heart disease events in men associated with a 0.6 mmol/L reduction in cholesterol (approximately 10%) by duration of trials. Reproduced with permission from BMJ Publishing Group

Trials	Time since entry to trial		
	<2 years	2.1–5 years	5.1–12 years
	(Percentage reduction in IHD events)		
All drug trials	10	21	22
All dietary trials	9	14	37
Trials of men without known ischaemic heart disease	11	25	24
Trials of men with ischaemic heart disease	6	20	24
All trials (95% confidence)	7 (0–14)	22 (15–28)	25 (15–35)

conclusions so that preventive action can be taken to confer the substantial health benefit of lowering average serum cholesterol concentrations in Western populations.

As well as assessing the potential hazards of low cholesterol and lowering cholesterol, Law and colleagues (1994a–c) provided an overview of cholesterol-lowering trials available up to 1994. The analysis is shown in Table 9.2. It concerned 28 randomized trials involving 46 254 men with 4241 reported CHD events. The trials chosen were randomized and controlled; they involved lipid lowering with diet and drugs and one trial of surgical intervention by partial ileal bypass. All the trials documented at least one death and were associated with a cholesterol reduction of at least 1 per cent. Trials that used what transpired to be noxious agents (oestrogen in men, and *d*-thyroxine) and that intervened on multiple risk factors were omitted.

The trials adopted similar diagnostic criteria for non-fatal myocardial infarction and CHD death and the assessment of these events was blinded as to treatment. All trials were analysed by intention to treat – that is, on the basis of the allocated treatment whether or not the treatment was actually taken. This is important to avoid bias.

As can be seen, the trials were analysed according to the nature of the intervention (diet or drug), the study population (with and without existing symptomatic coronary heart disease) and the duration of the trials. The results of meta-analysis were expressed as CHD risk reduction associated with a reduction of serum cholesterol concentration of 0.6 mmol/L. This figure was chosen because it represents approximately 10 per cent of the average cholesterol concentrations seen in Western countries.

As might be expected, the observed benefit of cholesterol lowering increased with increasing duration of cholesterol reduction and overall there was a highly significant reduction in non-fatal (21 per cent; $P < 0.001$) events and also in CHD death (10 per cent; $P = 0.004$) for a 0.6 mmol/L cholesterol reduction. Most trials excluded women but the small amount of data available from three of the trials that did include women showed significant reduction in CHD events of similar magnitude to that for men (Law *et al.*, 1994b).

PRIMARY PREVENTION TRIALS ▰▰▰▰▰▰▰

EARLY TRIALS

When these trials are critically evaluated, there is no doubt that they illustrate a learning curve with regard to the design, conduct, statistical analysis and reporting of clinical trials. Defects in clinical trial technology in the past have contributed to the cholesterol controversy.

It is important for the individual physician to be in a position to evaluate published trials. This skill was not taught when the authors were at medical school. Fortunately, this particular inadequacy has since been remedied and considerable attention is now paid to the design and evaluation of clinical trials in undergraduate clinical pharmacology courses. Nevertheless, it is worth a little general revision.

The writings of the Furbergs (Bengt and Curt) on the subject of clinical trials are thoroughly recommended – in particular, a book entitled *All That Glitters is not Gold: What clinicians need to know about clinical trials* (published by Dr Potata, Winston-Salem, USA, 1994). A distillation of what the Furbergs refer to as the 'road map for reading trial results' is shown in Table 9.3.

TABLE **9.3** • 'Road map' for evaluating clinical trial reports according to Furberg and Furberg (1994)

■ Is the scientific question clearly stated and are the results important to my patients and clinical practice?
■ What were the selection criteria and are they applicable to my patients?
■ Were the dosing and treatment periods adequate?
■ Was the trial of sufficient size to allow the detection of moderate but clinically meaningful differences?
■ Were the placebo and treated groups well matched at baseline and were data on concomitant other therapies and diseases described?
■ To minimize potential bias:
  – Was treatment allocation randomized and double-blind?
  – Was the assessment of treatment outcomes blinded to treatment groups?
■ Were all randomized patients accounted for in the final analysis?
■ Are the negative effects of the treatment thoroughly documented?
■ Are the results consistent with other similar, well conducted studies?
■ Do the benefits outweigh the risks and associated costs?
■ Are the authors sufficiently independent of any potential conflicts of interest that could cast doubt on the objectivity of the trial?

With regard to the cholesterol-lowering trials the principal defects over the years have been:

■ lack of statistical power to test effects on CHD death or overall mortality;
■ lack of effective intervention, leading to small differences in cholesterol between treated and placebo groups;
■ small numbers of observed CHD events and death due to exclusion of high-risk patients.

In the overview of the cholesterol-lowering trials by Law *et al.* (1994b), it is clear that the early primary prevention trials do demonstrate a significant reduction in CHD events. However, no reduction – or even a slight excess – of non-CHD events was observed. The increase in non-CHD deaths was not due to any particular cause. This fits with the hazards analysis by the same authors, which examined not only the trials but also international comparisons and cohort studies. The significant overall increase in non-CHD deaths in the early trials appeared for the most part to be due to the first fibrate drug, clofibrate, and the hormone trials (oestrogen and *d*-thyroxine) (Law *et al.*, 1994a).

It was the WHO clofibrate trial that was mainly responsible for the excess non-CHD deaths in the drug trials (Committee of Principal Investigators, 1978). In this trial the excess mortality was attributed to cancer and hepatobiliary disease. It is known that clofibrate increases the lithogenicity of bile and therefore gallstone formation. For this reason the drug is now largely redundant. Several of the deaths in the WHO trial were indeed associated with gallbladder surgery. This trial will be described in detail later.

Some of the major primary prevention trials using diet and drug therapy are discussed here to provide a flavour of the trials and to provide the background for the landmark trials using statins.

OSLO STUDY

The Oslo study (Table 9.4a) is a particularly attractive trial in the sense that it took as its study population a group of men considered to be at high CHD risk because of hypercholesterolaemia and intervened with dietary and anti-smoking advice – therapeutic options that are still first line for most physicians (Hjermann *et al.*, 1981). More than 16 000 men (aged 40–49 years) were screened for possible inclusion in this 5-year randomized trial and 1232 asymptomatic men were selected with total serum cholesterol concentrations of 7.5–9.8 mmol/L. Eighty per cent were smokers.

The 604 men randomly allocated to the treatment arm of the study were prescribed a cholesterol-lowering diet and were given anti-smoking advice. Over the course of the study there was an approximately 13 per cent reduction in serum cholesterol and a 45 per cent reduction in tobacco consumption. At the end of the study, 25 per cent of men had stopped cigarette smoking compared with 17 per cent in the non-intervention group.

Over the 5-year course of the study there was a 47 per cent reduction in the combined endpoint of fatal and non-fatal myocardial infarction and sudden death in the intervention group compared with the control group ($P = 0.028$). Two-thirds of this benefit was attributed to cholesterol reduction. Follow-up of the study participants at 42 months after the end of the trial showed a 40 per cent reduction in overall mortality, which was marginally significant.

The results of the Oslo study confirmed those of earlier dietary intervention trials, such as the Los Angeles Veterans Study (Dayton *et al.*, 1969) (Table 9.4b) and the Finnish

TABLE **9.4** • Primary prevention trials

(a) Oslo Primary Prevention Trial (Hjermann *et al.*, 1981)	(b) Los Angeles Veterans Study (Dayton *et al.*, 1969)	(c) Finnish Mental Hospitals Study (Turpeinen, 1979)
Study participants: men aged 40–49 years (*n* = 1232) with hypercholesterolaemia (≥7.5 mmol/L; 80% were smokers	Study participants: men, mean age ~ 65 years, (*n* = 846) resident in a Veterans Administration Hospital	Study participants: inpatients of two mental hospitals in Helsinki
Five-year randomized trial of cholesterol-lowering diet and anti-smoking advice	Eight-year randomized double-blind study of usual diet vs. modified fat diet (PS ratio 2.0)	Cross-over study of cholesterol-lowering, modified fat diet vs. usual diet. One group received experimental diet for 6 years and the other the usual diet and then changed over
In the intervention group, serum cholesterol was reduced by 13% and tobacco consumption fell by 65%. In the intervention group, 25% quit cigarette smoking, compared with 17% in the control group	Mean reduction in total serum cholesterol 13% on experimental diet	CHD deaths (experimental vs. usual diet): 3.0 vs. 6.1 per 1000 man-years (NS); CHD disease plus major ECG changes 4.2 vs. 12.7 per 1000 4.2 vs. 12.7 per 1000 man-years (*P* < 0.001)

Endpoint effects (number of episodes):

	Control (*n* = 628)	(*n* = 604)
Coronary heart disease	36	19*
All cardiovascular disease	39	22*
Total cardiovascular death	15	8
Sudden death	11	3*
Total deaths	24	16

Results (experimental vs. usual diet, *P* < 0.05): CHD deaths, 48 vs. 70; Atherosclerotic events, 66 vs. 96

Benefits greatest in younger men and those with higher cholesterol levels

Increase in non-cardiovascular deaths

This type of diet not now used

Confounding factors: patients were receiving a variety of psychotropic drugs; patients discharged from hospital were lost to the trial; patients admitted during the trial were enrolled

Applicability to 'free living' people

No excess of non-cardiovascular deaths

Mental Hospitals study (Turpeinen, 1979; Table 9.4c) which pointed to the potential benefit of the lipid-lowering diet. The Oslo study had the great advantage of a free-living population, as opposed to institutionalized participants in the other two studies.

WHO COOPERATIVE TRIAL OF CLOFIBRATE

This trial was the first major primary prevention trial of drug therapy and was initiated in the mid-1960s in three major European cities – Budapest, Edinburgh and Prague (Committee of Principal Investigators, 1978). About 30 000 men (aged 30–59 years) were screened for possible inclusion in the trial. Approximately 10 000 men whose cholesterol fell in the upper third of the distribution were randomly allocated to double-blind treatment with either clofibrate, 1.6 g/day (*n* = 5331), or placebo capsules containing olive oil (*n* = 5296).

Over the course of the study (5.3 years) clofibrate therapy was associated with a net cholesterol reduction of 8 per cent (the baseline cholesterol was $\cong 6.4$ mmol/L) and this was associated with an overall reduction in CHD events (167 events on clofibrate versus 207 on placebo), mainly attributable to a 25 per cent reduction in non-fatal events. There was no significant reduction in fatal events, though this would be difficult to show as the incidence of fatal infarction was very low at 0.7 per cent.

The favourable effect of clofibrate on CHD events was overshadowed by an increase in total deaths in the clofibrate-treated group (162 on clofibrate versus 127 on placebo). This was due to an increase in non-CHD deaths (94 versus 65) with no difference in CHD deaths (68 versus 62). It is important to note that no particular cause of death was found to be in excess. However, the causes of death relating to 'liver, gallbladder and intestines' and the increased frequency of cholecystectomy are likely to relate to the biliary lithogenic effect of clofibrate.

Withdrawals from the clofibrate group during the trial were more frequent than those from the placebo group (346 versus 327). Gallstone operations, weight gain, indigestion, diarrhoea, diabetes and impotence were significantly more frequent in the clofibrate group.

The design of the WHO trial has been much criticized, particularly with regard to the analysis of the mortality data. The study design did not allow for in-trial results to be presented on an intention-to-treat analysis. Furthermore, the out-of-trial mortality follow-up data were incomplete. Taking this into account, there is no doubt that the most reliable data from the study related to the numbers of non-fatal myocardial infarction as participants were withdrawn from the trial after these events. The principal investigators of the WHO Cooperative study did publish later an intention-to-treat analysis of the results (Heady et al., 1992). This analysis still showed an excess of non-cardiac deaths without any significant excess of particular causes of death. In relation to the excess non-CHD deaths in this study, it is worth considering the other large clofibrate trial, which formed one treatment arm of the Coronary Drug Project (CDP) secondary prevention trial (Coronary Drug Project Research Group, 1975). In the clofibrate group there was no significant increase in non-CHD mortality during 6 years of study.

LIPID RESEARCH CLINICS (LRC) CORONARY PRIMARY PREVENTION TRIAL (CPPT)

This large, well-designed trial was reported in 1984 (Lipid Research Clinics Programme, 1984) and its results prompted guidelines to be drawn up in the USA for the treatment of hypercholesterolaemia for the prevention of CHD.

The study population consisted of asymptomatic men aged 35–59 years with a cholesterol level greater than the 95th centile for the US population, approximately 6.8 mmol/L. The average baseline concentration was 7.5 mmol/L and individuals with triglyceride concentrations greater than 3.4 mmol/L were excluded.

A total of 3806 men were recruited and randomly allocated to the anion-exchange resin cholestyramine (24 g/day; $n = 1906$) or placebo ($n = 1900$). In addition to the study medication, all participants received lipid-lowering dietary advice, which produced a mean cholesterol reduction of 4 per cent.

Over the study period (mean follow-up 7.4 years) the net fall in serum cholesterol in the cholestyramine group compared with placebo was 9 per cent and for LDL cholesterol 13 per cent (Table 9.5). The power of the study was based on a 25 per cent reduction in serum cholesterol in the treated group but was not achieved because of compliance problems with the resin, which is difficult to take. Therefore, the power of the study was reduced. Nevertheless, there was a significant reduction in the primary endpoint of the study (definite CHD event – fatal or non-fatal), with 155 events in the cholestyramine group versus 187 events in the placebo group ($P < 0.05$).

TABLE **9.5** • Primary and secondary endpoints of Lipid Research Clinics (LRC) Coronary Primary Prevention Study

Endpoint	Placebo ($n = 1900$)		Cholestyramine ($n = 1906$)		Risk reduction (%)
	No.	%	No.	%	
(a) Primary endpoints					
Definite CHD death and/or definite non-fatal infarction	187*	9.8	155*	8.1	19
Definite or suspect CHD death or non-fatal infarction	256*	13.5	222*	11.6	15
All-cause mortality	71	3.7	68	3.6	7
(b) Secondary endpoints					
CHD:					
Positive exercise test	345	19.8*	260	14.9*	25*
Angina	287	15.1*	235	12.4*	20*
Coronary bypass surgery	112	5.9	93	4.9	21*
Congestive heart failure	11	0.6	8	0.4	28
Intraoperative myocardial infarction	7	0.4	5	0.3	29
Resuscitated coronary collapse	5	0.3	3	0.2	40
Cerebrovascular disease:					
Definite or suspect transient ischaemia attack	22	1.2	18	0.9	18
Definite or suspect atherothrombotic brain infarction	14	0.7	17	0.9	+21
Peripheral vascular disease:					
Intermittent claudication	84	4.4*	72	3.8*	15

*Statistically significant.
Study participants: men aged 35–59 years with primary hypercholesterolaemia; 7.4-year randomized controlled trial of cholestyramine, 24 g/day ($n = 1906$) vs. placebo ($n = 1900$), both groups receiving cholesterol-lowering diet. In treated group, net reduction of serum cholesterol = 9% and of LDL-C = 13%.
Source: Lipid Research Clinics Program (1984), *J Am Med Assoc* **251**, 351.

TABLE **9.6** • Compliance with cholestyramine and reduction of serum cholesterol: relationship to CHD risk

Packet count	No.	Total cholesterol and reduction	CHD events (% reduction)
0–2	439	4.4	10.9
2–5	496	11.5	26.1
5–6	965	19.0	39.3

Source: Lipid Research Clinics Program (1984), *J Am Med Assoc* **251**, 351.

The principal finding is supported by other data from the study, which show a pleasing consistency in relation to cholesterol lowering with cholestyramine. For instance, other secondary CHD endpoints showed similar reductions (Table 9.5) Furthermore, because of the variation in compliance already mentioned, it was possible to examine the relationship between the degree of LDL lowering and CHD events (Table 9.6). The one-third of individuals with LDL cholesterol reductions of more than 25 per cent showed a 64 per cent reduction in myocardial infarction.

There was no difference in overall mortality (68 deaths in the cholestyramine group versus 71 deaths in the placebo group). There was no difference in cancer deaths. As discussed elsewhere, some commentators made much of the small, non-significant excess of deaths from accidents and violence (11 on cholestyramine versus 4 on placebo).

Adverse effects encountered during the study were predictably (given the drug used) related to the gastrointestinal tract. In the first year, gastrointestinal symptoms were reported in 64 per cent of participants on cholestyramine compared with 43 per cent on placebo.

HELSINKI HEART STUDY (HHS)

This major primary prevention trial (Frick *et al.*, 1987) differs from the LRC trial in several respects. First, the trial drug used, gemfibrozil, is a second-generation fibrate and second, the lipid entry criteria (non-HDL cholesterol $\geqslant 5.2$ mmol/L) led to inclusion of individuals with lipoprotein phenotypes (28 per cent IIb; 9 per cent IV) (see Table 3.1) other than isolated hypercholesterolaemia (63 per cent IIa). Baseline lipid concentrations were: total cholesterol 6.9 mmol/L, total triglyceride 2.0 mmol/L and HDL cholesterol 1.2 mmol/L.

All participants (men aged 40–55 years) were advised on a lipid-lowering diet and 2051 men were randomly allocated to gemfibrozil (1.2 g/day) and 2031 to placebo. The lipid changes achieved in the study are shown in Table 9.7. Not surprisingly, these changes were in part dependent on the lipoprotein phenotype – apart from the increase in HDL cholesterol, which was roughly equivalent.

After a mean 5-year follow-up period, there was a significant 35 per cent reduction in the primary study endpoint of combined non-fatal and fatal myocardial infarction

TABLE **9.7** • Helsinki Heart Study (Frick *et al.*, 1987)

Study participants:
 men aged 40–55 years ($n = 4082$)
 with non-HDL-C $\geqslant 5.2$ mmol/L;
 63% were Type IIa, 28% Type IIb and 9% Type IV

Five-year randomized trial of gemfibrozil (1200 mg/day) vs. placebo

Lipid and lipoprotein changes in the gemfibrozil-treated group ($n = 2051$):
 Cholesterol   10% net reduction
 LDL-C   11% net reduction
 Triglyceride   35% net reduction
 HDL-C   11% net increase

Major endpoint: a combination of fatal and non-fatal myocardial
 infarction – 54 treated vs. 84 placebo ($P < 0.02$).

No difference in overall mortality:
 45 deaths on gemfibrozil
 42 deaths on placebo

(56 events on gemfibrozil versus 84 on placebo). As in the LRC study, there was no difference in overall mortality (45 deaths on gemfibrozil versus 42 deaths on placebo). However, as discussed elsewhere, the study did not have the statistical power to determine effects on mortality. Cancer deaths were identical (11 versus 11) and there was a non-significant excess of deaths from accidents and violence in the gemfibrozil group (5 versus 1).

Adverse effects in the gemfibrozil group during the study period were mainly related to the gastrointestinal tract (11 per cent versus 7 per cent). Of particular interest, in view of the findings of the WHO clofibrate study, was the incidence of gallbladder surgery. There were 18 operations in the gemfibrozil group compared with 12 in the placebo group, which did not reach statistical significance.

In multivariate regression analysis, the benefit observed in the HHS was related to both the reduction in LDL cholesterol and the increase in HDL cholesterol. In an interesting *post hoc* analysis it was found that much of the benefit of gemfibrozil occurred in individuals with cholesterol/HDL cholesterol ratios greater than 5 who were also hypertriglyceridaemic. This is discussed on page 217.

THE STATIN PRIMARY PREVENTION TRIALS

WEST OF SCOTLAND CORONARY PREVENTION STUDY (WOSCOPS)

This landmark study (Shepherd *et al.*, 1995) largely overcame the design defects in earlier primary prevention trials and provides invaluable assistance in assessing CHD risk in middle-aged men, allowing the targeting of drug treatment to those at higher risk.

The design of WOSCOPS (West of Scotland Coronary Prevention Study Group, 1992) built on the information available from the LRC and HHS studies. It was designed to have the statistical power to address the question of cholesterol lowering and the prevention of coronary events (combined incidence of non-fatal myocardial infarction and death from CHD). In order to achieve this, it was necessary to study a population with a higher event rate and to increase the sample size. In addition, with the advent of the statin class of drugs, it was possible to use a more powerful and better-tolerated drug.

Approximately 160 000 men were invited to attend cholesterol screening sessions in general practices in the West of Scotland district for possible inclusion in the trial and 81 161 attended. Of these, those whose non-fasting plasma cholesterol (using the Reflotron bench-top analyser) was greater than 6.5 mmol/L were given lipid-lowering dietary advice and asked to reattend 4 weeks later. At the second visit, 20 914 men had a fasting lipid profile. At this occasion, if LDL cholesterol was at least 4.0 mmol/L and there were no exclusion criteria, individuals were recalled after a further 4 weeks of diet. At the third visit, which involved 13 654 men, a further lipoprotein profile was performed together with an electrocardiogram. At the fourth visit, randomization to trial drug (pravastatin, 40 mg daily) or placebo was performed if:

■ fasting LDL cholesterol was at least 4.0 mmol/L, with one value of at least 4.5 mmol/L and one value below 6.0 mmol/L;
■ there were no serious ECG abnormalities;
■ there was no history of myocardial infarction.

The 6595 study participants were seen at 3-monthly intervals during the study, with a fasting lipid profile every 6 months and a physical examination every year. The mean study period was 4.9 years, providing 32 216 subject-years of follow-up.

The effects of pravastatin on LDL cholesterol achieved during the study are shown in Figure 9.1 both on an intention-to-treat and actual treatment basis.

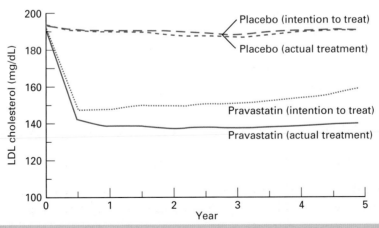

FIGURE **9.1** • Effects of pravastatin therapy on plasma LDL cholesterol concentrations in the West of Scotland Coronary Prevention Study (to convert values for cholesterol to mmol/L, multiply by 0.026). Source: Shepherd *et al.* (1995).

The primary endpoint of the study – death from CHD and definite non-fatal myocardial infarction – showed a 31 per cent reduction (95 per cent confidence intervals, 17–43 per cent; $P < 0.001$) in the pravastatin group as compared with placebo. This result and effects on other secondary endpoints are shown in Table 9.8. It can be seen that there was a significant reduction in CHD deaths and, importantly, this was not accompanied by an increase in non-cardiovascular deaths in the pravastatin group (56 versus 62), such that overall mortality was also reduced. There were 116 individuals with cancer (fatal and non-fatal) in the pravastatin compared with 106 in the placebo group.

Pravastatin therapy was well tolerated with little difference from the placebo group for myalgia or muscle pains. Four subjects (three pravastatin, one placebo) had asymptomatic episodes of high CPK levels ($\geqslant 10$ times normal). There were no cases of rhabdomyolysis and no significant differences in liver function tests between the pravastatin and placebo groups.

It is of interest that the same percentage benefits of pravastatin were seen whether or not LDL cholesterol or HDL cholesterol or triglyceride was above or below the median

TABLE **9.8** • West of Scotland Coronary Prevention Study – results (Shepherd *et al.*, 1995)

Events and causes	Placebo ($n = 3293$)	Pravastatin ($n = 3302$)	P	Risk reduction % (95% CI)
Definite coronary events				
Non-fatal MI or CHD death	248	174	<0.001	31 (17–43)
Non-fatal MI	204	143	<0.001	31 (15–45)
CHD death	52	38	0.13	28 (−10–52)
Other events				
Coronary angiography	128	90	0.007	31 (10–47)
PTCA or CABG	80	51	0.009	37 (11–56)
Fatal or non-fatal stroke	51	46	0.57	11 (−33–40)
Incident cancer	106	116	0.55	−8 (−41–17)
Death from other causes				
Other cardiovascular causes, including stroke	12	9	–	–
Suicide	1	2	–	–
Trauma	5	3	–	–
Cancer	49	44	0.56	11 (−33–41)
All other causes	7	7	–	–
Deaths from all cardiovascular causes	73	50	0.033	32 (3–53)
Deaths from non-cardiovascular causes	62	56	0.54	11 (−28–38)
Deaths from any cause	135	106	0.051	22 (0–40)

for the group. Furthermore, similar benefits were seen in smokers versus non-smokers; those aged less than 55 years compared with those older than 55 years; and those with multiple risk factors versus those without other risk factors.

This landmark trial has answered important questions on the benefit of lowering cholesterol in the prevention of CHD. This can be done safely with pravastatin and what is now needed is to identify a risk score for patients based on the WOSCOPS data which will identify those at higher risk, so that therapy can be targeted on a cost-effective basis.

AIR FORCE/TEXAS CORONARY ATHEROSCLEROSIS PREVENTION STUDY (AFCAPS/TEXCAPS)

This important study is complementary to WOSCOPs and extends the evidence base for primary prevention of CHD. Whereas WOSCOPs recruited hypercholesterolaemic middle-aged men, AFCAPS/TexCAPS recruited healthy men and women with average total and LDL cholesterol levels and below average HDL cholesterol levels (Table 9.9). The trial addressed the issue of the potential benefits of statin therapy in a healthy population (Downs *et al.*, 1998).

The study population consisted of 6605 healthy men ($n = 5608$; age 45–75 years) and women ($n = 997$; age 55–73 years), mean age 58 years, with no clinical evidence of CHD. Indeed, according to the NCEP guidelines current when the trial was planned, only 17 per cent of the cohort would have fulfilled criteria (LDL cholesterol concentrations plus other risk factors) for lipid-lowering treatment. Lipid and lipoprotein entry criteria are shown in Table 9.9. Baseline LDL cholesterol was 150 mg/dL (3.89 mmol/L) and HDL cholesterol 36.4 mg/dL (0.94 mmol/L). All participants received low-fat, low-cholesterol

TABLE **9.9** • AFCAPS/TexCAPS

Study design	Randomized, double-blind, placebo-controlled Lovastatin (20–40 mg/day) versus placebo
Study population	5608 men (age 45–73 years) and 997 postmenopausal women (55–73 years) with no evidence of vascular disease
Lipid entry criteria	Total cholesterol 4.65–6.83 mmol/L LDL-C 3.36–4.91 mmol/L HDL-C ≤ 1.16 mmol/L in men, < 1.22 mmol/L in women
Primary endpoints	Non-fatal myocardial infarction, sudden cardiac death, CHD death, and unstable angina
Baseline lipids (% change at 1 year) with lovastatin	Total cholesterol 5.71 mmol/L (−18%) Total triglyceride 1.84 mmol/L (−15%) LDL-C 3.88 mmol/L (−25%) HDL-C 0.96 mmol/L (+6%)
Average follow-up	5.2 years

dietary advice together with lovastatin 20–40 mg/day or placebo on a randomized, double-blind basis. The primary endpoint was the incidence of first acute major coronary event, combination of fatal and non-fatal myocardial infarction, sudden cardiac death and the development of unstable angina. This was a treat-to-target study and the starting dose of lovastatin could be increased to 40 mg/day to achieve an LDL cholesterol of <110 mg/dL (<2.9 mmol/L); approximately half the cohort needed the 40 mg dose and the mean daily dose was 30 mg/day. The goal of therapy was achieved only in 42.5 per cent. Lovastatin therapy was associated with a 25 per cent reduction in LDL cholesterol, a 6 per cent increase in HDL cholesterol and a 15 per cent reduction in triglyceride.

The primary endpoint of the study showed a relative risk reduction of 0.63 (95 per cent CI 0.50–0.79) in the lovastatin-treated group ($P < 0.001$) after 5.2 years of follow-up (Figure 9.2). Indeed, the trial was terminated early on efficacy grounds by the Data and Safety Monitoring Board following the second interim analysis (based on 267 events). Effects on the secondary endpoints were significant, with reductions in fatal/non-fatal myocardial infarction (35 per cent), unstable angina (34 per cent) and revascularization procedures (33 per cent). Treatment effects were consistent across population subgroups including women (−54 per cent), the elderly (−29 per cent), hypertensives (−43 per cent) and smokers (−59 per cent). Benefits were apparent across baseline tertiles of LDL cholesterol concentrations.

This important, well-conducted study complements and extends the information available from WOSCOPS on the benefits of statins to individuals (including women) with relatively normal cholesterol levels but with moderately low HDL cholesterol values. In addition, the trial provided substantial further safety and tolerability data for lovastatin with a very low rate of drug discontinuation for adverse events. The authors estimated that approximately 8 million Americans would fulfil the entry criteria for

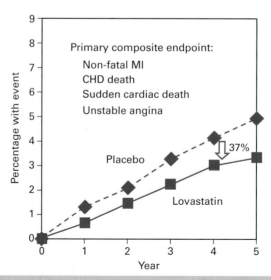

FIGURE **9.2** • AFCAPS/TexCAPS results.

AFCAPS/TexCAPS. Clearly, however, implementation of treatment strategies for primary prevention of necessity needs to take account of cost-benefit considerations.

SECONDARY PREVENTION TRIALS

There is now overwhelming clinical trial evidence to justify aggressive lipid lowering in individuals with established CHD. Unfortunately, as the results of recent audits confirm, much still needs to be done to ensure that all patients have the opportunity to benefit clinically from current knowledge.

In this section, an overview of the evidence linking cholesterol to outcome in those with manifest disease is provided. The exciting findings of the angiographic and clinical events trials that have 'closed the loop' and demonstrated unequivocal benefits are described.

Perhaps the early indication from trials such as the CDP that the degree of myocardial infarction is the major determinant of outcome post-infarction led to an impression that other factors, including cholesterol, were of little prognostic importance. There is no doubt of the importance of myocardial damage, particularly in the short term, but many studies in different populations have demonstrated that cholesterol is an important independent determinant of outcome in the long term.

Data from the LRC follow-up study (Pekkanen *et al.*, 1990) are shown in Figure 9.3. Increasing LDL cholesterol concentrations and decreasing HDL cholesterol concentrations are associated with risk of coronary death over 10 years of observation in men aged 40–69 years, both with and without clinical CHD. However, the observed relationships are stronger in CHD patients. For instance, LDL cholesterol concentrations greater than 4.1 mmol/L are associated with a sixfold increased risk compared with concentrations of less than 3.4 mmol/L in patients with CHD. Similar findings have been reported from the Framingham study (Wong *et al.*, 1991), where information is also

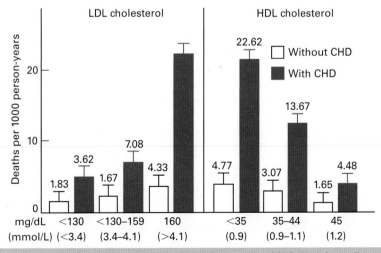

FIGURE **9.3** • Lipid Research Clinics Follow-up Study. Relative risk of CHD death (age-adjusted) in men (40–69 years) in relation to LDL and HDL cholesterol. Source: Pekkanen *et al.* (1990).

available on women. Cholesterol levels greater than 7 mmol/L were associated with a ninefold increased CHD risk in women and a threefold increased risk in men compared with levels of less than 5 mmol/L. In addition, all-cause mortality doubled with high cholesterol concentrations.

The potential for benefit of cholesterol reduction from observation studies such as the LRC and CDP is clear, as discussed by Rossouw *et al.* (1990) in an important overview in the *New England Journal of Medicine*. This article also provided a meta-analysis of lipid-lowering secondary prevention trials available up to that date. Using data from the LRC study, it was calculated that if all the benefits could be obtained by reducing cholesterol from above 6.2 mmol/L (10-year CHD death risk, 170 per 1000) to below 5.2 mmol/L (16 per 1000) the potential saving of CHD death would be 154 per 1000. Obviously this presupposes that cholesterol lowering with diet or hypolipidaemic drugs, or both, would indeed deliver such a benefit. This can only be determined from controlled clinical trials.

EARLY TRIALS

Early secondary prevention trials suffered from many of the deficiencies discussed at the beginning of this section. Rossouw and colleagues set various criteria for inclusion of trials in their meta-analysis: at least 100 subjects in each treatment arm; a duration of at least 3 years; randomized assignment to treatment; no confounding due to treatment of other risk factors and no trials which used compounds that were subsequently shown to be toxic, such as *d*-thyroxine and oestrogen (Rossouw *et al.*, 1990).

Baseline mean total cholesterol concentration varied between 6.3 and 7.6 mmol/L. Patients, on the whole, were not entered into the trials until at least 3 months following myocardial infarction. This is an important consideration, as early deaths due to severe myocardial damage would confound treatment effects due to cholesterol lowering.

The results of the meta-analysis are shown in Figure 9.4. Despite the fact that treatment differences were small due to the lack of efficacy or poor tolerability of early drugs (e.g. clofibrate and nicotinic acid) and the use of dietary therapy alone, there was a highly significant reduction in coronary death and non-fatal CHD events. Furthermore, there did not appear to be any excess of non-cardiovascular death.

ANGIOGRAPHIC TRIALS

With improvement in angiographic methods for visualizing the coronary arteries and the standardization of these techniques, it has become possible to assess the effect of lipid-lowering therapy on progression and regression of individual coronary artery atherosclerotic plaques. Early studies used a panel of radiologists (blinded to the treatment arm) to score angiograms. More recent studies have used sophisticated computerized techniques, which allow increased measurement precision.

Angiographic trials have provided a useful means of assessing the benefits of cholesterol lowering as they can be performed in a relatively short time (2–4 years) and on smaller numbers of patients than are required when clinical endpoints are studied.

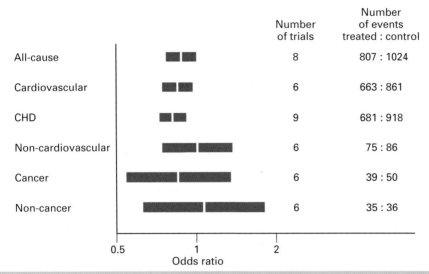

	Number of trials	Number of events treated : control
All-cause	8	807 : 1024
Cardiovascular	6	663 : 861
CHD	9	681 : 918
Non-cardiovascular	6	75 : 86
Cancer	6	39 : 50
Non-cancer	6	35 : 36

FIGURE 9.4 • Meta-analysis of early secondary prevention trials: CHD mortality and other-cause mortality. Sources: Rossouw *et al.* (1990) *N Engl J Med* **323**, 1112 and (1991) *N Engl J Med* **325**, 1813.

The most often quoted measurements in angiographic trials are the minimum lumen diameter and the percentage stenosis. Early angiographic trials are summarized in Table 9.10. To give a flavour of these trials, some of them are discussed in more detail illustrating dietary, combined drug and single drug regimens.

Diet and lifestyle angiographic trials

The Leiden Intervention Trial (LIT) published in 1985 was the first to use quantitative coronary angiography (Barth *et al.*, 1987). This was an uncontrolled study of a low-fat diet (P/S ratio ⩾ 2, dietary cholesterol, 100 mg) plus increased exercise (brisk walking for 20 minutes, three times per week) for 2 years in 39 CHD patients with greater than 50 per cent stenosis in at least one coronary artery. The mean baseline cholesterol was 6.9 mmol/L and LDL cholesterol fell by approximately 10 per cent during the trial period whilst HDL cholesterol increased by 4 per cent. Although these lipoprotein changes were only modest, 46 per cent of patients showed no new lesion growth at 2 years. Regression was seen in compliant individuals who showed a significant decrease in the LDL cholesterol/HDL cholesterol ratio.

Diet and lifestyle effects have also been studied in the St Thomas Atherosclerosis Regression Study (STARS) (Watts *et al.*, 1992), the Lifestyle Heart Trial (LHT) (Ornish *et al.*, 1990) and the small Heidelberg study (Hambrecht *et al.*, 1993). The intervention adopted in the LHT study of 96 subjects with symptomatic CHD was a very low-fat (<7 per cent total calories) and cholesterol (12 mg/day) diet together with behavioural modification – yoga, exercise and advice against smoking. Although 96 patients were originally recruited, only 48 completed the study; of these, 41 (22 intervention group and 19 controls) had analysable angiographic film pairs – this is an obvious criticism of the study. Nevertheless, a substantial reduction was observed in LDL

TABLE **9.10** • Summary of early angiographic trials

(a) Summary descriptions for nine reported angiographic lipid-lowering trials: lipid response to treatments

Study	n	Entry requirements	Control regimen[a]	Treatment Regimen	Response		Years
					LDL	HDL	
NHLBI II	143	CAD,LDLD	D	D + R	−31%	+8%	5
CLAS I	188	CABG	D (−)	D + R + N	−43%	+37%	2
POSCH	838	MI,CHOL	D	D + PIB ± R	−42%	+5%	9.7
Lifestyle	48	CAD	U	V + M + E	−37%	−3%	1
FATS (N + C)	146	CAD,Apo B	D + R	D + R + N	−32%	+43%	2.5
FATS (L + C)				D + R + L	−46%	+15%	2.5
CLAS II	138	CABG	D	D + R + N	−40%	+37%	4
UC-SCOR	97	FH	U	D + R + N ± L	−39%	+25%	2
STARS (D)	90	CAD,CHOL	U	D	−16%	0%	3
STARS (D + R)				D + R	−36%	−4%	3
SCRIP	300	CAD	U	D + (R/N/L/F/) + E,BP	−21%	+13%	4
Heidelberg	113	CAD	U	D + E	−8%	+3%	1

(b) Summary of arteriographic outcomes and frequencies of reported clinical events in nine lipid-lowering angiographic trials

Study	Control patients			Treatment patients			% 'Event' reduction[c]
	Progression (%)	Regression (%)	Δ (%S)[b]	Progression (%)	Regression (%)	Δ %S(P)	
NHLBI[II]	49	7	–	32	7	–	33%
CLAS	61	2	–	39	16	–	25%
POSCH (5 years)	65	6	–	37	14	–	35% (62%)*
Lifestyle	32	32	+3.4	14	41	−2.2 (0.001)	0 vs. 1
FATS (N + C)	46	11	+2.1	25	39	−0.9 (0.005)	80%*
FATS (L + C)				22	32	−0.7 (0.02)	70%
CLASII	83	6	–	30	18	–	43%
UC-SCOR	41	13	+0.8	20	33	−1.5 (0.04)	1 vs. 0
STARS (D)	46	4	+5.8	15	38	−1.1 (NS)	69%*
STARS (D + R)				12	33	−1.9 (0.01)	89%
SCRIP	–	10	–	–	21	–	50%
Heidelberg	42	4	+3.0	20	30	−1.0 (0.05)	
	53	8		26	26		

Apo B, apolipoprotein B ≤125 mg/dL; BP, blood pressure therapy; C, colestipol; CABG, coronary artery bypass graft surgery; CAD, coronary artery disease; CHOL, cholesterol >220 mg/dL; D, diet; E, exercise programme; F, fibrate-type drugs; FH, familial hypercholesterolaemia; HDL, high density lipoprotein; L, lovastatin; LDL, low density lipoprotein >90th percentile; M, relaxation techniques; MI, myocardial infarction; N, nicotinic acid; PIB, partial ileal bypass; R, resin (colestipol or cholestyramine); U, usual care; V, vegetarian diet <10% fat.

[a] Mean LDL-C response to control regimen, −7%; mean HDL-C response, 0%.

[b] Δ (%S) is usually reported as the average change in percentage stenosis over all the lesions measured per patient. A positive (+) value represents 'progression', negative (−) regression.

[c] Events are variably defined in these studies; in general, the frequency of cardiovascular events (death, myocardial infarction, unstable ischaemia requiring revascularization) in control and treated groups are compared using the sometimes sketchy details and definitions provided. Statistical comparison uses a lesion-based method.

*Studies for which the reduction in cardiovascular clinical events was statistically significant.

Source: Brown *et al.* (1993). Reproduced with permission.

cholesterol (37 per cent) from a baseline of 3.9 mmol/L in the intervention group compared with 6 per cent in the control group. Apoprotein B also fell by 24 per cent in the intervention group. As a result of the very low-fat and very high-carbohydrate diet, plasma triglyceride rose by 22 per cent in the intervention group.

After 1 year, repeat quantitative coronary angiography demonstrated a 2.2 per cent reduction in stenosis in the lifestyle intervention group compared with a 3.4 per cent increase in the control group ($P < 0.001$). In lesions of greater than 50 per cent stenosis, there was a 5.3 per cent reduction compared with 2.7 per cent increase in the control group. Although this study is open to criticism, it is nevertheless encouraging and does suggest it is possible to make an impact on atherosclerosis with lifestyle measures.

The findings of the LHT were confirmed in the diet limb of the STARS trial, which employed less strict dietary intervention likely to be more acceptable for the majority of patients. The diet consisted of a reduction in dietary fat to 27 per cent of daily energy (saturated fat 8–10 per cent; polyunsaturated fat 8 per cent) with a cholesterol intake of 100 mg/1000 kcal. Soluble fibre was increased. Baseline mean cholesterol was 7.2 mmol/L and during the trial period (39 months) was 6.93 in the control and 6.17 mmol/L in the diet group.

This dietary-induced change in plasma cholesterol was associated with an overall progression of coronary narrowing in 15 per cent of patients ($n = 26$ completed) compared with 46 per cent in the control group ($n = 24$ completed) as assessed with quantitative angiography. Furthermore, the proportion of patients who showed an increase in luminal diameter was 38 per cent of the diet group compared with 4 per cent in the control group. The mean absolute width of coronary segments decreased by 0.201 mm in controls compared with an increase in the diet group of 0.003 mm.

Combination drug therapy angiographic trials

The landmark Cholesterol Lowering Atherosclerosis Study (CLAS) was published by the late David Blankenhorn and colleagues (1987). The study population consisted of 188 non-smoking, diet-treated men (aged 40–59 years) who had undergone coronary artery bypass grafting. Patients were randomly allocated to receive the anion-exchange resin colestipol (30 g/day) and high-dose nicotinic acid (3–12 g/day) or placebo preparations. Additional entry criteria were a total plasma cholesterol between 4.79 and 9.07 mmol/L and a confirmed ability to comply with the proposed study medication, which is notoriously difficult to take. In the intervention group, there were impressive reductions in LDL cholesterol (43 per cent) and triglycerides (22 per cent), whilst HDL was substantially increased (37 per cent).

Coronary angiograms at zero and 2 years were assessed by a panel of experts and a global coronary score was arrived at, based on a comprehensive count of all lesions and an assessment of percentage diameter stenosis for each lesion in native coronary arteries and bypass grafts. The study was completed by 162 patients and in the intervention group there was a significant reduction in the average number of lesions per subject which progressed. In addition, both in native vessels and grafts, new plaque formation was significantly reduced. Using a global score analysis, regression was considered to have occurred in the treated group. This was the first angiographic trial to suggest that regression of atherosclerotic plaques could occur.

A subgroup of 103 patients completed a further 2 years of follow-up (CLAS-II) during which the lipid and lipoprotein alterations were maintained (Cashin-Hemphill *et al.*, 1990). After 4 years there were further observed effects on atherosclerosis progression and regression. Plaques remained unchanged ('non-progression') in 52 per cent of patients in the treated group compared with 15 per cent in the placebo group. Regression in native coronaries was observed in 18 per cent in the treated group compared with 6 per cent in the placebo group. Fewer drug-treated patients developed new lesions (14 per cent versus 40 per cent) in native vessels and in grafts (16 per cent versus 38 per cent). This highly encouraging study argued for early and vigorous lipid-lowering therapy in coronary bypass graft recipients.

The findings of the CLAS study received considerable support with the publication of the results of the Familial Atherosclerosis Treatment Study (FATS) (Brown *et al.* 1990). The study population consisted of 146 men (<62 years of age) with a family history of premature cardiovascular disease and angiographically demonstrable CHD with at least one coronary stenosis equal to or greater than 50 per cent or three lesions equal to or greater than 30 per cent. At baseline, Apo B levels were greater than 1.25 g/L.

There were three treatment arms: a conventional treatment group which received placebo; a group which received colestipol (30 g/day) and nicotinic acid (4 g/day); and a group which received colestipol (30 g/day) together with the HMG-CoA reductase inhibitor lovastatin (40 mg/day). Patients allocated to the placebo group received colestipol if LDL cholesterol exceeded the 90th percentile for the US population. In the group receiving colestipol and niacin, LDL cholesterol was reduced by 34 per cent and HDL increased by 41 per cent. In the colestipol/lovastatin group, LDL fell by 48 per cent and HDL cholesterol increased by 14 per cent.

Quantitative computer coronary angiography was performed at baseline and at 2.5 years. Nine standard proximal coronary artery segments were analysed and the two principal measures were minimum lumen diameter and percentage stenosis. In the control group, 46 per cent of patients showed definite lesion progression in at least one segment. In the intervention groups, 21 per cent of patients showed progression in the colestipol/lovastatin group and 25 per cent in the colestipol/niacin group. Regression of lesions was observed in 32 per cent of patients taking colestipol and lovastatin and 39 per cent in the colestipol/nicotinic acid group compared with 11 per cent in the control group. These differences were highly statistically significant.

Although an open study, the Specialized Center of Research (SCOR) Familial Hypercholesterolaemia Trial (University of California, San Francisco) is worthy of discussion as the study population consisted of FH heterozygote females as well as males (Kane *et al.*, 1990). Patients were randomized to conventional therapy (diet and low-dose resin) or aggressive therapy with combination drug therapy (colestipol, niacin and lovastatin). Percentage stenosis showed a mean change of +10.80, indicating progression, compared with −21.53 in the intervention group, which indicates regression ($P = 0.039$). When males and females were analysed separately, the lesion change was only significant in females.

The HDL Atherosclerosis Treatment Study (HATS)

Recently Brown and colleagues (2001) have reported on the effects of a combination of simvastatin and nicotinic acid on angiographic progression/regression of coronary atherosclerosis in 160 patients with CHD and low HDL cholesterol (<35 mg/dL, 0.91 mmol/L in men; <40 mg/dL, 1.03 mmol/L in women) with LDL cholesterol <145 mg/dL (3.75 mmol/L). Compared with placebo, the simvastatin/nicotinic acid combination therapy was associated with an LDL reduction of 42 per cent and an HDL increase of 26 per cent. In this group the average coronary stenosis regressed by 0.4 per cent compared with 3.9 per cent progression in the placebo group ($P < 0.001$). The investigators also reported on clinical events in this 3-year trial. The risk of the composite endpoint (death from coronary causes, confirmed myocardial infarction or stroke or revascularization for worsening ischaemic symptoms) was 90 per cent lower in the simvastatin/nicotinic acid group compared with placebo ($P = 0.03$) (Figure 9.5). In this trial the investigators also studied the potential benefit of an antioxidant cocktail (800 i.u. vitamin E, 1000 mg vitamin C, 25 mg of natural beta-carotene and 100 μg of selenium).

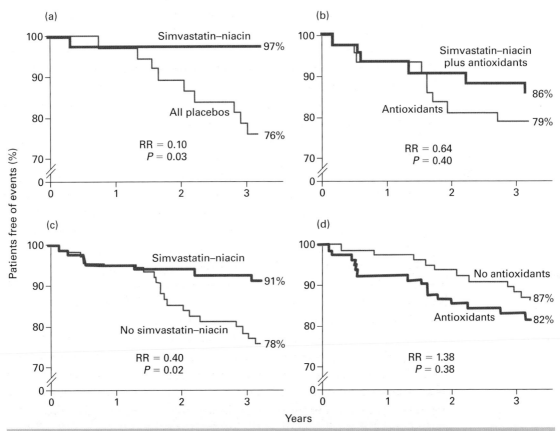

FIGURE 9.5 • Clinical events in the HATS trial: (a) simvastatin/niacin versus placebo; (b) simvastatin/niacin/antioxidants versus antioxidants; (c) all simvastatin/niacin patients versus non-simvastatin/niacin patients; (d) all antioxidant patients versus no antioxidant patients. Source: Brown *et al.* (2001).

Therapy with this cocktail of antioxidants was not associated with any difference in coronary stenosis compared with placebo. Importantly, when this cocktail was administered along with the simvastatin/nicotinic acid combination, there was a blunting of the increase in HDL and a blunting of the clinical benefits. The use of antioxidants is discussed elsewhere in this book (see page 186). This trial does not support their use.

Single drug angiographic trials

In the pre-HMG-CoA reductase era the anion-exchange resin cholestyramine ($n = 59$) was shown to delay lesion progression compared with a diet-treated control group ($n = 57$) in the National Heart Lung Blood Institute (NHLBI) Type II Study – 32 per cent of patients on cholestyramine (LDL reduction 26 per cent) compared with 49 per cent in the control diet group (LDL reduction 5 per cent) (Brensike et al., 1984). Similarly, in the cholestyramine arm of STARS, 12 per cent of patients showed lesion progression compared with 46 per cent in the control group ($P < 0.02$) (Watts et al., 1992).

Several randomized controlled trials have been performed with HMG-CoA reductase inhibitors, including the Monitored Atherosclerosis Regression Study (MARS) (Blankenhorn et al., 1993) and the Canadian Coronary Atherosclerosis Intervention Trial (CCAIT) (Waters et al., 1994); which used lovastatin. The Multicentre Anti-Atheroma Study (MAAS) used simvastatin (MAAS Investigators, 1994), and Pravastatin Limitation of Atherosclerosis in Coronary Arteries (PLAC-1) used pravastatin (Pitt et al., 1995). These studies showed remarkably similar results, with the percentage of patients showing progression ranging between 29 and 43 per cent and those showing regression ranging from 10 to 25 per cent. The treatment effects on plasma lipids in these trials were considerable, with LDL reductions of 29–38 per cent.

Less information is available in relation to fibrate drugs and effects on lesion progression/regression. A small, uncontrolled study involving 21 patients with minor coronary arterial narrowings showed some angiographic changes with diet and fenofibrate over 21 months of treatment. In this study the main lipid effects, as might be expected with a fibrate, were on triglycerides (-30 per cent) and HDL cholesterol ($+19$ per cent) though total cholesterol also fell (-19 per cent) (Hehmann et al., 1991).

The first controlled angiographic study using a fibrate was published in 1996: the Bezafibrate Coronary Atherosclerosis Intervention Trial (BECAIT) (Ericsson et al., 1996). The study population consisted of young male myocardial infarction survivors. Ninety-two patients entered the trial and were randomly allocated to bezafibrate (200 mg t.d.s.) or placebo after a 3-month period of dietary intervention. Median baseline cholesterol was 6.87 mmol/L in the bezafibrate group and 6.9 mmol/L in the placebo group.

Coronary angiographic data at baseline and at 2 and 5 years were available on 81 patients. In the bezafibrate group the minimum lumen diameter, as determined by quantitative angiography, decreased by 0.06 mm compared with 0.17 mm in the placebo group ($P = 0.049$).

These changes are of similar magnitude to those observed in the statin studies and it is of considerable interest that bezafibrate therapy was not associated with a significant reduction in LDL cholesterol, the main effects being on total triglycerides (-31.4 per cent), VLDL triglycerides (-37.17 per cent), VLDL cholesterol (-34.89 per cent) and HDL cholesterol ($+9.18$ per cent). This study raised the intriguing possibility that reduction of triglyceride and increase in HDL with bezafibrate may delay progression of atherosclerosis independently of effects on LDL cholesterol. Disappointingly, in the Bezafibrate Infarction Prevention (BIP) trial, there was no significant overall impact on clinical events, as discussed later in this chapter.

In the Diabetes Atherosclerosis Intervention Study (DAIS) the effect of the fibrate fenofibrate (micronized preparation, 200 mg/day) on angiographic endpoints in patients with type 2 diabetes ($n = 418$, aged 40–65 years, 113 women) was assessed. DAIS is a double-blind, randomized, placebo-controlled trial in 11 clinical centres in Canada, Finland, France and Sweden. Patients were selected on the basis of both metabolic and angiographic criteria. Lipid entry criteria (patients maintained on NCEP step 1 diet and after withdrawal of any lipid-lowering therapy) were total cholesterol/HDL cholesterol $\geqslant 4$ and either LDL cholesterol of 3.5–4.5 mmol/L and plasma triglyceride $\leqslant 5.2$ mmol/L or LDL cholesterol of $\leqslant 4.5$ mmol/L. Diabetic control was reasonable with mean glycated haemoglobin <170 per cent of the laboratory upper limit of normal. Eligible patients underwent an angiogram (731 patients screened) and at least one visible lesion was required for inclusion in the study. Fenofibrate, compared with placebo, reduced triglyceride by 29 per cent and increased HDL cholesterol by 6 per cent. LDL cholesterol was reduced by 7 per cent.

Baseline and post-study angiograms were assessed by computer-assisted quantitative analysis. Fenofibrate therapy was associated with a significant reduction (40 per cent) in progression of minimum lumen diameter ($P = 0.029$) and progression in percentage diameter stenosis (42 per cent, $P = 0.02$). When the study was planned, mean lumen diameter (MLD) was the primary endpoint and its decrease observed in a previous study used to calculate sample size. Changes in MLD were not significantly different between fenofibrate and placebo (Figure 9.6). Clinical events were few but the not significant 23 per cent reduction is in line with major event trials although clearly needs to be confirmed (DAIS investigators, 2001).

In the Lopid Coronary Angiographic Trial (LOCAT) the fibrate, gemfibrozil (Lopid SR, 1200 mg/day) was compared with placebo in 395 men (mean age 59 years) with previous coronary artery bypass surgery. Coronary angiography was performed at baseline and after a mean follow-up period of 32 months. Change from baseline to follow-up angiogram in average diameter of segments (ADS) and minimum luminal diameter (MLD) were assessed by quantitative computer-assisted angiography in native coronary arteries and bypass grafts (Frich et al., 1997).

Gemfibrozil produced a major reduction in plasma triglyceride (-36 per cent versus $+41.6$ per cent) and an increase in HDL cholesterol ($+21$ per cent versus $+7$ per cent) compared with placebo. As expected, only small changes were observed in total and LDL cholesterol (-5.5 per cent and -4.5 per cent, respectively, versus $+5.1$ per cent and $+5.3$ per cent). Gemfibrozil treatment was associated with a significant decrease in the progression of narrowing of the average diameter and minimum lumen diameter of

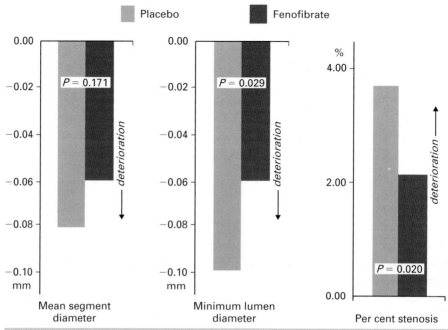

FIGURE **9.6** • Angiographic results in DAIS. Source: DAIS investigators (2001).

both graft-affected and non-graft-affected coronary segments. The appearance of new lesions was decreased by gemfibrozil in grafts and graft-affected coronary segments but not in non-graft-affected coronary segments. As is discussed later, a major endpoint trial in men with CHD, VA-HIT, has shown that the promise of gemfibrozil seen in this angiography trial translates into clinical benefit.

Programme on the Surgical Control of Hyperlipidaemias (POSCH) study

This unique large angiographic study employed partial ileal bypass surgery to lower cholesterol by interrupting the enterohepatic circulation of bile (Buchwald *et al.*, 1990). Of the 838 men (91 per cent) and women with previous myocardial infarction recruited, 421 were randomized to surgical treatment (5 per cent refused). Coronary angiography was performed at baseline and after 5–10 years. In the non-surgical group, some 32 per cent of patients were taking lipid-lowering drugs. LDL cholesterol fell by 38 per cent in the surgical group. Significantly less atherosclerosis progression was observed in the surgical group. Although this form of treatment is now largely redundant, this large trial gave the possibility of examining the effect of prolonged LDL cholesterol lowering on CHD morbidity, which was highly significantly reduced.

Post Coronary Artery Bypass Graft trial

This angiographic trial is important from several points of view (Post Coronary Artery Bypass Graft Trial Investigators, 1997). First, it confirms the beneficial effects of lipid-lowering therapy in decreasing the rate of progression of saphenous vein coronary artery

TABLE **9.11** • Post Coronary Artery Bypass Graft Trial Investigation (1997)

Study participants:
1351 men and women (~8%) aged 21–74 years with CABG between 1 and 11 years
  previously. Baseline LDL-C, 4 mmol/L.
4.3-year average follow-up; primary angiographic outcome – mean percentage per
  patient of grafts with a decrease of 0.6 mm or more in lumen diameter.
Two levels of treatment (diet, lovastatin ± cholestyramine) to achieve aggressive LDL
  lowering (2.4–2.5 mmol/L) or moderate LDL lowering (3.4–3.5 mmol/L).
Mean percentage of grafts with atherosclerosis progression was 27% in 'aggressive'
  group and 39% in moderate group ($P < 0.001$).
Revascularization procedures reduced by 29% – 6.5% versus 9.2%, ($P = 0.03$).

bypass grafts in a large group of patients (Table 9.11). In addition (and making this
trial a unique contribution), the investigators assigned patients to either 'moderate' or
'aggressive' treatment designed to achieve different levels of LDL cholesterol. In the
'aggressive' group, LDL cholesterol concentrations were reduced to between 93 and
97 mg/dL (2.4–2.5 mmol/L) and in the 'moderate' group to between 132 and 136 mg/dL
(3.4–3.5 mmol/L). This difference in LDL cholesterol was associated with a significantly lower percentage of grafts showing progression of atherosclerosis. Furthermore,
there was a reduction in the rate of revascularization procedures in the aggressive treatment group compared with the moderate treatment group.

The results of this study argue for aggressive lowering of LDL cholesterol in patients
with established CHD and this is in line with the recommendation of the NCEP in the
USA, which has a goal of therapy for such patients of LDL cholesterol less than
100 mg/dL (2.6 mmol/L).

Atorvastatin vs Simvastatin on Atherosclerosis Progression (ASAP) study

Further insights into the benefits of aggressive lipid lowering have come from the ASAP
study of atherosclerosis progression in familial hypercholesterolaemia. In this prospective,
randomized, double-blind trial of 325 patients (197 women) heterozygous for familial
hypercholesterolaemia, the effects of atorvastatin (80 mg/day) or simvastatin (40 mg/day)
on the change in carotid intima-media thickness (IMT) were measured by B-mode
ultrasound over a 2-year follow-up period (Smilde *et al.*, 2001). Atorvastatin treatment
reduced LDL cholesterol by 50.5 per cent and Apo B by 44.1 per cent whereas simvastatin treatment reduced LDL cholesterol by 41.2 per cent and Apo B by 34.9 per cent
($P = 0.0001$ for differences between treatment groups). Treatment with atorvastatin for
2 years resulted in a decrease in IMT (-0.031 mm; 95 per cent CI -0.007 to -0.055,
$P = 0.0017$). In the simvastatin group, IMT increased (0.036 mm; 95 per cent CI
0.014–0.058, $P = 0.0005$). These results are consistent with the benefits of more aggressive LDL cholesterol lowering. IMT measurements are, of course, a surrogate endpoint
for CVD. Nevertheless, IMT is acknowledged as a good marker of future CHD events
and regression in IMT is likely to lead to long-term clinical benefit.

Clinical events in the angiographic trials

A surprising but gratifying finding in many of the angiographic regression trials was a reduction in clinical events which in some studies was statistically significant. It is important to bear in mind that the trials were not designed to assess impact on clinical events (apart from POSCH). Nevertheless, this finding was impressive given the relatively short time course of the majority of the studies.

It is conceivable that the recorded changes in coronary plaques could explain the decreased number of events, though it seems unlikely that this could be the whole explanation. Brown and colleagues, using data from their own FATS, have hypothesized – with considerable supporting evidence – that the explanation for the relatively early impact of lipid lowering on events is likely to be due to stabilization of lipid-rich plaques (Brown et al., 1993). These plaques, which constitute less than 20 per cent of coronary lesions and are generally less than 50 per cent stenosis, have a thin fibrous cap and are prone to rupture, with consequent platelet thrombosis formation and blockage of the artery or at least rapid expansion of the plaque if the thrombosis is incorporated into it. Lipid-lowering therapy may result in mobilization of lipid from these plaques, thus allowing the fibrous cap to thicken. (This is discussed in more detail later.)

Stabilization of plaques is a very attractive hypothesis, but other mechanisms may play a role. It is now known, for instance, that abnormal arterial endothelial function – which is an important feature of atherosclerotic arteries – can be restored towards normal with lipid-lowering diet and drug therapy (Leung et al., 1993; Anderson et al., 1995; Treasure et al., 1995). The usual technique for demonstrating coronary artery endothelial dysfunction is to instil acetylcholine at the time of angiography. This mediator results in vasodilatation through release of endothelial-derived relaxing factor (EDRF), now known to be nitric oxide. In diseased arteries, acetylcholine produces a paradoxical vasoconstriction. Normal responses to acetylcholine in coronary arteries have been restored after 6–12 months of lipid-lowering therapy.

SCANDINAVIAN SIMVASTATIN SURVIVAL STUDY (4S)

The encouraging results of the angiographic trials, taken together with meta-analyses of the early diet and drug secondary prevention trials, suggested overall benefit for cholesterol lowering in secondary prevention. However, for many physicians what was required was a definitive clinical trial with sufficient statistical power to determine effects on overall mortality. Fortunately, such a landmark trial (4S) was published in 1994 (Scandinavian Simvastatin Survival Study Group, 1994).

The 4S recruited 4444 patients (872 females) aged 35–70 years with established CHD and total cholesterol concentrations between 5.5 and 8 mmol/L despite 8 weeks' dietary therapy. Originally, 7027 patients entered the dietary run-in period and of these, 4444 met the entry criteria and were randomized to the HMG-CoA reductase inhibitor simvastatin or placebo.

The impact of cholesterol lowering on overall mortality was the primary endpoint of the study and it was necessary to continue the study until 440 deaths had been observed, to meet statistical power calculations. Secondary objectives of the study were the impact on major coronary events, including fatal and non-fatal myocardial infarction and sudden cardiac death. In addition, important tertiary endpoints included hospitalization episodes for heart disease, the incidence of cerebrovascular disease and other atherosclerotic diseases and surgical interventions such as coronary artery bypass grafting and angioplasty.

Patients were recruited from 94 cardiac centres throughout the Nordic countries; most had a history of previous myocardial infarction (80 per cent) and a minority (20 per cent) had stable angina alone. Excluded from the study were patients at risk of early arrhythmic death including those with unstable angina, congestive heart failure, an enlarged heart or atrial fibrillation and those on anti-arrhythmic therapy.

In the simvastatin group, the goal of therapy was a total cholesterol concentration between 3.0 and 5.2 mmol/L. Most patients achieved this goal on 20 mg of simvastatin but 37 per cent of patients required 40 g daily. During the course of the study, substantial differences in lipid and lipoprotein concentrations were maintained with a 35 per cent reduction in LDL cholesterol, an increase in HDL cholesterol of 8 per cent and a reduction in triglyceride of 10 per cent.

The 4S trial finished in August 1994 after the requisite number of deaths had occurred and the median follow-up time was 5.4 years. It is quite remarkable that the vital status of all 4444 patients was available at the end of the trial. The principal results of the study were equally remarkable and had a major impact on the scientific community when they were announced at the American Heart Association in Dallas. There were also front page reports in major newspapers including the *Wall Street Journal* and the *New York Times*.

In the group receiving placebo there were 256 deaths whilst in the simvastatin group there were 182, giving a relative risk of 0.70 (95 per cent CI 0.59–0.85; $P = 0.0003$) (Table 9.12). Unfortunately, there were insufficient numbers of women recruited to the study to allow effects on overall mortality to be assessed, but a similar reduction in coronary events was observed in women. Furthermore, patients aged over 60 years showed similar benefit to younger patients. There was a 37 per cent reduction in the need for revascularization with coronary artery bypass grafting or angioplasty, which is of importance when the cost-effectiveness of cholesterol lowering in secondary prevention is assessed.

A follow-up report from the 4S investigators, and of relevance to clinical practice, has demonstrated that a similar relative risk reduction (35 per cent; 95 per cent CI 15–50) was observed with simvastatin therapy in those patients in the lowest LDL cholesterol quartile and those in the highest quartile (36 per cent; 95 per cent CI 19–49) (4S Study Group, 1995). Similar findings were observed for total cholesterol and HDL cholesterol. These findings argue that all CHD patients with total cholesterol concentrations greater than 5.5 mmol/L should be treated.

Subsequent reports from the 4S investigators have demonstrated the benefit of simvastatin on the development of signs and symptoms of ischaemia and the incidence of heart failure (Kjekshus et al., 1997; Pedersen et al., 1998). Significant reduction in the development of new angina and heart failure were observed.

TABLE **9.12** • Scandinavian Simvastatin Survival Study

Causes of death	Placebo (*n* = 2223)	Simvastatin (*n* = 2221)	Relative risk (95% CI)
Definite acute MI	63	30	
Probable acute MI	5	5	
Acute MI not confirmed			
Instantaneous death	39	29	
Death within 1 hour[a]	24	8	
Death within 1–24 hours	15	9	
Death >24 hours after onset	11	10	
Non-witnessed death[b]	23	13	
Intervention-associated[c]	9	7	
All coronary	189	111	0.58 (0.46–0.73)
Cerebrovascular	12	14	
Other cardiovascular	6	11	
All cardiovascular	207	136	0.65 (0.52–0.80)
Cancer	35	33	
Suicide	4	5	
Trauma	3	1	
Other	7	7	
All non-cardiovascular	49	46	
All deaths	256	182	0.70 (0.58–0.85)

[a] Following acute chest pain, syncope, pulmonary oedema or cardiogenic shock.
[b] With no likely non-coronary cause.
[c] Coronary death within 28 days of any invasive procedure.

The analysis of safety parameters in the 4S study provided strong reassurance of the long-term safety and tolerability of simvastatin. This is particularly pleasing given the degree of cholesterol lowering achieved. If cholesterol reduction is associated with increased non-cardiovascular disease, surely it should have been observed in 4S? However, there were no increases in other causes of death. Furthermore, the overall frequency of adverse events was similar in both simvastatin and placebo groups. Significant elevations in liver enzymes (greater than three times upper limit of normal) were seen in only small numbers (Pedersen *et al.*, 1996a). Major increases in CPK (greater than 10 times the upper limit of normal) were seen in seven patients (one on placebo and six on simvastatin). There was only one case of rhabdomyolysis (potentially the most serious side-effect of HMG-CoA reductase inhibitors), in a female patient on 20 mg/day simvastatin. The patient recovered when treatment was discontinued.

Details of cancer deaths during the study are shown in Table 9.12. There were no differences in non-fatal cancer cases, with 61 in the placebo and 67 in the simvastatin group.

The 4S authors concluded that the improvement in overall mortality observed with simvastatin therapy was achieved without any suggestion of an increase in non-CHD mortality. Simvastatin therapy was well tolerated and adverse events were similar in the placebo and treated groups. No previously unknown adverse effects were apparent in this trial.

The authors of the 4S study have published an important paper dealing with the implications of the study in terms of use of health-care resources. As discussed elsewhere in this book, the cost of health-care provision for cardiovascular disease is mammoth ($100 billion per year in the USA) and new therapies do need to be assessed in terms of their cost-effectiveness. In the 4S study there were 1905 hospitalizations (average duration 7.9 days) for coronary disease in 937 patients in the placebo group. In the simvastatin-treated group there were 1403 hospitalizations (average duration 7.1 days) in 720 patients. This is a highly significant difference ($P < 0.0001$). The difference in the number of hospital days was 15089 versus 9951 (34 per cent reduction; $P < 0.0001$). Based on US prices, the reduction in hospital costs over the course of the study (5.4 years) would be equivalent to $3872 per patient. This effectively reduces the cost of simvastatin to $0.28 day, a reduction of 88 per cent. So it can be concluded that the drug cost is largely offset by the reduction in the use of hospital services (Pedersen et al., 1996b; Johannesson et al., 1997).

CHOLESTEROL AND RECURRENT EVENTS STUDY (CARE)

CARE is a secondary prevention trial involving 4159 patients (14 per cent female) aged 21–75 years with a myocardial infarction 3–24 months prior to entry to the study (Sacks et al., 1996). This trial broke new ground in several respects:

- participants had 'normal' total (<6.2 mmol/L) and LDL cholesterol concentrations (3.0–4.5 mmol/L);
- 55 per cent of participants had previous coronary artery bypass grafts (CABG) or percutaneous transluminal coronary angioplasty (PTCA);
- participants were included with left ventricular dysfunction (left ventricular ejection fraction $\geqslant 25$ per cent);
- participants were included with entry total triglyceride concentrations up to 4 mmol/L;
- 83 per cent of participants were taking aspirin, 40 per cent beta-blockers and 39 per cent calcium antagonists.

Participants were randomly allocated to placebo or the HMG-CoA reductase inhibitor pravastatin, 40 mg/day. Lipid changes observed during the study were LDL cholesterol reduction of 28 per cent, HDL cholesterol increase of 5 per cent and triglyceride reduction of 14 per cent. The mean cholesterol concentration in the pravastatin group was 3.9 mmol/L and the mean LDL cholesterol 2.5 mmol/L.

The major endpoints were a combination of fatal and non-fatal myocardial infarction. These results (see Table 9.13) are quite remarkable, given the low lipid entry criteria, and give considerable strength to the argument that whatever the cholesterol level, it is 'too high' for the CHD patient and benefit will be observed if it is reduced. This conclusion is very much borne out by the HPS, as discussed later. When patient subgroups were analysed, similar risk reductions were observed in smokers, hypertensives, diabetics and those with low left ventricular ejection fractions. The CARE study

TABLE **9.13** • CARE study

Event	Placebo (n = 2078)		Pravastatin (n = 2081)		Risk reduction % (95% CI)	P value
	No.	%	No.	%		
CHD death or non-fatal infarction	274	13.2	212	10.2	24 (9–36)	0.003
CHD death	119	5.7	96	4.6	20 (−5–39)	0.10
Non-fatal infarction	173	8.3	135	6.5	23 (4–39)	0.02
Fatal infarction or confirmed non-fatal infarction	207	10.0	157	7.5	25 (8–39)	0.006
Fatal infarction	38	1.8	24	1.2	37 (−5–62)	0.07
CABG or PTCA	391	18.8	294	14.1	27 (15–37)	<0.001
Unstable angina	359	17.3	317	15.2	13 (−1–25)	0.07
Stroke	78	3.8	54	2.6	31 (3–52)	0.03

Source: Sacks *et al.* (1996).

contributed further to the case for secondary prevention as the population recruited was at lower risk than those in the 4S and had lower LDL cholesterol concentrations.

THE LONG TERM INTERVENTION WITH PRAVASTATIN IN ISCHAEMIC DISEASE (LIPID) STUDY

LIPID was a large, multicentre, randomized, double-blind trial carried out in Australia and New Zealand (LIPID Study Group, 1998). Patients ($n = 9014$; 17 per cent female; aged 31–75 years) with a previous history of acute myocardial infarction or hospitalization for unstable angina 3–36 months previously were randomly allocated to pravastatin (40 mg/day) or placebo. The entry criteria for plasma cholesterol was 4–7 mmol/L and plasma triglyceride up to 5 mmol/L. The primary study endpoint was CHD mortality.

Pravastatin therapy reduced LDL cholesterol by 25 per cent with a 5 per cent increase in HDL cholesterol and an 11 per cent reduction in triglyceride. Mean duration of the study was 6.1 years. These changes were associated with a significant reduction in CHD mortality, 6.4 per cent versus 8.3 per cent, a relative risk reduction of 24 per cent (95 per cent CI 12–35 per cent; $P < 0.001$) (Table 9.14). Overall mortality was 11 per cent in the pravastatin group compared with 14.1 per cent in the placebo group, a relative risk reduction of 22 per cent (95 per cent CI 13–31 per cent; $P < 0.001$). There was a consistent reduction in all cardiovascular outcomes including myocardial infarction, CHD death, non-fatal myocardial infarction and coronary revascularization. Analysis of pre-specified subgroups by age, gender, qualifying event, diabetes, hypertension, cigarette smoking and tertiles of lipid and lipoprotein concentrations did not demonstrate any significant heterogeneity of treatment effect. As with the other statin trials, the incidence of adverse clinical events was low. There were no differences in newly diagnosed cancers,

TABLE **9.14** • The LIPID Study Group, 1998

Outcome	No. (%) patients		Percentage risk reduction[a] (95% CI)	P value[b]
	Pravastatin (*n* = 4512)	Placebo (*n* = 4502)		
CHD death	287 (6.4)	373 (8.3)	24 (12–35)	<0.001
CVD death	331 (7.3)	433 (9.6)	25 (13–35)	<0.001
Death from all causes	498 (11.0)	633 (14.1)	22 (13–31)	<0.001
CHD death or non-fatal MI	557 (12.3)	715 (15.9)	24 (15–32)	<0.001
Total MI	336 (7.4)	463 (10.3)	29 (18–38)	<0.001
CABG	415 (9.2)	520 (11.6)	22 (11–31)	<0.001
PTCA	210 (4.7)	253 (5.6)	19 (3–33)	0.024
CABG or PTCA	585 (13.0)	708 (15.7)	20 (10–28)	<0.001
Unstable angina	1005 (22.3)	1106 (24.6)	12 (4–19)	0.005
Total stroke	169 (3.7)	204 (4.5)	19 (0–34)	0.048

[a] Percentage risk reduction and 95% confidence interval (CI) estimated using the hazard ratio in Cox regression analysis.
[b] Based on stratified log-rank test.

no differences in accidents, violence or attempted suicide. The incidence of adverse events attributable to study medication (3.2 per cent versus 2.7 per cent; $P = 0.16$) was not significantly different. In addition, liver function abnormalities (alanine aminotransferase greater than threefold increase) and elevated CK kinase levels did not differ. There were no differences in reported myopathy.

The LIPID investigators have provided further important evidence on the benefits of statin therapy in vascular beds other than the coronary circulation. A pre-specified endpoint in LIPID was stroke. There were 419 strokes (309 ischaemic) in 373 patients. The risk of stroke was 4.5 per cent in the placebo group compared with 3.7 per cent in the pravastatin group, a relative risk reduction of 19 per cent (95 per cent CI 0.34 per cent; $P = 0.05$). There was no difference in haemorrhagic stroke when analysed separately (White *et al.*, 2000).

The LIPID study adds a lot to the evidence base for secondary prevention. As the most recent of the statin trials to be reported in full, it is not surprising that background therapy represents up-to-date secondary prevention in the placebo and pravastatin-treated groups including aspirin (82 versus 83 per cent), beta-adrenergic blockers (48 versus 46 per cent), calcium antagonists (36 versus 35 per cent) and ACE inhibitors (16 versus 16 per cent). In addition, only 10 per cent of patients in the placebo group were current cigarette smokers. It is clear, therefore, that the benefits of statin therapy are over and above other therapies. It is likely that the absolute effects of statin therapy are underestimated in LIPID for a variety of reasons including crossover of therapy. It must be remembered that the results of 4S and CARE became available during this trial and as a consequence the use of statins in the secondary prevention of CHD was increasing. In the placebo group at 1 year, 3 years and end of study there were 3 per cent, 9 per cent and 24 per cent of patients taking open-label therapy with cholesterol-lowering drugs.

There was also considerable drop-out of treatment in the pravastatin group; at the same time-points, 6 per cent, 11 per cent and 19 per cent had stopped taking the medication. As a consequence the difference in total cholesterol between the placebo and pravastatin groups, which was 21 per cent at 6 months, fell to 13 per cent at 6 years.

The LIPID trial investigators (Tonkin *et al.*, 2000) have reported separately on the impact of pravastatin therapy in the 3260 patients recruited to the LIPID study with the diagnosis of unstable angina. In this large subgroup the relative risk reduction (26.3 per cent) in cardiovascular events was similar to that observed in the patients with previous myocardial infarction (20.6 per cent).

ATORVASTATIN VERSUS REVASCULARIZATION TREATMENT (AVERT) STUDY

This study set out to compare the effects of aggressive lipid lowering compared to PTCA and usual care for reducing the incidence of cardiac events in patients with ischaemic heart disease and stable angina pectoris (Pitt *et al.*, 1999). A total of 341 patients with mild-to-moderate stable angina (15–18 per cent were asymptomatic), a coronary stenosis of 50 per cent or more in at least one coronary artery and had been recommended for treatment with percutaneous revascularization, were recruited to this 18-month study. The patients were randomly assigned to medical treatment with atorvastatin (80 mg/day) or to undergo PTCA with usual care, which could include lipid-lowering therapy. The primary endpoint was a composite of incidence of death from cardiac causes, resuscitated cardiac arrest, non-fatal myocardial infarction, cerebrovascular accident, coronary artery bypass grafting, angioplasty and worsening angina with objective evidence resulting in hospitalization. Because of concern about the safety of patients who did not undergo PTCA, two interim analyses were performed and as a result the significance level for the final analysis of the incidence of ischaemic events was adjusted to 4.5 per cent from 5 per cent. In the atorvastatin group there was a 46 per cent reduction in LDL cholesterol [on treatment value 77 mg/dL (2 mmol/L)] compared with an 18 per cent reduction in the PTCA and usual care group [on treatment value 119 mg/dL (3 mmol/L)]. Twenty-two patients (13 per cent) developed ischaemic events in the atorvastatin group compared with 37 patients (21 per cent) in the PTCA group. This 36 per cent reduction ($P = 0.048$) was not statistically significant on the adjusted significance level following the two interim analyses. Time to first ischaemic event was longer in the atorvastatin group ($P = 0.03$). Two per cent of patients in the atorvastatin group had persistent elevation of liver transaminases (more than threefold upper limit of normal). No patients developed clinically important CK elevations or rhabdomyolysis.

This study provides evidence that aggressive lipid lowering is at least as effective as PTCA and usual care in low-risk patients with stable CHD. Clearly, PTCA is an important symptomatic measure and on current evidence should be combined with effective lipid lowering. Ongoing trials such as COURAGE (Clinical Outcomes Utilizing Revascularization and Aggressive Evaluation study; see page 281) will provide evidence as to whether PTCA adds any benefit in the presence of aggressive medical management in the reduction of ischaemic events. Perhaps a further reasonable conclusion from

AVERT is that in terms of LDL cholesterol and ischaemic event reduction, lower is better. This question is also addressed in ongoing trials such as TNT (Treat to New Targets) and SEARCH (Study of the Effectiveness of Additional Reductions of Cholesterol and Homocysteine; see page 280).

THE MYOCARDIAL ISCHAEMIA REDUCTION WITH AGGRESSIVE CHOLESTEROL LOWERING (MIRACL) STUDY

MIRACL is an interesting trial. On the one hand, it addressed an unanswered question with regard to statin therapy of importance to clinicians and on the other it enabled a trial with a newer statin, namely atorvastatin, to be performed in the context of secondary prevention with a placebo group comparison. The statin CHD secondary prevention trials, 4S, CARE and LIPID, which had shown conclusive benefit in the prevention of coronary events did not recruit patients with recent unstable angina or myocardial infarction. However, the highest rate of events is observed early after acute coronary syndromes. In addition, there are theoretical reasons why acute LDL cholesterol lowering with statins may have a beneficial outcome after acute coronary syndromes through effects on endothelial function, vascular inflammation and thrombosis formation. The MIRACL study therefore tested the hypothesis that acute aggressive statin therapy with atorvastatin (80 mg/day) in patients with unstable angina or non-Q-wave acute myocardial infarction would reduce early ischaemic events (Schwartz et al., 2001).

MIRACL was a randomized, double-blind, placebo-controlled trial in 3086 patients recruited from centres in North America, Europe, South Africa and Australasia. Patients (1074 women; mean age 65 years) received atorvastatin or placebo between 24 and 96 hours after hospital admission. The primary endpoint was a composite of death, non-fatal acute myocardial infarction, cardiac arrest with resuscitation or recurrent symptomatic myocardial ischaemia with objective evidence and requiring emergency rehospitalization at 16 weeks. The original power calculations for the study were based on a predicted event rate of 17 per cent. However, the event rate proved to be about 4 per cent less and it was decided to increase the sample size from $\cong$2100 to $\cong$3000 patients to maintain 95 per cent power to detect a 30 per cent relative treatment effect.

A primary endpoint was observed in 228 patients (14.8 per cent) in the atorvastatin group compared with 269 patients (17.4 per cent) in the placebo group. This represents a relative risk of 0.84 (95 per cent CI 0.70–1.00; $P = 0.048$). Of the composite primary endpoints, there were no significant differences in risk of death, cardiac arrest, non-fatal myocardial infarction – the main effect being a reduction in symptomatic myocardial ischaemia. The secondary endpoints, coronary revascularizations, worsening heart failure and worsening angina, showed no difference between atorvastatin and placebo but there was a reduction in the small number of strokes ($P = 0.045$).

There is no doubt that the definitive clinical conclusions from MIRACL are limited. However, the reduction in myocardial ischaemia is likely to translate into a reduction in more serious events in the longer term. Furthermore, high-dose atorvastatin in the acute situation appeared to be relatively free of adverse events. In the atorvastatin group, elevated liver function tests (greater than threefold increase in transaminases) were observed in 38 patients (2.5 per cent) compared with 9 patients (0.6 per cent) in the placebo group; 3 of the patients with abnormal liver function tests in the atorvastatin group were admitted with a diagnosis of hepatitis but recovered. Myositis was not observed.

What should be the take-home message from MIRACL? Clearly the trial provides no information on the appropriate dose of statin, having used only the maximum dose of atorvastatin. In the authors' view, MIRACL and other observational information (Aronow et al., 2001; Stenestrand and Wallentin 2001) suggest that early administration of statins should become an integral part of the management of all acute coronary syndrome patients. This approach is likely to improve outcome and also ensure that fewer patients fall into the treatment gap. The question of which dose of statin to use routinely remains unclear. Ongoing trials comparing different statin doses will help in this regard. Clearly, a lower dose of statin would have fewer adverse events. The lipid and lipoprotein data from MIRACL are unhelpful (given that they were taken in the acute situation) in determining statin dose. Perhaps in the short term it is best to use doses of statins equivalent to those used in the long-term secondary prevention trials and titrate up at a later date (if necessary) to achieve current guidelines goals of therapy.

THE GREEK ATORVASTATIN AND CORONARY HEART DISEASE EVALUATION (GREACE) STUDY

Publication of this study recently has provoked considerable interest, discussion and criticism (Athyros et al., 2002). It is an open-label study and there are considerable design faults; nevertheless the results are quite striking. GREACE is a prospective, randomized, open-label study comparing treatment with atorvastatin (10–80 mg/day) to achieve NCEP target (LDL cholesterol <2.6 mmol/L; 100 mg/dL) with usual care. One thousand and six hundred patients (344 women) with established CHD (prior myocardial infarction or >70 per cent stenosis of at least one coronary artery) were recruited over a 2-year period and followed for a mean period of 3 years. The mean dosage of atorvastatin was 24 mg/day and this was associated with a 36 per cent reduction in total cholesterol, a 46 per cent reduction in LDL cholesterol, a 31 per cent reduction in triglycerides and a 7 per cent increase in HDL cholesterol. The NCEP LDL cholesterol was achieved in 95 per cent of atorvastatin-treated patients. Statin use in the usual-care group was low; only 14 per cent received any hypolipidaemic agents and only 3 per cent reached the NCEP LDL cholesterol goal of therapy. The composite primary end-points (death, non-fatal myocardial infarction, unstable angina, congestive heart failure, revascularization and stroke) were reduced significantly in the atorvastatin group; 12 per cent of patients developed a recurrent CHD event versus 24.5 per cent in the usual-care group (relative risk 0.49, 95 per cent CI 0.27–0.73; $P < 0.0001$). The results of this study, in what is more or less a trial of highly effective statin treatment in high-risk patients compared to little or no lipid-lowering, point to the extraordinary benefits of LDL cholesterol lowering.

THE LESCOL INTERVENTION PREVENTION STUDY (LIPS)

This placebo-controlled, randomized, double-blind trial was designed to determine whether statin treatment with fluvastatin would reduce major adverse cardiac events in patients following percutaneous coronary intervention (PCI) (Serruys et al., 2001). One thousand, six hundred and seventy seven patients aged 18–80 years (271 women) were recruited between 1996 and 1998. These patients had undergone successful PCI (a reduction in the stenosis diameter to less than 50 per cent without evidence of myocardial necrosis, need for repeat PCI or CABG or death before hospital discharge) for stable or unstable angina or silent ischaemia. Patients were eligible for study if total cholesterol levels were between 3.5 and 7.0 mmol/L and plasma triglycerides were <4.5 mmol/L. Patients were randomized to fluvastatin 40 mg twice daily or matching placebo for at least 3 years and no longer than 4 years. The primary endpoint was survival time free of a composite of cardiac death, non-fatal myocardial infarction or re-intervention procedure. During the median follow-up period of 3.9 years, event-free survival was significantly longer in the fluvastatin group ($P = 0.01$); 2.4 per cent ($n = 181$) of the fluvastatin-treated patients ($n = 844$) developed a primary endpoint compared with 26.7 per cent ($n = 222$) in the placebo group ($n = 833$), relative risk 0.78 (95 per cent CI 0.64–0.95). These results were independent of baseline total cholesterol levels. On subgroup analysis, benefits of fluvastatin were observed in diabetic patients and in those with multivessel disease. No instances of significantly elevated creatinine phosphokinase (>10-fold) were observed and there were no cases of rhabdomyolysis (Serruys et al., 2002). This study provides evidence of benefit of statin therapy in PCI patients, which is of importance given the poor long-term outcome following these procedures, with only one-third of patients free of major cardiac events at 10 years.

SECONDARY PREVENTION TRIALS WITH FIBRATES

There have been two major endpoint trials in patients with established CHD using drugs of the fibrate class, the Veterans Administration HDL Intervention Trial (VA-HIT) and the Bezafibrate Infarction Prevention (BIP) studies. These are clearly of interest to the clinician but have not provided the consistent findings seen with the statins.

VA-HIT

VA-HIT was designed to test the potential benefit of therapy to increase HDL cholesterol in CHD patients where the primary lipid abnormality was a low HDL cholesterol (Rubins et al., 1999). A total of 2531 men with established CHD and HDL cholesterol (≤40 mg/dL, ≤1 mmol/L) and relatively normal LDL cholesterol (≤140 mg/dL, ≤3.6 mmol/L) were randomly allocated to gemfibrozil (1200 mg/day) or placebo. Gemfibrozil was chosen as this drug increases HDL cholesterol but has little or no effect on LDL cholesterol. Baseline lipid concentrations were LDL concentration 2.9 mmol/L, triglycerides 1.8 mmol/L and HDL cholesterol 0.8 mmol/L. At 1 year, gemfibrozil therapy was associated with a 6 per cent increase in HDL, no change in LDL cholesterol and a reduction in triglyceride of 31 per cent.

The primary outcome measure was the combined incidence of non-fatal myocardial infarction or CHD death. Secondary endpoints included stroke, transient ischaemic attack, revascularization procedures, carotid endarterectomy, hospitalization for unstable angina or congestive heart failure and death from any cause. Two hundred and seventy-five primary endpoints were recorded in the placebo group and 219 in the gemfibrozil group, a relative risk reduction of 22 per cent (95 per cent CI 7–35 per cent, $P = 0.006$). For the combined outcome measure of CHD death, non-fatal myocardial infarction and stroke, there was a 24 per cent reduction ($P < 0.001$). Although the study hypothesis of VA-HIT was that increasing HDL cholesterol would benefit outcome, it is clear that this could be the result of other factors including the reduction of triglyceride, which would also modulate postprandial lipaemia and result in a shift of LDL subfraction distribution to larger, more buoyant particles.

BIP

In this double-blind, randomized-controlled trial, 3090 patients (2825 men) with previous myocardial infarction or stable angina were randomized to bezafibrate (400 mg/day) or placebo (BIP Study Group, 2000). Lipid entry criteria were total cholesterol 180–250 mg/dL (4.7–6.5 mmol/L), LDL cholesterol $\leqslant$180 mg/dL (4.7 mmol/L), HDL cholesterol $\leqslant$45 mg/dL (1.2 mmol/L) and triglycerides $\leqslant$300 mg/dL (3.4 mmol/L). Baseline lipid and lipoprotein concentrations were total cholesterol 212 mg/dL (5.5 mmol/L), LDL cholesterol 148 mg/dL (3.8 mmol/L), HDL cholesterol 34.6 mg/dL (0.9 mmol/L) and triglycerides 145 mg/dL (1.6 mmol/L).

Bezafibrate treatment was associated with a reduction in triglycerides of 17 per cent, an increase in HDL cholesterol of 14.4 per cent, a decrease in total cholesterol of 4.7 per cent and in LDL of 5.2 per cent compared to placebo.

The primary endpoint of the study was the combination of fatal and non-fatal myocardial infarction or sudden death. The study had a power of between 62.5 and 85 per cent to detect a 20–25 per cent reduction in CHD incident rate with bezafibrate. Mean follow-up was 6.2 years and the cumulative probability of the primary endpoint was reduced by 7.3 per cent ($P = 0.24$). A *post hoc* analysis of patients with high baseline triglycerides ($\geqslant$200 mg/dL, 2.26 mmol/L) showed a 39.5 per cent reduction in the primary endpoint ($P = 0.02$). Clearly, this finding needs to be interpreted with caution given the *post hoc* nature of the analysis.

VA-HIT AND BIP – WHY THE DISCREPANT RESULTS?

Much has been written with regard to the explanation(s) for the discrepant results of VA-HIT and BIP (Robins, 2001). The populations studied were clearly different. VA-HIT included a large proportion of patients with diabetes, hypertension and obesity. Thirty-five per cent of patients had a BMI > 30. This points to the probability of a high proportion of patients with the metabolic syndrome and 30 per cent of the study population had plasma insulin levels in the hyperinsulinaemia range. The event rate was higher in VA-HIT because of the high-risk population and drop-in treatment was low (2 per cent). In the BIP study, drop in treatment was 15 per cent in the placebo group such that in the last 2 years of the study a change in the slope of the Kaplan–Meier curve became evident. Other possibilities include intrinsic differences between the drugs used or the play of chance. Haffner (2000) has pointed out that the 9 per cent reduction in events found in the BIP study falls within the 95 per cent confidence intervals of 7–35 per cent seen in VA-HIT. Although the explanation(s) of the different results of BIP and VA-HIT are unclear, it is certain that the evidence from clinical trials of fibrates is limited compared to that for statins.

COMBINED PRIMARY AND SECONDARY PREVENTION TRIAL

HEART PROTECTION STUDY (HPS)

The HPS is the largest clinical endpoint trial reported to date. The preliminary results were announced at the American Heart Association meeting in November 2001. This huge trial was designed to assess the effects on mortality and major morbidity of cholesterol-lowering therapy with simvastatin (40 mg/day) in a wide range of different categories of high-risk patients across a wide range of cholesterol levels (≥ 3.5 mmol/L) (Figure 9.7). A major thesis of the investigators was that cholesterol-lowering therapy would be shown to be worthwhile in individuals at high risk of CHD events irrespective of cholesterol levels (MRC/BHF Heart Protection Study Collaborative Group, 1999).

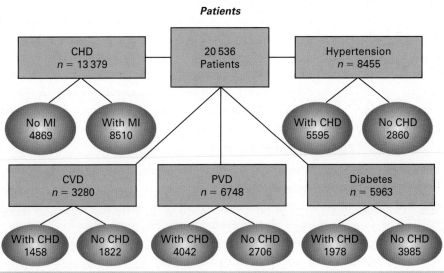

FIGURE **9.7** • Heart Protection Study patients.

Eligible participants for the HPS, which was conducted throughout the UK and organized by the Oxford Clinical Trial Service Unit, included men and women (aged 40–80 years) with a history of symptomatic vascular disease (myocardial infarction or other coronary heart disease, carotid artery disease or peripheral artery disease), diabetes mellitus or treated hypertension. Study participants were required to have no clear indication for the study drug simvastatin and no other predominant medical problem.

Of 32 145 participants who entered the pre-randomization run-in 11 609 were not randomized: for personal choice (65 per cent); deemed unlikely to be compliant long term (17 per cent); to have a low indication for statin (or contraindication); abnormal screening blood tests (10 per cent); problems with run-in treatment (9 per cent); vascular event during run-in (1 per cent); and other reasons (1 per cent). Between July 1994 and May 1997, 15 454 men and 5082 women were randomized: 8510 (41 per cent) had previous myocardial infarction, 4869 (24 per cent) had other CHD, 3288 (16 per cent) had cerebrovascular disease, 6748 (33 per cent) had peripheral vascular disease, 5963 (29 per cent) had diabetes mellitus and 8455 (41 per cent) had hypertension. Clearly, there is overlap between these diagnostic categories and 1822 of those with cerebrovascular disease, 3985 with diabetes and 2860 with hypertension did not have CHD. Forty-six per cent (9515) were aged over 65 years.

The study medications were simvastatin 40 mg or placebo. Using a two by two factorial design, the effects of an antioxidant cocktail were also studied. This is discussed elsewhere (page 187). Clearly, as this study was progressing the results of other statin trials were published and drop-in therapy occurred. Until 1998, trial participants prescribed non-statin therapy were routinely advised to stop their simvastatin or placebo tablets. Subsequently, non-study statin therapy was permitted equivalent to the lipid-lowering potency of 40 mg simvastatin. Simvastatin therapy was associated with a mean reduction in LDL cholesterol of 0.96 ($\pm$0.02) mmol/L over the duration of the trial ($\cong$ 5–5.5 years). This finding, based on intention-to-treat analysis, of course underestimates the effects of simvastatin because of drop-in therapy. The investigators estimated that actual use of simvastatin (40 mg/day) would have resulted in a reduction of 1.5 mmol/L.

The primary endpoints of the HPS were all-cause mortality, coronary heart disease mortality and all mortality from causes other than coronary heart disease. There were 791 (7.7 per cent) vascular deaths in the simvastatin group compared with 943 (9.2 per cent) in the placebo group, a 17 per cent reduction (SE 4.4), $P < 0.0002$ (Figure 9.8). There was no difference in non-vascular deaths between the two groups so that all-cause mortality was reduced by 12 per cent (1328, 12.9 per cent versus 1503, 14.6 per cent), $P < 0.001$. A very interesting finding from the HPS related to stroke. Previous meta-analyses of statin studies had shown a reduction in stroke but confirmatory clinical trial findings were needed. In the HPS there were 456 (4.4 per cent) strokes in the simvastatin group compared to 613 (6 per cent) in the placebo group, a 27 per cent (SE 5.3) reduction, $P < 0.00001$. In terms of major vascular events (total CHD, total stroke and revascularizations), there were a total of 2042 (19.9 per cent) events in the simvastatin group compared with 2606 (25.4 per cent) in the placebo group, a 24 per cent (SE 2.6) reduction, $P < 0.00001$ (Figure 9.9).

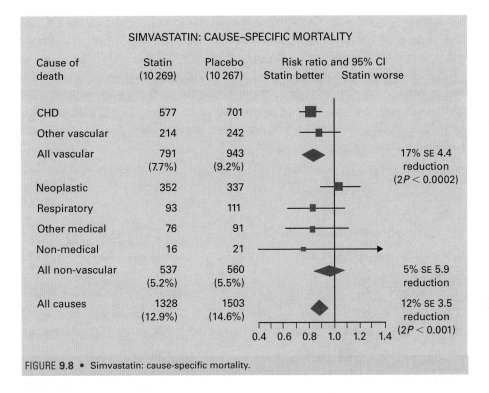

FIGURE **9.8** • Simvastatin: cause-specific mortality.

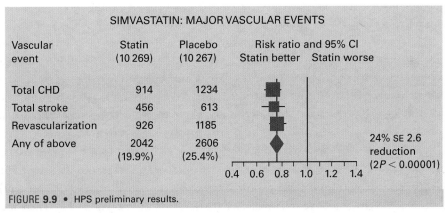

FIGURE **9.9** • HPS preliminary results.

It was clear from the HPS that benefit from simvastatin therapy extended to all subgroups, males and females and all age groups. Of particular interest and a finding likely to change current guidelines and clinical practice, relates to an analysis based on baseline LDL and total cholesterol concentrations. The relative risk reduction of vascular events when baseline LDL levels were below 2.6 mmol/L was the same as that seen at higher LDL levels. This suggests that patients at high risk, particularly those with existing disease, should receive statin treatment regardless of the LDL cholesterol concentration.

The database of the HPS provides very reassuring information with regard to the safety of simvastatin. Elevation of liver enzymes (greater than threefold × ULN alanine transaminase) was seen in 77 (0.8 per cent) individuals on simvastatin compared with 66 (0.6 per cent) on placebo. Similarly, CK elevations (>10-fold ULN) were seen in 9 (0.09 per cent) individuals on simvastatin compared with 5 on placebo (0.05 per cent).

The investigators concluded their presentation of the preliminary results of the HPS by calculations of the true potential benefits of simvastatin therapy after allowance for non-compliance: simvastatin (40 mg/day) safely reduces the risk of heart attack, of stroke and of revascularization by at least one-third. Five years of simvastatin would prevent major vascular events in:

- 100 of every 1000 with previous MI;
- 80 of every 1000 with other CHD;
- 70 of every 1000 with diabetes;
- 70 of every 1000 with previous stroke;
- 70 of every 1000 with other PVD;

irrespective of cholesterol level, age, sex or other treatments.

MECHANISMS OF BENEFIT OF LIPID LOWERING

The established atherosclerotic lesion, the raised fibrolipid plaque, consists of an atheromatous core (foam cells and smooth muscle cells with a necrotic core of free lipid and cell debris) covered by a fibrous cap. The extent of these lesions in the coronary arteries and aorta predict the development of CHD. The fibrous cap, rich in collagen, is crucial in separating the highly thrombogenic materials in the lipid core of the plaque from the bloodstream. In the majority of acute coronary syndromes it is plaque rupture following fissuring, erosion or ulceration of the fibrous cap which is the initiating event. The thrombogenic plaque contents are exposed to luminal blood with subsequent thrombosis. Although all plaques are composed of essentially the same constituents (lipid-rich core and fibrous cap), they vary in the relative proportions of these components. The plaque at high risk of rupture, the candidate lesion, is characterized by a large lipid pool (>40 per cent of the plaque volume) and a relatively thin fibrous cap. In addition, these plaques are rich in inflammatory cells, macrophages and T lymphocytes. Increased production and release of matrix metalloproteinase enzymes by macrophages has been implicated in collagen degradation, weakening of the fibrous cap and increased predisposition to rupture. Expression of inflammatory cytokines (e.g. interleukin-1β and tumour necrosis factor α) leads to apoptosis (cell death) of smooth muscle cells and endothelial cells. Smooth muscle cells are important in collagen synthesis. Candidate lesions show a reduction in the ratio of smooth muscle cells to lipid-laden macrophages. Plaque rupture with intraplaque haemorrhage is not inevitably associated with clinical events. It is clear that these lesions may be subject to repair processes and contribute to progression of the plaque and increased stenosis.

How does lipid lowering influence the atheromatous process and reduce coronary events and death? Clearly, there is no doubt of the benefits of statin therapy, but what are the mechanisms? These questions have prompted a considerable amount of research activity, which has provided new insights into plaque dynamics and in the future should point to new therapeutic targets.

Atherosclerosis progression/regression studies using angiographic techniques to delineate coronary lesions or B-mode ultrasound to measure intima-media thickness in the carotid arteries to assess statin therapy showed undoubted but small effects. In the main, the findings showed reduced progression of disease rather than regression. For example, in one of the largest trials (Regression Growth Evaluation Statin Study, REGRESS) involving men ($n = 885$) with stable angina and cholesterols ranging from 4 to 8 mmol/L, statin therapy (pravastatin, 40 mg/day) was associated with less disease progression. In the statin group, mean segment diameter reduced by 0.06 mm compared with 0.1 mm in the placebo group (Jukema et al., 1995). The relatively small quantitative changes clearly underestimate the observed clinical benefits not only in acute coronary events but also the need for revascularization procedures (Cobbe, 2002). Given the above discussion on the role of atherosclerotic plaque rupture in the generation of acute coronary syndromes, the question arose as to whether lipid-lowering therapy was associated with qualitative changes in plaques that would render them less likely to rupture or rapidly progress. Both in vitro effects of statins and experiments in animal models of atherosclerosis (e.g. the Watanabe heritable hyperlipidaemic rabbit, WHHL) support this view. In these experiments statin therapy was associated with decreases in plaque lipid and macrophages with no change in smooth muscle cells. Along with reductions in macrophages, reductions in the activities of various collagen-degrading matrix metalloproteinases were observed, together with reduced tissue factor expression and an increase in interstitial collagen. These sorts of studies are obviously difficult to perform in patients. However, carotid endarterectomy specimens from a randomized trial of statin pre-treatment showed reductions in lipid-content, inflammatory cells and apoptosis with an increase in vascular smooth muscle cells and collagen content (Crisby et al., 2001). No doubt in the future new imaging techniques, such as intravascular ultrasound and nuclear magnetic resonance, which not only show the quantitative nature of plaques but also qualitative characteristics, will enable the impact of various therapies including lipid lowering to be determined in vivo.

A further important mechanism of benefit to lipid-lowering therapy relates to arterial endothelial dysfunction (Davignon and Laaksonen, 1999). Endothelial function can be measured non-invasively using B-mode ultrasound to measure brachial artery dilatation in response to flow or other stimuli. In coronary arteries, endothelial function can be measured at the time of angiography, usually in response to acetylcholine. In addition, myocardial blood flow during maximal vasodilative response to adenosine can be measured by positron emission tomography. Lipid-lowering therapy has been shown in many studies to improve these parameters relatively quickly – a matter of weeks rather than months. Indeed, an abrupt reduction in LDL cholesterol of 58 per cent after a single LDL apheresis was associated with a 30 per cent improvement in coronary vasodilatation capacity within 24 hours (Mellwig et al., 1998). Effects on endothelial function may explain the relatively early benefits of statin therapy as seen in the MIRACL study, for example. This argues for the early administration of statins to patients with acute coronary syndromes. Clearly, many mechanisms may be involved in this improvement in endothelial function. Of recent interest is the role of caveolae, which are cholesterol-rich invaginations in the plasma membrane (Kinlay et al., 2001). These organelles play an integral role in endothelial function through association with nitric oxide synthase. Caveolae contain the transmembrane protein caveolin, which suppresses nitric oxide. High cholesterol levels increase the interaction between caveolin and nitric oxide synthase, thus reducing nitric oxide production. Furthermore, LDL cholesterol stimulates caveolin expression. Statin drugs reduce the expression of caveolin but LDL cholesterol reverses this direct effect, suggesting that it is primarily cholesterol reduction that is responsible for the inhibition of caveolin production.

A surprising benefit observed in the statin studies was the reduction in stroke. Clearly, the impact of statins on candidate atherosclerotic plaques is likely to contribute to this benefit but improvement in endothelial function is also likely to be of importance. Interesting insights on this possibility come from experiments in mice treated with statins. In these animals there was an increase in cerebral blood flow of 25–30 per cent and after cerebrovascular occlusion the statin-treated animals showed 50 per cent smaller infarct sizes. These effects were not observed in mice deficient in nitric oxide synthetase, pointing to the likely role of nitric oxide in this effect of statins. Interestingly, cholesterol levels were not affected by the statin treatment (Endres et al., 1998).

FUTURE DIRECTIONS

Ongoing trials will provide further information which will inform clinical practice in various patient groups. Many of these trials, together with completed trials, are part of The Cholesterol Treatment Trialists' Collaboration (CTT Collaboration, 1995). This protocol, based on prospective trials, is designed to provide reliable information (based on large numbers and avoiding methodological problems of retrospective analyses) about the effect of lipid-lowering therapy on morbidity and mortality in a wide range of patient populations and risk groups. The HPS, the preliminary results of which were announced at the American Heart Association in November 2001 and published in 2002, will contribute hugely to this project.

Other ongoing trials will provide further important information on how low to lower LDL cholesterol. Treat to New Targets (TNT), Incremental Decrease in Endpoints Through Aggressive Lipid Lowering (IDEAL), Study of the Effectiveness of Additional Reductions of Cholesterol and Homocysteine (SEARCH) and Pravastatin or Atorvastatin Evaluation and Infection Therapy (PROVE-IT) compare standard with more aggressive statin therapy in high-risk patients. This possibility would be supported by international epidemiological studies and also by the Post Coronary Artery Bypass Graft Trial (page 262) and the AVERT trial (page 270).

Ongoing trials will provide further evidence of the benefits of early statin therapy following acute coronary syndromes and also whether angioplasty confers any additional benefit in CHD patients on optimal aggressive medical therapy. The Aggrastat to

Zocor (A to Z) study, in its lipid-lowering arm compares simvastatin 40 mg (1–4 days after the event then rising to 80 mg at 1 month) with simvastatin 20 mg (4 months after the event) in ~4500 patients with acute coronary syndromes. This is an event-driven trial (termination of the study after 970 events) and is expected to run for about a year after the final patient is recruited.

In the Clinical Outcomes Utilizing Revascularization and Aggressive Drug Evaluation (COURAGE) study, ~3200 CHD patients are randomized to simvastatin 80 mg versus balloon angioplasty and usual care versus both. The primary endpoint is all-cause mortality and non-fatal myocardial infarction. The trial is expected to take 6 years.

The Prospective Study of Pravastatin in Elderly at Risk (PROSPER) focuses, unlike previous trials, on the elderly population (age 70–82 years). Analyses of previous statin trials including the recent HPS, do indicate that older patients show benefit similar to younger patients. PROSPER will contribute significantly to these analyses. It is likely given the high event rates in the elderly that the absolute benefit of statin therapy will be high. Clearly, however, this needs to be documented in a specific clinical trial and cost-benefit calculated, particularly for the elderly without symptomatic disease. PROSPER compares pravastatin (40 mg/day) versus placebo in ~5500 subjects (3000 women) with total cholesterol of 4.0–9.0 mmol/L and triglycerides <6.0 mmol/L. Roughly half of the patients will have symptomatic vascular disease. The primary endpoint is a composite of CHD death, non-fatal myocardial infarction and fatal/non-fatal stroke. Important substudies include effects on cognitive function and brain MRI.

The Stroke Prevention by Aggressive Reduction in Cholesterol Levels (SPARCL) compares atorvastatin (80 mg/day) to placebo in ~4000 patients with previous TIA or stroke and baseline LDL cholesterol concentrations of 100–190 mg/dL (2.6–4.9 mmol/L). The primary endpoint of this study, which is scheduled to run for 5 years, is a combination of fatal and non-fatal stroke. This trial will provide more useful information on the secondary prevention of stroke.

Two large hypertensive trials, the Antihypertensive Lipid Lowering Treatment to prevent Heart Attack Trial (ALLHAT) and the Anglo-Scandinavian Cardiac Outcomes Trial (ASCOT) have lipid-lowering arms. ALLHAT involves 20 000 hypertensive men and women over 65 years with or without CHD; pravastatin 20 mg/day is compared with placebo and the primary endpoint is total mortality. ASCOT is recruiting ~9000 hypertensive patients and the lipid-lowering arm compares atorvastatin to placebo.

Major trials are under way in specific diabetic populations. The Collaborative Atorvastatin Diabetes Study (CARDS) in the UK compares atorvastatin to placebo in ~2750 type 2 diabetic patients (aged 40–75 years) with at least one other risk factor – hypertension, retinopathy, microalbuminuria or macroalbuminuria, or cigarette smoking. Baseline LDL cholesterol must be 4.14 mmol/L (160 mg/dL) or less and fasting serum triglyceride 6.78 mmol/L (600 mg/dL) or less. CARDS is a primary prevention trial such that patients with a past history of cardiovascular disease are excluded. The primary endpoint is a composite of fatal or non-fatal myocardial infarction (including silent myocardial infarction), unstable angina, heart failure, coronary revascularization, stroke and severe peripheral vascular disease warranting surgery. The Atorvastatin as

Prevention of Coronary Heart Disease in Patients with type 2 Diabetes (ASPEN) carried out in the USA, Europe and Australia also compares atorvastatin 10 mg to placebo in ~2250 patients. This is a combined primary and secondary prevention trial. The lipid entry criteria are the same as in CARDS. The similarity means that combined subgroup analyses will be feasible.

The Fenofibrate Intervention and Event Lowering in Diabetes (FIELD) trial aims to recruit approximately 8000 patients with type 2 diabetes in Australia, New Zealand and Finland. This trial compares micronized fenofibrate (200 mg/day) with placebo. Lipid entry criteria are total/HDL cholesterol ratio of 4 or over or a fasting triglyceride concentration of 1.0 mmol/L or over and less than 5 mmol/L. Total cholesterol concentrations are 3.0–6.5 mmol/L (5.5 mmol/L in Finland). The trial will provide additional information on the potential benefits of fibrate therapy where currently there is conflicting evidence from endpoint trials.

REFERENCES

Anderson, T.J., Meredith I.T., Yeung, A.C. *et al.* (1995) The effect of cholesterol lowering and antioxidant therapy on endothelium-dependent coronary vasomotion. *N Engl J Med* **332**, 488–93.

Aronow, H.D., Topal, E.J., Roe, M.T., Houghtaling, P.L., Wolski, K.E. and Lincoff, A.M. (2001) Effect of lipid-lowering therapy on early mortality after acute coronary syndromes: an observational study. *Lancet* **357**, 1063–8.

Athyros, V.G., Papageorgious, A.A., Mercouris, B.R. *et al.* (2002) Treatment with atorvastatin to the National Cholesterol Educational Program Goal versus 'usual' case in secondary coronary heart disease prevention. *Curr Med Res Opin* **18**, 220–8.

Barth, J.D., Arntzemus, A.C. and Kromhout, D. (1987) Follow up on the Leiden Trial. *N Engl J Med* **316**, 881–2.

The BIP Study Group (2000) Secondary prevention by raising HDL-cholesterol and reducing triglycerides in patients with coronary artery disease: the Bezafibrate Infarction Prevention (BIP) Study. *Circulation* **102**, 21–7.

Blankenhorn, D.H., Nession, S.A., Johnson, R.L. *et al.* (1987) Beneficial effects of combined colestipol–niacin therapy on coronary atherosclerosis and coronary venous bypass grafts. *J Am Med Assoc* **257**, 3233–40.

Blankenhorn, D.H., Azen, S.P., Karmsch, D.M. *et al.* (1993) Coronary angiographic changes with lovastatin therapy. The Monitored Atherosclerosis Regression Study (MARS). *Ann Intern Med* **119**, 969–76.

Brensike, J.F., Levy, R.I., Kelsey, S.F. *et al.* (1984) Effects of cholestyramine on progression of coronary atherosclerosis: results of the NHLBI Type II Coronary Intervention Study. *Circulation* **69**, 313–24.

Brown, G., Albers, J.J., Fisher, L.D. *et al.* (1990) Regression of coronary artery disease as a result of intensive lipid lowering therapy in men with high levels of apolipoprotein B. *N Engl J Med* **323**, 1289–98.

Brown, G., Zhao, Z.-Q., Sacco, D.J. *et al.* (1993) Lipid lowering and plaque regression: new insights into prevention of plaque disruption and clinical events in coronary disease. *Circulation* **87**, 1781–91.

Brown, B.G., Zhao X.-Q., Chait, A., Fisher, L.D., Cheung, M.C., Morse, J.S. *et al.* (2001) Simvastatin and niacin, antioxidant vitamins, or the combination for the prevention of coronary disease. *N Engl J Med* **345**, 1583–92.

Buchwald, H., Varco, R.L., Matts, J.P. *et al.* (1990) Effect of partial ileal bypass surgery on mortality and morbidity from coronary heart disease in patients with hypercholesterolaemia: report of the Programme on the Surgical Control of the Hyperlipidaemias (POSCH). *N Engl J Med* **323**, 946–55.

Cashin-Hemphill, L., Mack, W.J., Pogoda, J.M. *et al.* (1990) Beneficial effects of colestipol niacin on coronary atherosclerosis. A 4-year follow up. *J Am Med Assoc* **264**, 3013–17.

Cobbe, S.M. (2002) How best to combat the enemies? Lipid lowering. *Eur Heart J Suppl* **4**(Suppl. A), A48–52.

Committee of Principal Investigators (1978) Report on a cooperative trial in the primary prevention of ischaemic heart disease using clofibrate. *Br Heart J* **40**, 1069–118.

Coronary Drug Project Research Group (1975) The Coronary Drug Project: clofibrate and niacin in coronary heart disease. *J Am Med Assoc* **231**, 360–81.

Crisby, M., Nordin-Fredriksson, G., Shah, P.K., Yano, J., Zhu, J., Nilsson, J. (2001) Pravastatin treatment increases collagen content and decreases lipid content, inflammation, metalloproteinases, and cell death in human carotid plaques: implications for plaque stabilization. *Circulation* **103**, 926–33.

Davignon, J. and Laaksonen, R. (1999) Low-density lipoprotein-independent effects of statins. *Curr Opin Lipidol* **12**, 543–59.

Dayton, S., Pearce, M.L., Hashimoto, S. *et al.* (1969) A controlled clinical trial of a diet high in unsaturated fat in preventing complications of atherosclerosis. *Circulation* **39**(Suppl. II), II-1–II-60.

Diabetes Atherosclerosis Intervention Study Investigators (2001) Effect of fenofibrate on progression of coronary-artery disease in type 2 diabetes: the Diabetes Atherosclerosis Intervention Study, a randomized study. *Lancet* **357**, 905–10.

Downs, J.R., Clearfield, M., Weis, S. *et al.* (1998) Primary prevention of acute coronary events with lovastatin in men and women with average cholesterol levels. *JAMA* **279**, 1615–22.

Endres, M., Laufs, U., Huang, Z. *et al.* (1998) Stroke protection by 3-hydroxy-3-methylglutaryl (HMG)-CoA reductase inhibitors mediated by endothelial nitric oxide synthase. *Proc Natl Acad Sci USA* **95**, 8880–5.

Ericsson, C.G., Hamsten, A., Nilsson, J. *et al.* (1996) Angiographic assessment of effects of bezafibrate on progression of coronary artery disease in young male postinfarction patients. *Lancet* **347**, 849–53.

Frick, M.H., Elo, O., Haapa, K. *et al.* (1987) The Helsinki Heart Study: primary prevention trial with gemfibrozil in middle-aged men with dyslipidaemia. Safety of treatment, changes in risk factors and incidence of coronary heart disease. *N Engl J Med* **317**, 1237–45.

Frick, M.H., Syvanne, M., Nieminen, M.S. *et al.* (1997) Prevention of the angiographic progression of coronary and vein-graft atherosclerosis by gemfibrozil after coronary bypass surgery in men with low levels of HDL-cholesterol. *Circulation* **96**, 2137–43

Furberg, B. and Furberg, C. (1994) What clinicians need to know about clinical trials. In *All That Glitters is Not Gold*. Dr Potata, Winston-Salem, USA.

Haffner, S.M. (2000) Secondary prevention of coronary heart disease. The role of fibric acids. *Circulation* **102**, 2–4.

Hambrecht, R., Niebauer, J., Marburger, C. et al. (1993) Various intensities of leisure time physical activity in patients with coronary artery disease: effects on cardiorespiratory fitness and progression of coronary atherosclerotic lesions. *J Am Coll Cardiol* **22**, 468–77.

Heady, J.A., Morris, J.N. and Oliver, M.F. (1992) WHO clofibrate/cholesterol trial: clarifications. *Lancet* **340**, 1405–6.

Hehmann, H.W., Bunt, T., Hellwig, N. et al. (1991) Progression and regression of minor coronary arterial narrowings by quantitative angiography after fenofibrate therapy. *Am J Cardiol* **67**, 957–61.

Hjermann, I., Holme, I., Velve Byre K. and Leren, P. (1981) Effect of diet and smoking intervention on the incidence of coronary heart disease: report from the Oslo Study Group of a randomised trial in healthy men. *Lancet* **2**, 1303–10.

Holme, I. (1990) An analysis of randomized trials evaluating the effect of cholesterol reduction in total mortality and coronary heart disease incidence. *Circulation* **82**, 1916–24.

Johannesson, M., Jonsson, B., Kjekshus, J. et al. (1997) Cost effectiveness of simvastatin treatment to lower cholesterol levels in patients with coronary heart disease. *N Engl J Med* **336**, 332–6.

Jukema, J.W., Bruschke, A.V.G., van Boven, A.J. et al. (1995) Effects of lipid lowering by pravastatin on progression and regression of coronary artery disease in symptomatic men with normal to moderately elevated serum cholesterol levels: the Regression Growth Evaluation Statin Study (REGRESS). *Circulation* **91**, 2528–40.

Kane, J.P., Malloy, M.J., Ports, T.H.A. et al. (1990) Regression of coronary atherosclerosis during treatment of familial hypercholesterolemia with combined drug regimens. *J Am Med Assoc* **264**, 3007–12.

Kinlay, S., Libby, P. and Ganz, P. (2001) Endothelial function and coronary artery disease. *Curr Opin Lipidol* **12**, 383–9.

Kjekshus, J., Pederson, T.R., Olsson, A.E., Faergeman, O., Pyorala, K. (1997) The effect of simvastatin on the incidence of heart failure in patients with coronary heart disease. *J Cardiac Failure* **3**, 249–54.

Law, M.R., Thompson, S.G. and Wald, N.J. (1994a) Assessing possible hazards of reducing serum cholesterol. *Br Med J* **308**, 373–9.

Law, M.R., Wald, N.J. and Thompson, S.G. (1994b) By how much and how quickly does reduction in serum cholesterol concentration lower risk of ischaemic heart disease? *Br Med J* **308**, 367–72.

Law, M.R., Wald, N.J., Wu, T. et al. (1994c) The Cholesterol Papers I–III. *Br Med J* **308**, 363–79.

Leung, W.-H., Lau, C.-P. and Wong, C.-K. (1993) Beneficial effect of cholesterol-lowering therapy on coronary endothelium-dependent relaxation in hypercholesterolaemic patients. *Lancet* **341**, 1496–500.

Lipid Research Clinics Programme (1984) The Lipid Research Clinics Coronary Primary Prevention Trial Results I. Reduction in incidence of coronary heart disease. *J Am Med Assoc* **251**, 351–64.

The long-term intervention with pravastatin in ischaemic disease (LIPID) study group (1998) Prevention of cardiovascular events and death with prevastatin in patients with coronary heart disease and a broad range of initial cholesterol levels. *N Engl J Med* **339**, 1349–57.

MAAS Investigators (1994) Effect of simvastatin on coronary atheroma: The Multicentre Anti Atheroma Study (MAAS). *Lancet* **344**, 633–8.

Mellwig, K.P., Baller, D., Gluchmann, U., Moll, D., Betker, S., Weise, R., Notohamiprodjo, G. (1998) Improvement of coronary vasodilitation capacity through single LDL-apheresis. *Athersclerosis* **139**, 173–8.

MRC:BHF Heart Protection Study Collaborative Group (1999) MRC:BHF heart protection study of cholesterol-lowering therapy and antioxidant vitamin supplementation in a wide range of patients at increased risk of coronary heart disease death: early safety and efficacy experience. *Eur Heart J* **20**, 725–41.

Muldoon, M.F., Manuck, S.B. and Mathews, K.A. (1990) Lowering cholesterol concentrations and mortality: a quantitative review of primary prevention trials. *Br Med J* **301**, 309–14.

Ornish, D., Brown, S., Scherwitz, L.W. *et al.* (1990) Can lifestyle changes reverse coronary heart disease? The Lifestyle Heart Trial. *Lancet* **336**, 129–33.

Pedersen, T.R., Berg, K., Cook, T.J. *et al.* (1996a) Safety and tolerability of cholesterol lowering with simvastatin during 5 years in the Scandinavian Simvastatin Survival Study. *Arch Intern Med* **156**, 2085–92.

Pedersen, T.R., Kjekshus, J., Berg, K. *et al.* (1996b) Cholesterol lowering and the use of Healthcare Resources. Results of the Scandinavian Simvastatin Survival Study. *Circulation* **93**, 1796–802.

Pedersen, T.R., Kjekshus, J., Pyorala, K., Olsson, A.E., Cook, T.J., Musliner, T.A. *et al.* (1998) Effect of simvastatin on ischaemic signs and symptoms in the Scandinavian Simvastatin Survival Study(4S). *Am J Cardiol* **81**, 333–5.

Pekkanen, J., Linn, S., Heiss, G. *et al.* (1990) Ten year mortality from cardiovascular disease in relation to cholesterol level among men with and without pre-existing cardiovascular disease. *N Engl J Med* **322**, 1700–7.

Pitt, B., Mancini, G.B.J., Ellis, S.B. *et al.* (1995) Pravastatin Limitation of Atherosclerosis in the Coronary Arteries (PLAC 1): reduction in atherosclerosis progression and clinical events. *J Am Coll Cardiol* **26**, 1133–9.

Pitt, B., Waters, D., Brown, W.V. *et al.* (1999) Aggressive lipid-lowering compared with angio-plasty in stable artery disease. *N Engl J Med*, **341**, 70–6.

Post Coronary Artery Bypass Graft Trial Investigators (1997) The effect of aggressive lowering of low density lipoprotein cholesterol levels and low dose anticoagulation on obstructive changes in saphenous vein coronary artery bypass grafts. *N Engl J Med* **336**, 153–62.

Ravnskov, U. (1992) Cholesterol lowering trials in coronary heart disease: frequency of citation and outcome. *Br Med J* **305**, 15–19.

Robins, S.J. (2001) PPAR α ligands and clinical trials: cardiovascular risk reduction with fibrates. *J Cardiovasc Risk* **8**, 195–201.

Rossouw, J.E., Lewis, B. and Rifkind, B.M. (1990) The value of lowering cholesterol after myocardial infarction. *N Engl J Med* **323**, 1112–19.

Rubins, H.B., Robins, S.J., Coillins, D., Fye, C.L., Anderson, J.W., Elam, M.S. *et al.* (1999) Gemfibrozil for the secondary prevention of coronary heart disease in men with low levels of high density lipoprotein cholesterol. *N Engl J Med* **341**, 410–18.

Sacks, F.M., Pfeffer, M.A., Moye, L.A. *et al.* (1996) The effects of pravastatin on coronary events after myocardial infarction in patients with average cholesterol levels. *N Engl J Med* **335**, 1001–9.

Scandinavian Simvastatin Survival Study Group (1994) Randomised trial of cholesterol-lowering in 4444 patients with coronary heart disease: the Scandinavian Simvastatin Survival Study (4S). *Lancet* **344**, 1383–9.

Scandinavian Simvastatin Survival Study Group (1995) Baseline serum cholesterol and treatment effect in the Scandinavian Simvastatin Survival Study (4S). *Lancet* **345**, 1274–5.

Serruys, P.W., de Feyter, P.J., Benghozi, R., Hugenholtz, P.G., Lesaffre, E. for the LIPS Investigators (2001) The Lescol Intervention Prevention Study (LIPS): a double-blind, placebo-controlled, randomized trial of the long term effects of fluvastatin after successful transcatheter therapy in patients with coronary heart disease. *Int J Intervent Cardiol* **4**, 165–72.

Serruys, P.W., de Feyter, P., Macaya, C., et al. (2002) Fluvastatin for prevention of cardiac events following successful first percutaneous coronary intervention: A randomized controlled trial. *J Am Med Assoc* **287**, 3215–22.

Shepherd, J., Cobbe, S.M., Ford, I. et al. (1995) Prevention of coronary heart disease with pravastatin in men with hypercholesterolaemia. *N Engl J Med* **333**, 1301–7.

Smilde, T.J., van Wissen, S., Wollersheim, H., Trip, M.D., Kastelein, J.J.P. and Stalenhoef, A.F.H. (2001) Effect of aggressive versus conventional lipid lowering on atherosclerosis progression in familial hypercholesterolaemia (ASAP): a prospective randomised double-blind trial. *Lancet*, **357**, 577–81.

Smith, G.D. and Pekkanen, J. (1992) Should there be a moratorium on the use of cholesterol lowering drugs? *Br Med J* **304**, 431–4.

Stenestrand, U., Wallentin, L. (2001) Early statin treatment following acute myocardial infarction and 1-year survival. *JAMA* **285**, 430–6.

Tonkin, A.M., Colquhoun, D., Emberson, J., Hague, W., Keech, A., Lane, G. et al. for the LIPID Study Group (2000) Effects of pravastatin in 3260 patients with unstable angina: results from the LIPID study. *Lancet* **355**, 1871–5.

Treasure, C.B., Klein, J.L., Weintraub, W.S. et al. (1995) Beneficial effects of cholesterol lowering therapy on the coronary endothelium in patients with coronary artery disease. *N Engl J Med* **332**, 481–7.

Turpeinen, O. (1979) Effect of cholesterol-lowering diet on mortality from coronary heart disease and other causes. *Circulation* **59**, 1–7.

Waters, D., Higginson, L., Gladstone, P. et al. (1994) Effects of monotherapy with an HMG-CoA reductase inhibitor on the progression of coronary atherosclerosis as assessed by serial quantitative arteriography. The Canadian Coronary Atherosclerosis Intervention Trial. *Circulation* **89**, 959–68.

Watts, G.F., Lewis, B., Brunt, J.N.H. et al. (1992) Effects on coronary artery disease of lipid-lowering diet, or diet plus cholestyramine in the St Thomas' Atherosclerosis Regression Study (STARS). *Lancet* **339**, 563–8.

West of Scotland Coronary Prevention Study Group (1992) A coronary primary prevention study of Scottish men age 45–64 years: trial design. *J Clin Epidemiol* **45**, 849–60.

White, H.D., Simes, R.J., Anderson, N.E., Hankey, G.J., Watson, J.D.G., Hunt, D. et al. (2000) Pravastatin therapy and the risk of stroke. *N Engl J Med* **343**, 317–26.

Wong, N.D., Wilson, P.W.F., Kannel, W.B. (1991) Serum cholesterol as a prognostic factor after myocardial infarction: the Framingham Study. *Ann Intern Med* **115**, 687–93.

Wysowski, D.K. and Gross, T.P. (1990) Deaths due to accidents and violence in two recent trials of cholesterol-lowering drugs. *Arch Intern Med* **150**, 2169–72.

PRACTICAL CONSIDERATIONS AND SPECIAL AREAS

MEETING THE CHALLENGE

EVIDENCE OF UNDER-TREATMENT

Despite the compelling nature of the evidence base and widespread endorsement of the principles, there remains a wide therapeutic gap between recommendations for preventative cardiovascular interventions and their implementation. The failure to achieve the potential of evidence-based interventions in the secondary prevention of coronary heart disease in hospital practice in the UK was highlighted in the ASPIRE study (Action on Secondary Prevention through Intervention to Reduce Events) published in 1996. Between 1994 and 1995 the notes of more than 2400 patients undergoing revascularization or experiencing a myocardial infarction were examined and it was found that only a tiny minority were receiving lipid-lowering treatment (8 per cent) and that even when treated, the majority were inadequately controlled according to national guidelines. In mitigation, the landmark 4S trial, with its seminal impact on practice, was not published until November 1994.

Subsequently, as part of a European-wide strategy, the European Society of Cardiology (ESC) launched the EUROASPIRE study to survey current practice in nine other European countries: the Czech Republic, Finland, France, Germany, Hungary, Italy, the Netherlands, Slovenia and Spain. A total of 4863 consecutive male and female patients <70 years old with CHD were identified from hospital records and after deaths and non-responders were excluded; 3569 patients received a follow-up interview and examination at least 6 months after the index event. With data collection between May 1995 and April 1996, the impact of new information was evident, but the overall results were tremendously disappointing. The results are shown with those of EUROASPIRE 2, the most recent survey, where the results of data collection between September 1999 and February 2000 were announced at the ESC meeting in Amsterdam in August 2000 (Table 10.1).

An equally gloomy picture is seen in the USA where Pearson and colleagues found in the Lipid Treatment Assessment Project (LTAP, published 2000) that amongst 4888 patients, only 38 per cent achieved target NCEP LDL cholesterol goals at all and that of 1460 CHD patients, only 18 per cent achieved the goal of <100 mg/dL.

TABLE **10.1** • Results of EUROASPIRE 1 and 2 (% patients)

Audit criterion (European Task Force recommendations)	EUROASPIRE 1	EUROASPIRE 2
Smoking persistence	19.4	20.8
BMI >30 kg/m²	25.3	32.8
BP >140/90 mmHg	55.4	53.9
Aspirin Rx	81.2	83.9
Beta blocker Rx	53.7	66.4
ACE inhibitor Rx	29.5	42.7
Lipid-lowering Rx	32.0	62.9
Total cholesterol >5.0 mmol/L	86.2	58.8

Source: EUROASPIRE I and II Group (2001).

The situation is no better in primary care where the continuous nature of patient contact should afford greater opportunities for implementing long-term strategies. In 1998, Campbell *et al.* surveyed 1921 patients with CHD aged less than 80 years from a random sample of general practices in the Grampian region of Scotland. Most patients undertook little physical activity, one-fifth continued to smoke and two-thirds were overweight. Aspirin usage was high in patients with recent MI (85 per cent) but only 32 per cent took beta-blockers and ACE inhibitor usage in those with heart failure was low at 40 per cent. Lipid management was largely neglected, despite the existence of local guidelines, and only 17 per cent achieved a goal of <5.2 mmol/L. Ninety-three per cent of patients had at least one aspect of their medical management that would benefit from change and half had at least two modifiable risk factors.

OBSTACLES TO PREVENTION

The reasons for the failure of health professionals to implement preventative interventions are multiple. Influences are active not only at the levels of individual health professionals and patients, but also within the structure of care wherein both consult. The influences range from historical, cultural and ideological to attitudinal, organizational and fiscal.

For **health professionals**, time constraints are common. It takes time to coordinate and enact CHD prevention strategies. Health professionals are busy and the responsibility for these activities is not always demarcated. Hospital practitioners rightly concentrate on the acute event, as to fail the patient then is obvious and potentially tragic. The failure to implement long-term strategies is, however, just as tragic but is deferred to the future and the failing practitioner feels no immediate guilt. At its worst, lack of communication at the primary/secondary care interface can lead to a collusion of anonymity whereby nobody assumes responsibility for implementing long-term strategies. In addition, hospital doctors exert a strong influence on general practice prescribing. The effect of not prescribing a statin at discharge post-MI might be to devalue the intervention in the eyes of the receiving general practitioner. Guidelines can facilitate the resolution of these issues but they need to be simple, consistent, evidence-based and cost-effective as well as reflective of local priorities and agreement to ensure ownership and uptake.

Health professionals also differ in their knowledge base, beliefs and the acknowledgement of their preventative role in what they may perceive as a complex scenario. There is evidence of selection bias in the choice of which individuals receive treatment and age, gender, race, weight, educational attainment, socioeconomic status, payment source, geographic region and physician specialty all strongly influence lipid management decisions. CHD prevention is a major undertaking to achieve systematically across the range of risk factors and health professionals may be concerned about their existing workload or resistant to change. They may still be influenced by past controversy, concerned about adverse effects, or naturally nihilistic and conservative. For many, budgetary constraints are important and tend to encourage older approaches, particularly in countries where levels of atherosclerosis are high. Resource constraints mean that many practitioners lack the infrastructure, in terms of ancillary personnel, information technology and models of care, to provide appropriate support and follow-up to patients for CHD prevention. Support for health professionals should also include appropriate education and training and the development of systems of quality monitoring.

Barriers to the implementation of CHD prevention strategies also arise within **patients**. Patients tend to overestimate their health and incompatible health beliefs are commonly juxtaposed with cultural influences. For example, increased abdominal girth and a cigar to match are universal symbols of wealth, power and prosperity. The influences of family members, friends, the media and even, unfortunately, different health professionals all affect the knowledge, fears and perceptions that each individual brings to the negotiation.

The National Cholesterol Education Program in America helpfully lists tactics for enhancing compliance and these are shown below.

- Teach the patient about the treatment regimen – instructions should be simple but complete.
- Help the patient to remember to take the medication – tailor doses to daily habits.
- Reinforce compliance – ask about it, chart lipid responses, provide encouragement.
- Anticipate common problems and teach the patient how to manage them.
- Involve a family member or friend in the patient's therapy programme.
- Establish a supportive relationship with the patient – provide ongoing updates and information about the patient's illness and treatment.
- Provide individualized services for patients who avoid compliance.
- Assess barriers:
  - (a) Physical, e.g. poor vision, forgetfulness;
  - (b) Access, e.g. transportation, income and time;
  - (c) Attitude, e.g. fatalism;

(d) Therapy, e.g. complexity, side-effects;

(e) Social, e.g. family instability;

(f) Faulty perceptions, e.g. denial, looks to symptoms to prompt treatment.

CHD PREVENTION IN THE COMMUNITY

Community-based prevention programmes generally use the population approach to risk factor modification and utilize professionals from many disciplines in a variety of settings to communicate, usually, multiple health messages. As well as health-care professionals, educators, nutritionists, exercise facilitators, the media and government agencies may all be involved. Large-scale CHD prevention programmes were initiated in the 1970s following the epidemiological identification of the key risk factors by cohort studies such as Framingham. The discovery by Keys in the analysis of the Seven Countries Study (page 34) that eastern districts of Finland had very high rates of CHD led to the foundation of a community-based project in North Karelia to target CHD. Activities included media campaigns to urge people to eat more fruit and vegetables and stop smoking, the training of health professionals, teachers, social workers and volunteers to provide lifestyle advice, the reorganization of hypertension services, changes in food labelling and composition and increased tobacco taxation. After 10 years, cigarette smoking in men had fallen by 34 per cent, cholesterol by 11 per cent and mean diastolic blood pressure by 6 per cent, compared with controls in Kuopio, where levels fell by 8 per cent, 9 per cent and 4 per cent, respectively. Between 1974 and 1979, North Karelia experienced a 24 per cent reduction in CHD mortality in men and 51 per cent in women, compared with 12 per cent and 24 per cent for the rest of Finland. The results of the study in the 1980s were less convincing and this may have been due to natural population effects producing declining rates of CHD, obscuring the effects of the interventions.

Although most community-based interventions have tended to show small improvements in risk factors, the results of others have been more equivocal and the conclusions disputed, as interventions compared with baseline or control communities do not have the evidential strength of randomized controlled trials. Overall, the evidence for benefit is mixed and, given the high cost of intensive programmes like the North Karelia project, there is little likelihood that similar large-scale programmes will be replicated.

CHD PREVENTION IN PRIMARY CARE

In the UK in 1982, Fullard, Fowler and Gray initiated the Oxford Prevention of Heart Attack and Stroke project. A systematic approach by nurses greatly improved the recording of cardiovascular risk factors compared with opportunistic activity by GPs. In the early 1990s, the contract for UK GPs favoured health promotion activity for the first time and nurse involvement running 'OXCHECK' well-person and new-patient medicals was financially rewarded. There was much scepticism, however, surrounding the efficacy of the checks in relation to health gain and a study in Powys, Wales (1993), suggested that well-person clinics were ineffective.

TABLE **10.2** • Oxcheck Trial and British Family Heart Study (BFHS): summary of results (1994)

Risk factor	Reduction in risk factors (%) Oxcheck		
	Year 1	Year 2	BFHS
Total cholesterol	2.3	3.1 (>)	4.0
Systolic BP	2.5	1.9	7.0
Diastolic BP	2.4	1.9	
Smoking	0	0	5.0
BMI	0	1.4	
Diet	Improved (not significant)	Improved (significant)	

The results of two large randomized, controlled, nurse-led screening and intervention programmes have been published and the results are shown in Table 10.2.

■ The **OXCHECK Trial** (The OXCHECK Study Group 1994–95). Participants aged 35–64 years were drawn from the patients of five group practices in three towns in Bedfordshire, England. After a 45-minute initial interview in 1989, the patients were followed up 1 year and 3 years later.
■ The **British Family Heart Study** (Family Heart Study Group, 1994). In the BFHS, lifestyle screening and advice were given to men and their partners from 26 practices across 13 towns. Each town had a control practice as well as the intervention practice. The interviews were longer and more intensive and the results were compared at 1 year.

Much publicity surrounded the publication of the results, which were considered disappointing considering the effort, the level of motivation of the researchers and the high expectations of benefit. However, when examined in terms of CHD risk reduction, OXCHECK showed a reduction of 6 per cent in males and 13 per cent in females due to cholesterol alone. The drop in blood pressure over time could be an 'acclimatization' effect (noted in other studies), but if significant would further reduce CHD risk by 7 per cent. The BFHS researchers calculated a 12 per cent CHD risk reduction in men and almost the same in women. Small but significant benefits are thus evident. It is interesting to note that the results are comparable to the 1-year results of the North Karelia project, which eventually demonstrated a 40 per cent CHD reduction over 20 years.

Cost-effectiveness data were published in 1996 by Langham *et al.* and Wonderling *et al.* In terms of life-years gained, the more intensive BFHS intervention was more effective but less cost-effective than the OXCHECK trial. The OXCHECK programme is cost-effective if the effect were to last for 5 years but the effect must last for about 10 years if the extra cost associated with the BFHS were to be justified.

Both of these studies extended invitations randomly to screening candidates irrespective of their cardiovascular risk factor profiles. Undoubtedly, targeting specifically those patients at high risk would have proved more cost-effective.

NURSE-LED CLINICS IN PRIMARY CARE

As up to 5 per cent of patients on general practitioners' lists have CHD, the implementation of a comprehensive range of intervention strategies is a daunting remit. A multidisciplinary, team-based approach is more likely to be effective. The extended role of nurses has been further examined in a randomized controlled trial from North East Scotland.

A total of 1343 patients with CHD were identified from 19 practices through searches of morbidity registers and nitrate-prescribing records and randomized to intervention and control groups. Patients in the intervention group attended nurse-run clinics where attention was given to aspirin usage, blood pressure and lipid control (according to established guidelines) and the encouragement of increased exercise, the consumption of a low-fat diet and the cessation of smoking. The clinics ran for 1 year, preliminary visits averaging 45 minutes and follow-up visits (every 2–6 months) around 20 minutes.

The intervention improved all aspects of secondary prevention except smoking and percentage improvements and odds ratios comparing the groups are shown in Table 10.3.

The improvement in lipid parameters in both groups is striking and probably reflects the effect of emerging data during the course of the trial. The study clinics, however, still produced more effective lipid control.

These findings contrast markedly with the results of OXCHECK and the Family Heart Study. The differences lie in the large element of medical treatment implicit in secondary prevention, in comparison to lifestyle advice, which is much more difficult to implement in a lower risk population. The importance of this study is that it demonstrates that significant interventions can be achieved within a short space of time in primary care for patients whose absolute risk of a further event is high.

Investigators have taken a different approach in the Southampton Heart Integrated Care Project (SHIP). A total of 597 patients with newly diagnosed CHD were identified in hospital and randomized. Three specialist liaison nurses were recruited to coordinate secondary prevention by improving communication between hospital and general practice and to encourage practice nurses to provide structured follow-up. The liaison nurse telephoned the practice prior to hospital discharge to speak to the practice nurse and book the first follow-up appointment. Practice nurses were encouraged to use

TABLE **10.3** • Percentage improvements and odds ratios for CHD interventions in nurse-led clinics

	% Improvement intervention group	% Improvement control group	Odds ratio
Aspirin uptake	11.7	3.2	3.22
Blood pressure control	9.8	0.2	5.32
Lipid control	29.2	7.8	3.19
Exercise	4.4	−1.1	1.67
Low fat diet	7.5	0.0	1.47
Non-smoking	0.2	1.9	0.78 NS

TABLE **10.4** • Changes in CHD risk factors in SHIP

	Control group	Intervention group
Cholesterol (mmol/L)	5.93	5.80
SBP (mmHg)	139.1	136.9
DBP (mmHg)	85.0	83.7
Distance walked in 6 minutes (m)	433	443
BMI (kg/m^2)	28.2	27.4
Stopped smoking (%)	20	19

the liaison nurses for advice on clinical or organizational issues. Recommendations for clinical management were attached to each discharge communication and each patient held their own record, prompting follow-up at standard intervals. The liaison nurses had further educational and support roles to the primary care teams. Outcome measures at 1 year are shown Table 10.4.

Although all parameters are improved, none is statistically significant. In addition, there were no significant differences in prescribing, but 18 per cent more patients in the intervention group attended cardiac rehabilitation sessions and this was significant.

The findings are disappointing and suggest that the benefit of nurse liaison interventions is limited. The position of practice nurses in primary care teams may limit their effectiveness in coordinating and monitoring prescribing. A unified strategy, involving the whole primary care team, is urged with a register, clear quality standards, follow-up and routine audit of care.

Such a strategy emerged in the UK in March 2000 with the publication of the National Service Framework for Coronary Heart Disease (see box).

THE UK NATIONAL SERVICE FRAMEWORK FOR CORONARY HEART DISEASE

In the UK, National Service Framework statements are part of the government's initiative to improve the quality of health care. The statement on CHD outlines an ambitious programme to reduce the incidence of CHD in the UK over the subsequent decade. The document itemizes explicit standards for health professionals to achieve at all organizational levels and success will demand new structures of care with both integral monitoring systems and accountability for the quality of care at the core. As a 'blueprint for tackling heart disease', it stands as a model statement to improve the overall health of a high-risk population and reduce variations and inconsistencies in service provision.

Twelve standards cover:

- Population approaches to CHD reduction: standards 1 + 2
- Preventing CHD in high-risk patients: standards 3 + 4
- Myocardial infarction and other acute coronary syndromes: standards 5 + 6 + 7

STATEMENTS ON CHD

- Stable angina: standard 8
- Revascularization: standards 9 + 10
- Heart failure: standard 11
- Cardiac rehabilitation: standard 12.

Standards 3 and 4 describe the care to be provided by primary care teams for people with established cardiovascular disease (standard 3) and for those who have yet to develop symptoms but whose CHD risk exceeds 30 per cent over 10 years (standard 4). The standards define specific criteria to focus data recording and enhance the usefulness and quality of clinical audit within the health service at practice, locality and wider levels. It is likely that these performance indicators will ultimately contribute to assessment of the primary care team's performance and potentially, its remuneration. The criteria for standards 3 and 4 are shown in Table 10.5.

To accommodate primary care teams at different stages of development, the expectations of the National Service Framework are staged in a series of milestones. However, by 2003, all primary care teams will be expected to:

- develop local protocols and provide register-based, structured care for all high-risk patients;
- audit care annually;
- meet regularly to discuss clinical issues and discuss audit results.

TABLE **10.5** • Criteria for standards 3 and 4

Criterion	Primary prevention	Secondary prevention
Advice about how to stop smoking including NRT	+	+
Advice about other modifiable risk factors including exercise, diet, alcohol consumption, weight and diabetes	+	+
Advice and treatment to maintain BP <140/80 mmHg	+	+
Statins and dietary advice to lower serum cholesterol below 5 mmol/L (LDL-C <3 mmol/L) or by 20–25% (LDL-C by 30%) – whichever is the greater	+	+
Meticulous control of BP and glucose in diabetics	+	+
Low-dose aspirin		+
ACE inhibitors for patients with left ventricular dysfunction		+
Beta-blockers for patients with a history of MI		+
Warfarin or aspirin for people >60 years with AF		+

MANAGING LIPIDS IN PRIMARY CARE

It is perhaps anachronistic, in this age of multifactorial CHD risk reduction to focus unilaterally on a single risk factor but the confident management of lipid disorders still eludes many primary care team members.

Primary care teams are now organizing integrated CHD prevention services, specifically targeting high-risk patients such as those with multiple risk factors, bad family histories, genetic hyperlipidaemia, hypertension, diabetes and, above all, those with pre-existing atherosclerosis.

The management of lipids in primary care does not require a formal stand-alone clinic (cf. the antenatal clinic) but can be incorporated seamlessly into everyday practice as part of an integrated programme (in the same way that antenatal patients can be seen individually in normal surgeries). There is considerable scope for a multidisciplinary approach involving other primary care team members with different team members contributing according to their skill mix. To ensure uniformity of approach, it is essential to establish agreed guidelines or, more formally, a practice protocol. Constructed from the available evidence, this can set standards, specify data recording and facilitate clinical audit. An example is shown below.

Whom to test

Cholesterol screening should be offered to:

1. All patients with a history of atherosclerosis [coronary heart disease (CHD), peripheral arterial disease (PAD) and cerebrovascular disease (CVD)]. Intervention is justified for individuals with reasonable life expectancy and quality of life.
2. Patients aged up to 75 years with
   - A family history of – CHD (especially before 55 years)
                          – PAD or CVD
                          – Hyperlipidaemia
   - Diabetes mellitus – HPS would suggest up to 80 years
   - Hypertension
   - Physical stigmata of hyperlipidaemia
   - Smoking habits
   - Obvious obesity
   - Chronic renal disease

What to test

A random non-fasting cholesterol is adequate on most occasions

For patients known to be at high-risk, e.g. secondary prevention, the full 12–14-hour fasting profile should be measured to estimate total serum cholesterol (TC), HDL cholesterol (HDL-C) and triglycerides (TG). LDL-C is calculated from these values, using the Friedewald equation.

Taking blood

Sitting, after 10 minutes rest.
Preferably uncuffed.
After minor illness (e.g. 'flu)
postpone 3 weeks

After major illness (e.g. MI or surgery) take
blood within 24 hours or postpone 3 months

CLINICAL AUDIT

Interpretation of results

Taking several readings helps to overcome biological and laboratory variation.

	Acceptable	Abnormal	Very high
Total cholesterol	<5.0	5.0–7.8	>7.8
HDL-C	Higher levels	<0.9 men	Lower levels
		<1.1 women	

The fasting profile (12–14 hours) enables accurate assessment of triglyceride levels and delineates the pattern of dyslipidaemia. Higher TG levels (>1.5) are associated with low HDL-C and changes in LDL-C, producing a more atherogenic profile. TG > 5.0 carries an increasing risk of pancreatitis.

Does the patient have secondary hypercholesterolaemia?

Common secondary causes	Less common causes
1. Obesity	6. Chronic renal failure (and nephrosis)
2. Diabetes mellitus	7. Chronic liver disease (e.g. primary
3. Alcohol abuse	biliary cirrhosis)
4. Hypothyroidism (esp.	8. Anorexia/bulimia
post-menopausal females)	9. Myeloma
5. Drugs – thiazides, beta-blockers,	
cimetidine, steroids,	
immunosuppressives, e.g. cyclosporin	

Investigations might include: urinalysis, fasting glucose, T4, TSH, creatinine, liver function.

Primary hypercholesterolaemia

1. Common polygenic hypercholesterolaemia (99%)
2. Familial hypercholesterolaemia (0.2%)
3. Familial combined hypercholesterolaemia (0.3%)

(6 + 7 – pancreatitis risk not CHD)

4. Familial dysbetalipoproteinaemia (0.04%)
5. Familial hyperalphalipoproteinaemia (longevity)
6. Familial hypertriglyceridaemia
7. Familial hyperchylomicronaemia

Adult FH criteria: **TC > 7.5 mmol/L** (LDL > 4.9 mmol/L) **plus either**:
Tendon xanthomata in patient or relative or proven DNA mutation *(definite)*
or: Family history of MI < 50 y (2° relative) or < 60 y (1° relative) or raised cholesterol (1°) or TC > 7.5 mmol/L (2°) *(possible)*

Assessment of global risk

Informed clinical judgement of a patient's risk of cardiovascular disease is necessary for:

■ Choosing suitable treatment
■ Prognosis

Sources of high cardiovascular risk

■ Presence of pre-existing atherosclerosis (CHD, PAD or CVD)
■ Presence, severity or weighting and number of risk factors

Risk factors for coronary heart disease

Modifiable	Non-modifiable
Hyperlipidaemia	
Hypertension/LVH	Family history CHD
Smoking	Personal history CHD
Diabetes	Increasing age (esp. male >55, female >65)
Obesity	Male sex
Lack of exercise	Ethnic origin
Thrombogenic factors	

Priorities for treatment

1. Patients with pre-existing atherosclerosis (2° prevention)
2. ■ Patients with an absolute CHD risk >20% over 10 years (30% in UK) assessed using Framingham based risk calculator, e.g. Joint British or European (1° prevention)
   ■ Patients with genetic hyperlipidaemia

INTERVENTION

Non-lipid risk factor optimization

Risk factor	Goal of treatment	Comments
Hypertension	Systolic BP <140 mmHg Diastolic BP <85 mmHg	Combination therapy more likely to achieve these targets. Thiazides and beta-blockers may worsen co-existing hyperlipidaemia. Ca antagonists and ACE inhibitors lipid neutral. Alpha-blockers may

CLINICAL AUDIT

		improve lipid profiles. Beta-blockers and ACE inhibitors to be used with caution in PAD
Cigarette smoking	Cessation of smoking	*Repeated* counselling and reinforcement may be required
Diabetes mellitus	Optimization of lipids, BP, weight and glycaemic control.	BP <130/80 mmHg
Alcohol consumption	Men ≤ 21 units/week Women ≤ 14 units/week	
Obesity	Reduction ideally to BMI 20–25 kg/m^2	Truncal obesity worse than gynaecoid obesity
Lack of exercise	30 minutes moderate intensity exercise most days	Level of activity tailored to the individual

Diet

Cardioprotective diet. Optimize body weight. Maximizes benefit of drugs if prescribed. Ideally individual consultation with dietitian or trained practice nurse. Particularly consider benefits of fish, plant sterols and soya.

Drugs

Drug	Side-effects	Interactions	Comments
1. Hypercholesterolaemia (raised LDL)			
HMG-CoA reductase Inhibitors **(statins)** (lovastatin, simvastatin, pravastatin, fluvastatin, atorvastatin, rosuvastatin)	GI symptoms Occasionally myositis and liver damage	Risk of myositis with fibrates. CYP 450 3A4 inhibitors: PPIs, imidazole antifungals, macrolide antibiotics, calcium antagonists, SSRIs, amiodarone, protease inhibitors, cyclosporin and grapefruit juice. Potential interactions with warfarin, digoxin	Predominant effect is to reduce LDL-C. Take after food at night (unless long half-life). Monitor liver function tests (LFTs) first year, CK if indicated. Stop if AST × 3 or CPK × 10 ULN

Bile acid sequestrants **(resins)** (colestipol, cholestyramine, colesevelam)	GI symptoms especially constipation	Can prevent GI absorption of other drugs, e.g. digoxin, thyroxine, folic acid, anticoagulants, Fe	GI side-effects less likely, if introduced slowly. Most effective with or just before food. May increase TG. Give other drugs 1 hour before or 4–6 hours after

2. Mixed hyperlipidaemia (raised LDL + TG)

Statins			TG lowering effect = LDL-C reduction where TG raised
Fibrates (gemfibrozil, bezafibrate, fenofibrate, ciprofibrate)	GI symptoms Rarely myositis, impotence	Anticoagulants, statins	Best taken after food. Reduce TG, raise HDL-C. Newer agents reduce LDL-C.
Nicotinic acid drugs (nicotinic acid, acipimox, nicofuranose)	Flushes and pruritis. GI symptoms. Rarely liver damage and rashes		Aspirin alleviates. May worsen gout, diabetes and peptic ulcer

3. Hypertriglyceridaemia

Fibrates, nicotinic acid drugs.	GI symptoms
Omega-3 fatty acids	(Maxepa Omacor)

Combinations

Safe combinations include resins with statins or fibrates. The risk of myositis is increased when statins and fibrates are used together, but with careful monitoring this is possible in specialized circumstances. Plant sterol spreads may produce significant additional LDL-C reduction. Other cholesterol absorption blockers, such as ezetimibe, are due to be launched soon.

Target levels for cholesterol and LDL-C

■ TC < 5.0 mmol/L
■ LDL-C < 3.0 mmol/L (US < 2.6 mmol/L)

For all adults including the elderly and those with diabetes.

Follow-up

6-weekly fasting sample (with liver function if statin or fibrate) until target levels achieved.
Once stable, monitor lipids (can be non-fasting) every 6–12 months.
Discontinue if AST > ×3 normal.
Check CK if symptoms suggestive of myositis (abnormal-ULN ×10).

Referral

Consider referral with

■ Severe hyperlipidaemia (TC > 8.0 ± TG > 5.0)
■ Familial syndromes
■ Failure to achieve target levels

Special situations

Women
■ CHD events occur 10 years later than in men. This reduces the absolute risk of CHD except in the presence of diabetes.
■ In high-risk individuals there is no evidence to suggest that the benefits of lipid lowering are any less in women compared with men.
■ Continue HRT if already prescribed but do not consider as an adjunct to treatment in postmenopausal women.
■ The use of lipid-lowering drugs in pregnancy is best monitored in hospital lipid clinics.

Children
■ Screening can be undertaken early where genetic hyperlipidaemias are suspected.
■ Balanced low-fat diet has been shown to be safe beyond 5 years. Drug therapy generally commenced after 16 years. Best monitored in hospital lipid clinics.

Elderly	■ Value of primary prevention in patients without diabetes over 73 years is unknown.
	■ Those up to 80 years with established CHD, PAD, CVD or diabetes should be considered for intervention, according to life expectancy and quality of life.
	■ Hypothyroidism is common.
	■ Lower doses of drugs may be effective.
	■ Renal function may be compromised.
Targeting high-risk patients	■ All patients with MI should be targeted for risk factor screening and lipid lowering intervention, ideally within hospital (<24 hours) or in 1° care.
	■ Families of patients with MI under 50–60 years should be screened for genetic hyperlipidaemia.
	■ Patients with angina, post-CABG or -angioplasty have been much neglected.
	■ The CHD risk of diabetic patients is at least 3 × normal.
	■ The typical diabetic dyslipidaemia of low HDL-C/high TG is also much ignored.

CLINICAL AUDIT

COMMENTARY ON THE GUIDELINES

The illustrated primary care guidelines are an example of locally produced guidelines influenced by the recommendations of the Second Joint European Task Force and the Joint British Societies. They adopt a flow chart design from screening and result interpretation, through diagnosis and assessment, to interpretation and follow-up. All aspects are covered in greater detail in the wider context of this book.

Patients can be identified in a number of ways, either opportunistically or by systematic screening or from the scrutiny of disease registers or prescription databases (e.g. to identify patients for secondary prevention).

Whom to test

At initial interview, a decision can be made using the selective screening list to identify those patients who may be offered cholesterol testing. A history or symptoms of CHD, PAD (peripheral arterial disease) or CVD (cerebrovascular disease) should be elicited and an enquiry made into family history and other risk factors for CHD. Lipid stigmata can be identified and baseline measurements of height, weight and blood pressure taken and recorded.

As the evidence base extends the benefit of cholesterol lowering in patients beyond the age of 75, the age criteria can be extended in the secondary prevention situation, according to the patient's general state of health and their ability to survive long enough to benefit from the intervention.

What to test

In most instances, a random non-fasting cholesterol sample is adequate. There may be situations, however (for example, in secondary prevention), where there is an advantage in having as much information as possible and a fasting profile is preferred.

Taking blood

There is a need to standardize phlebotomy conditions and to be mindful of the effect of intercurrent illness.

Interpretation of results

Repeated testing is required before management decisions can be taken, reflecting the biological and laboratory variation from which cholesterol estimation suffers. Patients without other risk factors and with serum cholesterol levels <5.0 mmol/L can be reassured but should be screened again in 5 years.

LDL cholesterol levels are calculated using the Friedewald formula:

LDL cholesterol = Total cholesterol − HDL cholesterol − (triglyceride/2.19)

where triglyceride concentration is below 4.5 mmol/L.

Other causes of hypercholesterolaemia are excluded by asking the question 'Does the patient have secondary hypercholesterolaemia?' and an attempt at diagnosing **primary hypercholesterolaemia** can be made. In most cases the diagnosis will be the 'essential hypercholesterolaemia' of lipid metabolism: *common polygenic hypercholesterolaemia*.

Assessment of global risk and risk factors for coronary heart disease

In primary prevention, having established that a patient is dyslipidaemic, an attempt must be made to assess the overall risk of CHD using a CHD risk calculator. Risk assessment tools, such as those discussed in Chapter 5, are derived from analyses of Framingham data.

Priorities for treatment

There is international consensus that high-risk patients benefit most and should be targeted first in any CHD prevention initiative. Above all, those with pre-existing atherosclerosis and high-risk conditions like diabetes or genetic hyperlipidaemia should be identified and offered optimal treatment.

Intervention

Intervention involves **non-lipid risk factor optimization** and **diet** for all. CHD is a multifactorial disease and requires health professionals to optimize the plurality of risk factors for an individual to maximize health gain. New blood pressure targets are difficult to achieve but trial data suggest this can be achieved without compromising a patient's quality of life with adverse drug reactions.

A healthy diet involves far more than just lowering fat or cholesterol and the cardioprotective diet is outlined in Chapter 7. Whilst the effect on lipid parameters may sometimes be disappointing, other cardioprotective mechanisms are active and the right diet is complementary to subsequent interventions. Establishing good dietetic principles is time consuming, typically taking 3–6 months. Diet sheets abound but the personal approach of a health professional with nutrition skills is more effective.

Drugs and combinations

Large numbers of the adult population who have either already experienced an atherosclerotic event or have a high absolute cardiovascular risk profile would benefit from lipid lowering with medication. Although the bulk of the evidence relates to treatment with statins, other drugs may have roles, either separately or in combination, according to the pattern of the lipid profile on fasting analysis.

Target levels for cholesterol and LDL

Until ongoing trials identify the optimum target levels to which total and LDL cholesterol should be reduced, the goals of treatment are consensus derived. The goals of 5.0 mmol/L and 3.0 mmol/L for total cholesterol and LDL cholesterol, respectively, are easy to remember. The evidence base for the American LDL cholesterol goal of <2.6 mmol/L is not yet particularly strong.

Follow-up and referral

Suggestions for drug monitoring are included. Not all patients are straightforward and some need to be referred for secondary care assessment.

Throughout the programme it is important to contain the patient's anxiety, to explain problems, negotiate and outline time limits in which to achieve realistic objectives. Accurate record keeping is required and several specific record cards are available. Computerization of records facilitates audit.

The communication of results should be effective and a call/recall system could be devised to eliminate defaulters and facilitate appropriate follow-up and rescreening.

ROLE OF THE HOSPITAL LIPID CLINIC

With the advent of national and international guidelines for lipid-lowering therapy based on an impressive evidence base derived from placebo-controlled clinical endpoint trials, management of lipid lowering, including drug therapy, is rightly the province of general physicians (both in hospital and primary care), cardiologists, diabetologists, neurologists and others responsible for management of individuals at risk of vascular disease. Given the increased awareness of the benefits of lipid lowering and the availability of well tolerated and highly effective drugs, principally the statins, is there still a role for the specialist lipidologist? Clearly the role of the lipidologist is changing. Following the paradigm of hypertension where previously patients were investigated and treated by specialists but now only more complex cases are referred to secondary care, most patients with dyslipidaemia can be investigated and treated effectively without referral to a specialist. The lipidologist increasingly is referred patients who have failed to show an effective response to therapy either because of the severity of the lipid abnormality or intolerance of first-line agents. In the author's experience non-specialists feel less secure in managing patients with severe hypertriglyceridaemia and mixed hyperlipidaemia than they do with pure hypercholesterolaemia. The lipidologist can offer help and advice on drug dosage. Often statin usage is still restricted to starting doses and combination therapy, e.g. with statins and fibrates. The familial dyslipidaemias, familial combined hyperlipidaemia, familial hypercholesterolaemia, type III (remnant particle disease) and type I and V disease are all probably best treated in secondary care. Often in these patients high drug dosage or combination therapy is required, together with expert dietetic support. Special investigations (ultracentrifugation, enzyme testing, apoproteins, DNA genotyping) are available in specialist centres enabling detailed diagnostic work-up. Family screening is an important component of the management of these disorders and often this is easier to organize from secondary care. This enables the identification of family pedigrees, which not only provide the opportunity for earlier therapy but also a research database for further study. Many patients with inherited dyslipidaemia are at high risk of premature vascular disease. Non-invasive assessment of coronary ischaemia (exercise tolerance test, stress thallium) and other imaging techniques such as carotid intima-media thickening enable appropriate work-up of at-risk patients.

In specialist centres it is possible to conduct additional specialist services, such as joint paediatric clinics. In addition, easy access to other specialists in cardiology, diabetology, nephrology, gastroenterology, neurology and vascular surgery is important for the management of some patients. An increasingly important group of patients is those with complex metabolic abnormalities secondary to antiretroviral therapy for HIV/AIDS. This clearly is the province of the specialist, due not only to the complex dyslipidaemia, lipodystrophy and insulin resistance but also the potential of drug interactions.

REFERENCES AND FURTHER READING

Anonymous (1998) Recommendations of the Second Joint Task force of the European and other Societies on Coronary Prevention. Prevention of coronary heart disease in clinical practice. *Eur Heart J* **19**, 1434–503.

Anonymous (2001) Third Report of the National Cholesterol Education Program (NCEP) Expert Panel on Detection, Evaluation and Treatment of High Blood Cholesterol in Adults (Adult Treatment Panel III). *J Am Med Assoc* **285**, 2486–97.

ASPIRE Steering Group (1996) A British Cardiac Society survey of the potential for the secondary prevention of coronary heart disease – ASPIRE (Action on Secondary Prevention through Intervention to Reduce Events). *Heart* **75**, 334–42.

Campbell, N.C., Ritchie, L.D. and Thain, J. (1998) Secondary prevention in coronary heart disease: a randomized trial of nurse led clinics in primary care. *Heart* **80**, 447–52.

Campbell, N., Thain, J., Deans, H. *et al.* (1998) Secondary prevention in coronary heart disease: baseline survey of provision in general practice. *Br Med J* **316**, 1430–4.

EUROASPIRE I and II Group. (2001) Clinical reality of coronary prevention guidelines: a comparison of EUROASPIRE I and II in nine countries. *Lancet* **357**, 995–1001.

Family Heart Study Group. (1994) Randomized controlled trial evaluating cardiovascular screening and intervention in general practice: principal results of British family heart study. *Br Med J* **308**, 313–20.

Imperial Cancer Research Fund OXCHECK Study Group. (1995) Effectiveness of health checks conducted by nurses in primary care: final results of the OXCHECK study. *Br Med J* **310**, 1099–104.

Jolly, K., Bradley, F., Sharp, S. *et al.* (1999) Randomised trial of follow up care in general practice of patients with myocardial infarction and angina: final results of the Southampton heart integrated care project (SHIP). *Br Med J* **318**, 706–11.

Pearson, T.A., Laurora, I, Chu, H. and Kafonek, S. (2000) The Lipid Treatment Assessment Project (L-TAP): a multicenter survey to evaluate the percentages of dyslipidemic patients receiving lipid-lowering therapy and achieving low-density lipoprotein goals. *Arch Intern Med* **160**, 459–67.

Wood, D., Durrington, P., Poultner, N. *et al.* (1988) Joint British recommendations on prevention of coronary heart disease in clinical practice. *Heart* **80**(Suppl. 2), 1–29S.

SPECIAL AREAS

CHAPTER 11

THE PATIENT WITH ESTABLISHED CHD

Patients with symptomatic CHD – previous myocardial infarction, revascularization procedure or angina – are top priority for assessment and intervention with lipid-lowering therapy. If hospital physicians or primary care teams do little else in the lipid field, they should at least identify and manage effectively these very high-risk patients. There remains a worrying treatment gap in this area throughout Europe (EuroAspire Group, 2001) and even in the USA (Pearson *et al.*, 2000) (Figure 11.1).

Statin therapy in the secondary prevention of CHD represents one of the strongest and most complete evidence-based interventions in medicine. In addition to the

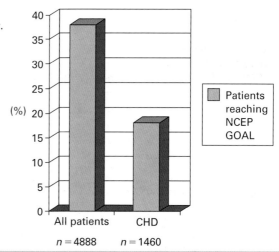

Patients

4888 patients (20–75 years, mean age 60.4 years) receiving lipid-lowering therapy.
23% <2 risk factors
47% 2 or more
30% CHD
606 primary care physicians across USA

FIGURE **11.1** • The Lipid Treatment Assessment Project (LTAP). Source: Pearson *et al.* (2000)

numerous angiographic studies (see Chapter 9) there is the massive data base of the endpoint trials (see Chapter 9) recently substantially enhanced by HPS. Statin therapy is highly cost-effective (Jönsson, 2001) and compares well with other important interventions (Table 11.1). In the 4S study, for example, the number needed to treat for 5 years was just six to prevent an event (death, coronary event, coronary artery bypass graft, angioplasty or stroke).

It is clear that all patients with new-onset CHD should be identified for potential statin therapy. In the past it was traditional to assess CHD patients 3 months following the acute event. This approach was adopted because of the changes that occur in the lipid profile following acute myocardial infarction – the decrease in cholesterol and increase in triglyceride. However, cholesterol can be measured on the first admission sample; though clearly not ideal, at least it draws attention to cholesterol and the need

TABLE **11.1** • Benefits of long-term strategies for prevention of CHD in post-myocardial infarction survivors

(a) Events prevented per 1000 patient-years of treatment

Treatment/strategy	Deaths prevented	Non-fatal events prevented
Aspirin[a]	7 vascular deaths	9 non-fatal reinfarctions, 3 non-fatal strokes
Beta-blocker[b]	21 deaths	21 reinfarctions
HMG-CoA reductase inhibitor (simvastatin)[c]	7 deaths	11, revascularizations, 12 non-fatal infarctions, 3 strokes, 4 congestive heart failures
Smoking cessation[d]	15 deaths	46 reinfarctions

(b) Number of patients who need to be treated for 5 years (NNT)

Treatment/strategy	Events prevented	NNT to prevent one event
Aspirin[a]	CHD death, stroke or infarction	12
HMG-CoA reductase inhibitor (simvastatin)[c]	CHD death, coronary event, CABG/PTCA or stroke	6
ACE inhibitor for left ventricular dysfunction:		
SAVE study[d]	CHD death or hospitalization for heart failure	10
SOLVD study[d]	CHD death or hospitalization for heart failure	21
CABG[e] for left main stem disease	CHD death	6

[a] Antiplatelet Trialists' collaboration (1994) *Br Med J* **308**, 81.
[b] Norwegian Multicentre Study Group (1981) *N Engl J Med* **304**, 801.
[c] 4S Study (1994) *Lancet* **344**, 1383.
[d] Young (1994) *Heart Lung Transplant* **13**, 2135.
[e] Laupacis (1988) *N Engl J Med* **318**, 1728.
Adapted from Sivers, F. (1996) *Evidence Based Strategies for Secondary Prevention of Coronary Heart Disease*. Science Press.

for modification of this essential risk factor. Starting therapy at the time of the acute event gives necessary credence and importance to this therapy, which no doubt will help reduce the treatment gap. Furthermore, although ongoing studies will provide further evidence, existing information obtained from register sources, retrospective analysis of statin use in other CHD trials and the MIRACL study point to the benefits of early treatment. Locally adopted protocols are clearly needed which may differ in detail but should include the statin prescription before discharge (e.g. if total cholesterol >5), with an indication to titrate therapy as necessary or instigate therapy based on a fasting lipid profile at 3–4 months. It is the authors' practice to use the NCEP ATP-III goal of therapy of LDL <2.6 mmol/L. An important contributory factor to the treatment gap is the use of inappropriately low statin doses. In CHD patients with mixed lipaemia, the authors adopt the NCEP ATP-III secondary goal of therapy, i.e. non-HDL cholesterol (<130 mg/dL; 3.37 mmol/L). This may involve high-dose statin therapy and occasionally combination therapy.

A substantial minority of patients with CHD have low HDL cholesterol as the primary lipid abnormality. This situation is seen more commonly in the Far East. The VA-HIT trial (see Chapter 9) certainly provides evidence of benefit for gemfibrozil therapy in men with CHD and low HDL cholesterol. In CHD patients with wider lipid inclusion criteria, bezafibrate therapy did not significantly reduce events. In retrospect, a statin comparator drug arm would have been of interest in VA-HIT. However, it is clear from the massive database of HPS that simvastatin therapy was beneficial across a wide total cholesterol range, in the presence of low HDL cholesterol and in the presence of increased triglyceride concentrations. There is no doubt that when all the results and detailed analyses are available from HPS, current guidelines will need thorough re-thinking and revision. A strong argument could be made that all CHD patients should receive statin therapy whatever the lipid profile. Indeed, in the euphoria following the announcement of the HPS results at the AHA meeting in November 2001, it was suggested – and this was not necessarily 'tongue in cheek' – that lipid measurements were no longer required; after all, platelet function is not measured before aspirin or clopidogrel therapy! The question then arises of which statin and what dose. Furthermore, HPS does not inform the physician of how low to lower LDL for maximum benefit. This question is the subject of ongoing trials (see Chapter 10). It will be the authors' practice in the short term to stick to NCEP ATP-III guidelines but in those with moderate LDL cholesterol elevations ensure at least a 1 mmol/L reduction. This policy will also be adopted in the presence of a low HDL cholesterol together with dieting and lifestyle measures to help increase HDL. If, despite attaining the LDL goal, hypertriglyceridaemia (>200 mg/dL; 2.3 mmol/L) remains, the secondary goal of non-HDL cholesterol (<130 mg/dL; <3.37 mmol/L) should be pursued (as discussed in Chapter 5), which may involve combination therapy. It is the authors' opinion that for safety reasons gemfibrozil therapy as used in VA-HIT should not be used in combination with a statin.

Care should be exercised when statin therapy is prescribed in patients taking anti-coagulants because of the possibility of drug interactions. This does not affect the authors' choice of statin but they arrange more frequent monitoring of anticoagulant dosage.

The role of statin therapy in heart failure is not clear as there is at present no available information from controlled clinical trials. In the authors' opinion, statins are likely to be of benefit given the importance of ongoing ischaemia in many of these patients.

In addition to optimizing statin therapy, it is important for physicians and primary care teams to ensure that other well-established, evidence-based therapies shown to improve outcome are implemented in CHD patients. In the authors' experience, the implementation of the findings of the GISSI trial showing benefits of one fish-oil capsule daily, rich in omega-3 fatty acids (Omacor) in men with previous myocardial infarction has not been high. There has been considerable interest in the role of homocysteine as a CHD risk factor in recent years (see Chapter 5). A recent study from the USA for the first time to our knowledge points to the benefits of homocysteine-lowering medication. In patients following successful angioplasty, treatment with a combination of folic acid (1 mg), vitamin B12 (400 μg) and pyridoxine (10 mg) was associated with a significant reduction in re-stenosis at 6 months (Schnyder et al., 2001).

CHILDREN AND ADOLESCENTS

Early lesions of atherosclerosis have been described in post mortems of adolescents and correlate with the presence of multiple risk factors including LDL and HDL cholesterol (Berenson et al., 1998). From a public health perspective it would be a reasonable proposition to initiate prevention measures for CHD in childhood and adolescence, when dietary and exercise habits are developing. Furthermore, anti-smoking advice and education is imperative.

Severe genetic lipid disorders, such as familial hypercholesterolaemia and familial defective apoprotein B, which markedly increase CHD risk, are expressed from birth. In addition, familial combined hyperlipidaemia is identifiable in adolescents from affected families. Familial chylomicronaemia syndrome may present in childhood, with risk of pancreatitis.

Approaches to screening children and adolescents for lipid disorders vary from country to country and there are marked differences between the two sides of the Atlantic. Recommendations from the US National Cholesterol Education Program (NCEP) Expert Panel on Blood Cholesterol Levels in Children and Adolescents advocate a comprehensive screening strategy with LDL cholesterol cut-points for intervention with dietary and drug therapy (National Cholesterol Education Program, 1992). In the UK, the practice has been a more selective approach designed to identify major inherited disorders of lipoprotein metabolism, particularly familial hypercholesterolaemia.

The main recommendations of the NCEP panel are as follows:

- A lipid profile should be performed if parents or grandparents developed coronary atherosclerosis leading to need for intervention therapy below the age of 55 years.
- A lipid profile should be performed if parents or grandparents or aunts and uncles developed myocardial infarction, angina, peripheral vascular

disease, cerebrovascular disease or sudden cardiac death below the age of 55 years.

▓ Screen for hypercholesterolaemia in offspring of a parent found to have a plasma cholesterol concentration greater than 240 mg/dL (6.5 mmol/L).

▓ When history is unavailable on parents or grandparents, children and adolescents who have two or more cardiovascular disease risk factors may be screened at the physician's discretion.

These screening measures may be performed after 2 years of age. The NCEP LDL cholesterol cut-points for children from high-risk families are shown in Table 11.2.

The British Hyperlipidaemia Association's recommendations for screening for hyperlipidaemia in childhood (Neil *et al.*, 1996a, b) can be summarized as follows:

▓ The principal aim of screening should be to identify children with FH.

▓ A selective screening strategy should be used.

▓ Selection should be based on a family history of FH or premature coronary disease.

▓ A non-fasting total cholesterol measurement is a suitable screening test.

▓ If the cholesterol concentration is above 5.5 mmol/L, fasting measurement of total cholesterol, HDL cholesterol and triglycerides is required.

▓ The diagnosis of FH in a child under 16 years should be based on finding a total cholesterol concentration above 6.7 mmol/L and an LDL cholesterol concentration above 4.9 mmol/L and requires at least two measurements, to be made more than 1 month apart.

TABLE **11.2** • National Cholesterol Education Program Expert Panel on blood cholesterol in children and adolescents

(a) Cut-points for total and LDL cholesterol

Level	Total cholesterol		LDL-C	
	mg/dL	mmol/L	mg/dL	mmol/L
High	≥200	5.2	30	3.4
Borderline high	170–199		110–129	
Acceptable	≤170	4.4	≤100	2.6

(b) Guidelines for use of drug therapy: children 10 years or older

Risk factors for vascular disease	Post-dietary LDL-C	
	mg/dL	mmol/L
None	≥190	4.9
Positive family history for premature CHD or two or more other CHD risk factors	≥160	4.1

■ Children should not usually be screened before the age of 2 years, but the aim should be to diagnose heterozygous FH before the age of 10 years.

■ Affected children should be referred for specialist care.

Not surprisingly, we incline towards the UK view on screening in children, with the major emphasis on identifying FH. The mainstay of therapy in FH children is diet. Low-fat diets appear to be safe, as long as sufficient calories are provided and generally started at age 5 years.

The use of hypolipidaemic drug therapy in children remains a matter of judgement for the specialist. The main factor that argues for drug therapy is early-onset CHD in the family. If a first-degree relative developed CHD in the third decade, then drug therapy should be started after the age of 10 years. Girls with FH are less likely to require intervention with drugs unless there is premature CHD in a female relative. We also measure lipoprotein(a) as a further indicator of risk.

The drugs of choice have been the anion-exchange resins, which are not systemically absorbed. There has been no reported evidence of vitamin deficiencies, fat malabsorption or adverse effects on calcium or vitamin D metabolism. Folic acid levels decrease and supplements are advised. These drugs cause problems with compliance, as they are tiresome to take. The HMG-CoA reductase inhibitors may be considered. As a general rule, we do not start therapy with statins till late teenage. Lovastatin in adolescent boys with FH ($n = 110$) at increasing doses to 40 mg/day reduced LDL cholesterol by up to 27 per cent. There were no differences in growth, hormonal or nutritional factors between active and placebo groups (Stein *et al.*, 1999). The functional foods containing stanol ester or plant sterols are useful in this age group, as is soya protein.

In addition to diet and drug therapy for the hypercholesterolaemia, strong anti-smoking advice should be given together with general advice on a healthy lifestyle, particularly the benefits of regular exercise. Children are best managed in a special clinic run in conjunction with a paediatrician.

WOMEN AND CHD

The discovery in the early American epidemiological studies of the increased prevalence of CHD in middle-aged men has led to the erroneous assumption that CHD is predominantly a male condition. The stereotypic victim of CHD remains, in the eyes of most people, the 45-year-old stressed businessman. For largely economic reasons, cardiovascular research, prevention and intervention have often been targeted at men and relatively few studies incorporate data on women. Even treatment recommendations arise by extrapolation from the data on men.

The presentation of the symptoms of CHD varies between the sexes. Women tend to present with angina more commonly than myocardial infarction and their symptoms are often atypical. There is a bias towards non-cardiac diagnosis, especially in younger women. In addition, the incidence of vasospastic or microvascular angina (syndrome X) is increased and as a result, exercise ECG testing is less reliable. Thallium perfusion scanning is also less accurate because of the smaller size of the heart and breast attenuation of the signal. Stress echocardiography is more promising but under-used.

During the last decade there has been considerable debate concerning CHD in women, with accusations of misogyny and neglect being levelled at health professionals. Women suffer higher mortality after myocardial infarction and at the time of coronary artery revascularization and they attend less for cardiac rehabilitation. Whilst there is evidence for increased delay in reaching hospital and reduced thrombolysis rates, it may be that much of the difference between the sexes relates to the fact that presenting women are older, with more advanced disease in biologically smaller arteries.

Around the world the distribution of CHD in women closely mirrors that of men, with remarkably constant sex differences. In the UK, the chance of dying from CHD before the age of 65 for a man is 3.5 times that for a woman, but after 65 the rates are more equal. As we have seen, the onset of CHD in women is delayed about 10 years compared with men. With an ageing population, more female CHD deaths are to be expected. CHD has already become the commonest cause of death for women in the UK and the USA, responsible for one in four deaths, and in the USA, CHD is now responsible for proportionately more deaths in women than men. More women die of cardiovascular disease than cancer, trauma and diabetes combined and CHD exceeds the much feared breast cancer fourfold in white women and sixfold in black women.

There have been many attempts to explain these differences and discussion has centred on:

- sex roles
- parity
- hormonal effects
- risk factors.

SEX ROLES

Gender stereotyping weakens the impact of sex roles and their contribution to CHD risk. For example, the innate aggressive, hostile, competitive, coronary-prone behaviour of men is contrasted with the compliant, supportive, nurturing behaviour of women. Every housewife disputes the assertion that leaving home to work imparts extra stress to men and this is supported by data, which show reduced CHD in women who work away from home.

PARITY

Having more than five children is associated with a 20 per cent increased CHD risk. Possible causes discussed include lower socioeconomic status, the effect of hormonal influences in pregnancy or the stress engendered by child-rearing. Data from the Rancho Bernado study in the USA, however, suggest that the effect is obesity-mediated.

TABLE **11.3** • The protective effects of oestrogen

Antioxidant properties
Calcium channel blocking properties
Reduced LDL-C and Lp(a)
Increased HDL-C
Reduced fibrinogen and PAI-1
Reduced homocysteine
Increased vascular reactivity
Variably improved glucose tolerance

HORMONAL EFFECTS

Data from Framingham and the Nurses' Health Study convincingly demonstrate that the risk of CHD in women is increased after the menopause. In 1959, Robinson suggested that a hormonal effect, through endogenous oestrogen, might be active, when women who had premature oophorectomies were shown to suffer increased rates of CHD. Oestrogen is biologically plausible as a cardioprotective agent and documented effects are shown in Table 11.3.

The attraction of the hormonal theory is diminished by the lack of support from serial laboratory measurements of oestrogen for a protective effect. It is further undermined by the fact that CHD still occurs before the menopause; indeed, one in four CHD deaths in women under 65 years old occur before the age of 45.

RISK FACTORS FOR CHD IN WOMEN

The risk factors for CHD in women tend to be the same as for men but with quantitative differences in their effects. Women tend to have higher levels of blood pressure, cholesterol and fibrinogen, a greater incidence of diabetes and hypertension, but reduced central obesity and smoking levels and increased HDL cholesterol.

Lipids

The same lipoproteins that are risk factors in men are also risk factors in women. It is commonly supposed that LDL cholesterol levels suddenly increase at the menopause, but Figure 2.11 shows that LDL cholesterol starts to increase at about 30 years of age, increases steadily to 55 and then plateaus. By 55 years old in the UK, one in three women have cholesterol levels exceeding 7.8 mmol/L. Mean HDL cholesterol levels tend to be higher in women throughout life compared with men and, because of the inverse relationship with CHD, HDL cholesterol provides another popular explanation for the observed sex difference. That HDL cholesterol cannot be the sole explanation is shown by the observation that when men and women with the same HDL cholesterol levels are compared, women still fare better. In women, HDL cholesterol values <1.1 mmol/L are associated with increased risk. Ratios comparing total cholesterol or LDL cholesterol to HDL cholesterol can be useful in evaluating risk.

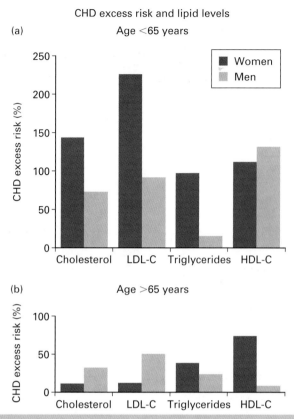

FIGURE **11.2** • Univariate relative risk of high cholesterol, LDL cholesterol and triglyceride levels and low HDL cholesterol levels in (a) middle-aged and (b) older women and men. Adapted from pooled data from 13 cohort studies in women and 25 in men. All results were statistically significant except those for LDL cholesterol in older women and HDL cholesterol in older men.

It is often thought that HDL cholesterol and triglycerides are more important predictors of CHD in women than LDL cholesterol. The best estimate of the overall univariate risks associated with lipid risk factors comes from Manolio's analysis of 13 cohort studies in women and 25 in men (Manolio et al., 1992). The data show that, if anything, the risks associated with high total cholesterol, LDL and triglyceride levels are more pronounced in women than in men and that the impact of low HDL levels appears to be about equal (Figure 11.2). When adjusted for HDL, the excess risk for high triglycerides is halved but is still significantly significant. The mediator for the effect of high triglycerides is likely to be small dense LDL and this is discussed elsewhere. In the elderly, the risks associated with lipids are attenuated but because of the greater burden of CHD, the impact of modification is likely to be as cost-effective as in younger persons.

High Lp(a) levels are associated with a higher risk for CHD in both women and men. In angiographic studies Lp(a) has been strongly associated with CHD in women and less so in men. Further corroboration is needed.

Although under-represented in the main outcome trials of cholesterol lowering, the benefits in women generally equalled, or even exceeded, those seen in men (Table 11.4).

TABLE **11.4** • CHD events in primary and secondary statin trials in women

Trial	Treatment		Control		Odds ratio
	CHD events	No. of patients	CHD events	No. of patients	
AFCAPS/TexCAPS	7	499	13	498	0.54 NS
4S	59	407	91	420	0.62
CARE	46	286	80	290	0.51
LIPID	90	756	104	760	0.85 NS

Studies of regression and progression of atheroma that have included women have also shown similar benefits from lipid-lowering therapy to those achieved in men. The newly published Heart Protection Study included 5082 female subjects and confirms that high-risk women respond just as well as men when they require a statin to prevent cardiovascular events. The Women's Health Initiative trial in the USA will provide more information on primary prevention but there is already no doubt that the data favour aggressive lipid lowering in women with evidence of CHD.

Obesity

Obese women are four times more likely to die of CHD than lean women. The predictive capacity of obesity measured in terms of weight or BMI is reduced in women. The distribution of adipose tissue seems more important and measures of central obesity (e.g. WHR > 0.8) are more powerful predictors. As in men, obesity itself contributes little to the increased risk of CHD but it is the relationship with associated risk factors such as diabetes, dyslipidaemia and hypertension that promotes the risk.

Hypertension

After the age of 50, hypertension is more prevalent in women than in men and after 75 years of age, up to 85 per cent of women are hypertensive. The benefits of treating mild to moderate hypertension in younger women of low absolute cardiovascular risk are controversial.

Diabetes

Diabetes provides the greatest example of gender difference, the presence of diabetes increasing the CHD risk in women threefold and completely neutralizing any protective sex advantage. Diabetes causes a dramatic increase in mortality after a myocardial infarction.

Smoking

Although smoking levels are generally lower than in men, dose-dependent increased CHD risk is still evident in women. Smoking more than 40 cigarettes a day increases CHD risk 20-fold. There is concern at the levels of smoking in younger women who, already victims of social stresses and targeted advertising, may also smoke to control weight.

Oral contraceptives

Most early epidemiological studies found an increased risk of myocardial infarction in current users of the combined oral contraceptive pill (COC). This was not unexpected, given the effect of ethinyl oestradiol on CHD risk markers, but reduction in dose, together with avoidance of use in high-risk groups, have improved safety. A recent large case–control study involving 448 women who had an MI and 1728 matched controls found no association and, additionally, no difference between the risk of second- and third-generation pills. The MI risk does increase with smoking, hyperlipidaemia, hypertension, diabetes, obesity and an adverse family history. COCs increase the small, 5/100 000, risk of ischaemic stroke by 1.5.

Third-generation COCs, containing ethinyl oestradiol and gestodene or desogestrel, were marketed on the basis of an improved cardiovascular risk profile but became controversial when increased rates of venous thromboembolism (VTE) were noted. The baseline rate of VTE is 5/100 000 in non-pill-takers and this is increased to 15/100 000 with second-generation COCs and 25/100 000 with third-generation COCs. The rates may be confounded by physicians prescribing third-generation COCs to women at higher risk but this may not be the complete answer and factor V Leiden may be involved.

COCs also cause a significant rise in BP (mean 2.6/1.8 mmHg) and this supports usual clinical practice to monitor patients at regular intervals.

PREGNANCY

During pregnancy the main change in the lipoprotein profile is a gradual two- to threefold rise in triglycerides. Despite this, pancreatitis is uncommon and when it occurs is usually due to biliary disease. LDL cholesterol is reduced in early pregnancy but at term is increased by 50–60 per cent. HDL cholesterol is also increased at term by 15 per cent. Postpartum lipid determinations should be postponed for 6 months in those who were not dyslipidaemic before pregnancy. As the safety of lipid-lowering drugs is not established in pregnancy, they are usually stopped, if possible, before conception. A report of 134 women inadvertently exposed to lovastatin and simvastatin showed no adverse fetal outcome.

MENOPAUSE AND HORMONE REPLACEMENT THERAPY (HRT)

In 1991, Stampfer and Colditz published 10-year data from the Nurses' Health Study, which showed that postmenopausal HRT with oral oestrogen almost halved the risk of CHD (RR 44 per cent). A subsequent meta-analysis of 25 observational studies by Barrett-Connor and Grady attenuated this figure to 30 per cent for users of oestrogen versus never users and 34 per cent for opposed preparations. It was reasonable to assume that this was largely mediated through the actions of HRT on lipoproteins and the effects of both the menopause and oestrogen replacement therapy on lipoproteins are summarized in Figure 11.3.

At the menopause there is an increase in total cholesterol, LDL cholesterol (particularly of the small dense atherogenic variety), Lp(a) and triglyceride. HDL cholesterol is slightly reduced but this disguises a large reduction in HDL_2 cholesterol with a slight rise in HDL_3 cholesterol and a consequent increase in CHD risk. Adding oestrogen reverses these changes, producing a fall in total cholesterol and LDL cholesterol (by 10–15 per cent) and a rise in HDL cholesterol (chiefly HDL_2 cholesterol) and triglycerides. Progestogens are necessary for endometrial protection but androgenic progestogens, such as norethisterone and levonorgestrel, commonly used in the UK, oppose the effect of oestrogens, raising LDL cholesterol and reducing HDL cholesterol. Medroxyprogesterone acetate is the leading progestogen used in the USA and its effect in combination with oestrogen is summarized as HDL cholesterol ↑, LDL cholesterol ↓, TG slightly ↑, Lp(a) ↓, factor VII ↑ and fibrinogen ↓.

The prospect of reducing CHD in postmenopausal women by up to 50 per cent with HRT is tantalizing and would seem to suggest 'oestrogen for all'. Many women were advised to use HRT to improve their cardiovascular and lipid profiles. Doubts began to appear when it was noticed that women who take HRT tend to be a generally healthier cohort, better educated and of higher social class than women who do not. In addition, they are leaner, have more medical supervision and therefore are at lower CHD risk before the benefits of HRT are added. To add to this selection bias, a large compliance bias may have also produced a strong effect in the observational studies.

The answer to these doubts was, of course, an intervention trial and the first randomized trial to publish produced surprising results. The Heart and Estrogen/ Progestin Replacement Study (HERS) enrolled 2763 postmenopausal women 44–79 years old with a history of CHD who had not had a hysterectomy. HRT was given in continuous combined form using conjugated equine oestrogens (0.625 mg) plus medroxyprogesterone acetate (1 mg) daily over an average follow-up period of

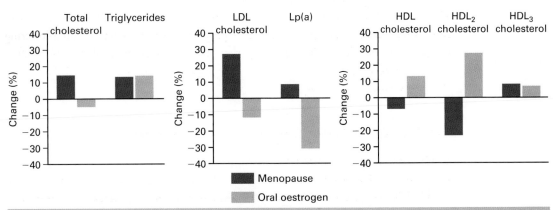

FIGURE 11.3 • Effects of the menopause and conjugated equine oestrogen (0.625 mg) on lipoproteins. Source: Crook and Stevenson (1996) *Lipids: Current Perspectives*, p. 179, using data from Stevenson, Lobo and Jenner.

4.1 years. A comprehensive gynaecological service was offered to all participants and at 3 years, 75 per cent of those assigned to HRT were still taking it.

Despite an 11 per cent reduction in LDL cholesterol and a 10 per cent increase in HDL cholesterol, 172 women in the treatment group had a non-fatal myocardial infarction or CHD death compared to 176 women in the placebo group. Predictions based on these changes in lipid parameters should have resulted in a reduction in CHD events of 30 per cent. In addition, there were no significant differences in other cardiovascular outcomes. Unfortunately, thromboembolic disease (34 versus 12) and gallbladder disease (84 versus 62) were significantly increased in the treatment group. Despite a trend, there was no significant increase in mortality (131 versus 123).

A time trend was observed in the treatment group with more CHD events being observed in the first year of the trial than in years 4 and 5. The authors postulate that prothrombotic, proarrhythmic or proischaemic effects of HRT may predominate in the early treatment phase but that an anti-atherosclerotic effect may emerge later. This mirrors the delayed positive effect seen in trials of lipid lowering and allows the authors to recommend that women with CHD who are already using HRT can continue its use.

There have been criticisms of the study. The event rate in the placebo group was lower than expected and undermines the power calculations. The lower event rate may relate to significantly greater use of statins in the placebo group after year 1, which may disguise a greater treatment benefit of HRT. In addition, the analysis after 1 year was *post hoc* and therefore to be treated with caution.

Subsequently, corroborative findings have been announced by the ERA study (Herrington *et al.*, 2000) but definitive data will not be available until 2005 when the large Womens' Health Initiative trial is complete. More trials are needed with different hormone combinations that reflect current usage. Until then it may not be sensible to initiate hormone therapy in postmenopausal women with CHD and they should receive instead the benefit of known secondary prevention interventions such as aspirin, beta-blockade, lipid lowering and smoking cessation.

Trends in hormone replacement therapy

Given the array of hormones and the ingenuity of the pharmaceutical industry, it should be possible to design the ideal preparation, the most likely candidate at present being an oestradiol/dydrogesterone combination. From a cardiovascular point of view, oral oestrogen remains the best answer and it is interesting to speculate whether more lives would be saved using oestrogen alone to prevent CHD than lost by abandoning endometrial protection with progestogens.

The effect of different HRT preparations is shown in Table 11.5.

Transdermal delivery

Transdermal delivery (skin patches) negates the rise in triglycerides seen with oral replacement and this may be important for those with hypertriglyceridaemia. Unfortunately, the fall in LDL and rise in HDL are also reduced.

TABLE **11.5** • The effect of different types of hormone replacement therapy on serum lipids (% changes)

	Oral oestrogen	Transdermal combined	Combined HRT	Tamoxifen	Raloxifene	Tibolone
Total cholesterol	↓4–8	–	↓8	↓12	↓6.4	↓12–17
LDL-C	↓12–19	↓7	↓14	↓20	↓10–12	↓6–27
HDL-C	↑9–30	↑4	↑11	–	–	↓27
Triglycerides	↑25	↓13	↑20	–	–	↓34
Lp(a)	↓20	–	↓19	↓32	↓8	↓26–48
Fibrinogen	↓10	–	↓10	↓24	↓12–14	↓15–20

Continuous combined HRT

In an effort to minimize the nuisance of menstruation by continuous endometrial suppression, continuous combined regimens have been marketed. Unfortunately, most use androgenic progestogens, which reduce HDL. It is not known whether this has any significance in the frequency of outcome events.

Tibolone

Tibolone is a synthetic steroid with oestrogenic, androgenic and progestogenic properties. Unfortunately, HDL can be markedly reduced.

Selective oestrogen receptor modulators (SERMs)

With the emergence of doubts concerning the risks of conventional HRT, the development of compounds with selective actions on oestrogen receptors has aroused much interest. Two of these SERMs, tamoxifen and raloxifene, have been examined for their effects on cardiovascular risk factors. Although the lipid effects of SERMs are significant, evaluation of the Breast Cancer Prevention Trial, where 13 388 women were treated for 5 years with tamoxifen, showed no reduction in CHD. More information will come from large outcome trials such as the Raloxifene Use for the Heart (RUTH) study.

Phytoestrogens

Many women are concerned about taking HRT and there is much interest in phytoestrogens from plants such as soya (see page 193).

Statins and osteoporosis

In 1999, Munday and colleagues published the remarkable finding that oophorectomized rats given simvastatin could develop new trabecular bone. By 2000, the findings were extended to humans when Chung *et al.* noted significant increases in bone mineral density at the femoral neck in 36 Korean patients with diabetes and hypercholesterolaemia, who had used statins over 15 months. Bauer's group examined the results of two prospective studies, the Study of Osteoporotic Fractures and the Fracture Intervention Trial, and again found differences in hip and non-spine fractures between statin users and non-users, albeit that the associations were not quite significant. As interest grew, Chan *et al.* performed a population-based case–control study, which again suggested a decreased risk of osteoporotic fracture in women, over the age of 60 years, taking a statin. If validated, there is no doubt that the findings would have major implications for women's health.

The exact mechanism whereby statins could exert this action remains unclear and because of the risks of confounding factors, randomized controlled trials in osteoporotic patients are needed. *Post hoc* analysis of the LIPID study, HPS and informal communications from the 4S investigators show no reduction in the fracture rate and offer no support for the hypothesis.

THE ELDERLY

The authors are often asked about their policy towards the elderly. Should statin treatment be stopped at a certain age? Should statin therapy be started for primary or secondary prevention in the elderly? This begs the question as to what constitutes 'elderly'. The definition will change as questioners (and indeed the authors) advance in years!

Important issues to address when considering lipid-lowering therapy in the elderly are:

- biological versus chronological age
- life expectancy
- concomitant morbidity
- predictive value of lipid and lipoprotein concentrations in older age groups
- clinical trial evidence.

It is the authors' view that the elderly should be treated for secondary prevention as benefits can be seen relatively early. In the major statin trials of secondary prevention, benefit was observed when the results were analysed by age. In 4S, for example, which included men and women up to the age of 70 years, similar benefits of therapy were observed in those aged more than 60 years as in those below 60 years. In the CARE study, which included men and women up to the age of 75 years, therapy benefits, in this case with pravastatin, were seen in the older subgroup. The most recent statin study, HPS, included 9515 men and women older than 65 years, 6575 with established CHD and 2940 without CHD but at high risk because of non-CHD vascular disease or hypertension or diabetes. Indeed, 5805 trial subjects were aged 70 years or over at baseline. This huge trial enabled detailed analyses by age of the benefits of simvastatin therapy. Similar benefit in terms of relative risk reductions for major vascular events were observed in those aged 65–69 years, 70–74 years and ≥75 years compared to those <65 years. Clearly, HPS has contributed enormously to the clinical trial database in the elderly. More information is available from the Prospective Study of Pravastatin in the Elderly at Risk (PROSPER) study, which involves 5804 elderly subjects (70–82 years) in Scotland, Ireland and the Netherlands treated with pravastatin (40 mg/day) or placebo. The primary outcome includes CHD events (coronary death, non-fatal MI), fatal and non-fatal stroke (Shepherd et al., 2002). Pravastatin reduced the incidence of the primary endpoint; hazard ratio 0.85, $P = 0.014$.

What is the case for primary prevention in the elderly? Antihypertensive therapy is now clearly established in the elderly based on clinical trial data. In the authors' opinion in the not-too-distant future a similar approach will be adopted to lipid lowering. Epidemiological evidence linking lipid and lipoproteins to vascular risk in the elderly (and particularly the very old) demonstrates less strong relationships than seen in younger people. However, as the burden of CHD increases with age, so the attributable risk increases despite the fact that the relative risk with increasing cholesterol levels diminishes. This important concept is demonstrated in Figure 11.4. With increasing information as to the benefit of statin therapy on stroke reduction as well as CHD, the intervention is likely to be highly cost-effective. Further analysis of HPS and PROSPER are awaited with interest.

An intriguing possibility that statin therapy may be associated with reduced dementia risk came from a case control study based on the General Practice Research Database in the UK (Jick et al., 2000). Clearly, this observation may be open to considerable bias but it fits with increasing evidence linking atherosclerosis with vascular dementia and risk factors for Alzheimer's disease. This observation needs to be confirmed by clinical trials. In PROSPER, in addition to stroke and CHD endpoints, annual neuropsychological tests were performed to assess the effects of statin therapy on cognitive decline (Shepherd et al., 1999). No impact on cognitive function was observed with pravastatin (Shepherd et al., 2002). Similar results were seen in HPS. These findings cast doubt on the observational studies.

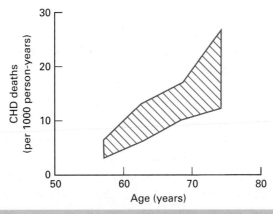

FIGURE 11.4 • Risk for CHD mortality with age in the top cholesterol quartile (upper line) versus bottom quartile (lower line). Shaded area is the attributable risk due to cholesterol, which can be seen to increase with age. Source: Rubin et al. (1990) Ann Intern Med **113**, 916–20.

Special areas

THE HYPERTENSIVE PATIENT

Hypertension is an important risk factor for atherosclerotic vascular disease. It has been known for many years that the major CHD risk factors interact to multiply risk. This is illustrated in Figure 11.5 with data taken from the Framingham study. It can be seen that the relative risk of CHD in relation to hypertension depends on both the concomitant LDL and HDL cholesterol concentration (Kannel, 1983).

Hypertension and dyslipidaemia commonly occur together in the same individual. Depending on the population studied and the definition adopted, the prevalence of

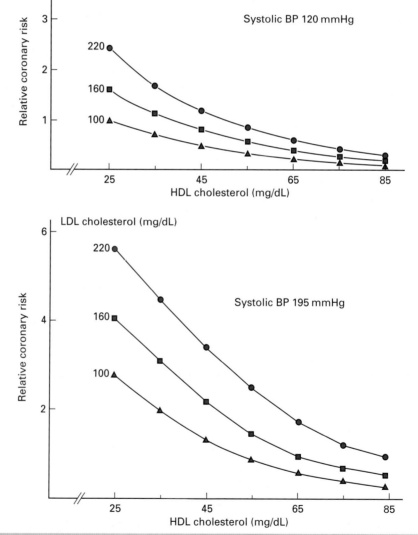

FIGURE **11.5** • Relative coronary risk in relation to HDL cholesterol at different levels of LDL cholesterol in normotensive and hypertensive individuals. Source: Kannel (1983).

hypercholesterolaemia in hypertensives ranges from 28 to 43 per cent (MacMahon *et al.*, 1985). This is perhaps not surprising since dyslipidaemia and hypertension share common environmental determinants, such as obesity. Furthermore, these factors are both components of the insulin resistance syndrome which no doubt involves the interplay of genetic and environmental factors, such as obesity and lack of physical activity. Williams and colleagues in Utah, USA, have described the familial association of essential hypertension and dyslipoproteinaemia in a study of 58 families. These authors have suggested that the association may occur in about 12 per cent of hypertensives (Williams *et al.*, 1988).

Trials of antihypertensive therapy have demonstrated unequivocal benefit in terms of stroke reduction but the impact on CHD (which in quantitative terms is a much more significant cause of death and morbidity) was less. Nevertheless, when the trials were combined in meta-analysis by Collins and colleagues, it was apparent that there was a reduction of 14 per cent in total CHD (Collins *et al.*, 1990). This reduction is less than would be expected from the observational data linking hypertension to CHD risk.

The discrepancy between the observed and expected benefit of blood pressure lowering on CHD has received much discussion. A possible contributing factor is the potential for adverse metabolic effects of antihypertensive agents used in the trials, particularly high-dose thiazides and beta-blockers (Krone and Müller-Wieland, 1990). In a cross-sectional study of hypertensives performed in Australia, the prevalence of dyslipidaemia was indeed higher in patients established on treatment compared with newly presenting untreated patients (MacMahon *et al.*, 1985).

There have been many trials of the effects of various antihypertensive agents on plasma lipid and lipoprotein concentrations (Tomlinson, 2000). A summary of these findings based on a meta-analysis of 474 trials involving over 65 000 patients is shown in Figure 11.6. It should be remembered that many of the studies used what are now recognized to be excessive doses, e.g. bendrofluazide 10 mg. It is likely that metabolic effects are minimal at low doses, e.g. bendrofluazide 2.5 mg. A further point to remember is that these studies were not performed in dyslipidaemic subjects. It is likely that antihypertensives with adverse metabolic effects will produce more marked changes where dyslipidaemia or glucose intolerance already exists. In fact it has been reported that the use of beta-blockers so exacerbated hypertriglyceridaemia as to precipitate pancreatitis. The metabolic effects of some antihypertensives are mainly attributed to adverse effects on insulin sensitivity and lipoprotein lipase activity.

Subgroup analyses of the statin secondary prevention trials, e.g. 4S, CARE and LIPID, demonstrate that hypertensive patients showed similar benefits to non-hypertensives. The question arises as to whether dyslipidaemia should be treated in the hypertensive. CHD risk is multiplied when more than one risk factor is present, which argues for an aggressive policy towards concomitant dyslipidaemia with lifestyle changes and, if necessary, hypolipidaemic drugs. Evidence of benefit of cholesterol lowering for primary prevention in hypertensives comes from subgroup analysis of AFCAPS/TexCAPS and WOSCOPS. Recent data from HPS has provided further evidence of benefit of statin therapy in hypertensive patients. HPS included a total of 7012

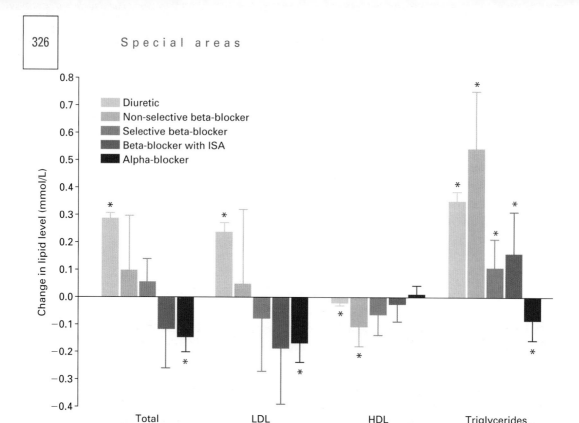

FIGURE **11.6** • Effects of different antihypertensive drugs on lipid levels in meta-analysis of 56 randomized controlled clinical trials. ACE inhibitory, dihydropyridine calcium antagonists, non-dihydropyridine calcium antagonists and sympatholytic drugs had no significant effect in this analysis. Values are means with 95% CI. *Significant changes exceeding 95% CI. Source: Kasiske, B.L., Ma, J.Z., Kalil, R.S. and Louis, T.A. (1995) *Ann Intern Med* **122**, 133–41.

hypertensive men and women, 2860 of whom were free of CHD. Ongoing trials such as ALLHAT and ASCOT will provide further evidence in hypertensives.

THE PATIENT WITH DIABETES

In his preface entitled 'A Time Bomb' to the recent International Diabetes Federation (IDF) publication *Diabetes and Cardiovascular Disease: Time to Act*, Sir George Alberti, the IDF President, points to the double jeopardy of diabetes and cardiovascular disease:

> the IDF considers cardiovascular disease to be one of the most serious problems facing people with diabetes. (International Diabetes Federation, 2001).

A current estimate puts the number of people with diabetes in the world at 150 million – a figure expected to double in the next 25 years. People with diabetes are two to four times more likely to develop cardiovascular disease than the general population, making it the most common complication. The observed overall decline in CHD mortality rates

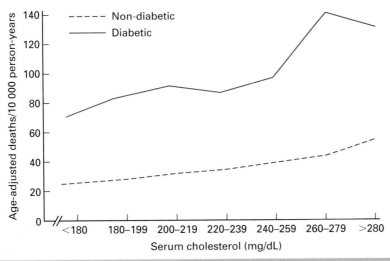

FIGURE **11.7** • Diabetic and cardiovascular disease in MRFIT: CVD death rates by serum cholesterol (mg/dL). Source: Stamler *et al.* (1993).

in developed countries is significantly less apparent in the diabetic population with even a possible increase in women. People with diabetes have approximately the same CHD risk as people without diabetes who have already had a heart attack and have a higher case fatality. Outcome after revascularizations is less good and diabetes remains an independent risk predictor in patients with heart failure.

Diabetes is a major risk factor for disease outside the coronary vasculature. Stroke (twofold increase) and transient ischaemic attack (two- to six-fold increase) are more common in people with diabetes. Lower limb amputation is dramatically increased, being 15- to 40-fold higher than in the general population.

It is clear that the major risk factors, cigarette smoking, hypertension and dyslipidaemia, contribute to vascular risk in diabetic populations and for each risk factor present the risk of cardiovascular disease is approximately threefold greater than in non-diabetics (Stamler *et al.*, 1993) (Figure 11.7). In the United Kingdom Prospective Diabetes Study (UKPDS), more intensive management of hyperglycaemia was associated with a significant reduction in diabetes-related endpoints. This reduction was mainly in microvascular disease and the impact on macrovascular disease was of borderline significance (UKPDS, 1998). A reasonable conclusion from this study, taken together with epidemiological and clinical trial data, is that reductions in cardiovascular disease will require aggressive and early modification of the other major risk factors.

Dyslipidaemia, common in the diabetic population, is a major risk factor for CHD and is open to therapeutic intervention (Betteridge, 2001a). It is present at the diagnosis of type 2 diabetes and largely persists despite treatment of hyperglycaemia requiring attention in its own right. It is an integral feature of the insulin resistance syndrome and correlates strongly with parameters of insulin resistance. It is characterized principally by moderate hypertriglyceridaemia and low HDL cholesterol concentrations. Total and LDL cholesterol concentrations are similar to non-diabetic populations. In the past these characteristics may have contributed to therapeutic nihilism amongst physicians along the lines that the relationship of triglycerides to CHD is controversial and hypercholesterolaemia is not a feature of diabetes. This position clearly is no longer tenable. Total and LDL cholesterol are major risk factors for cardiovascular disease in people with diabetes just as in the general population. Furthermore, the LDL distribution is shifted towards smaller, denser particles, which are thought to be highly atherogenic. The independent relationship between increasing plasma triglycerides and vascular risk has been a controversial issue over the years. Although a recent analysis has pointed to triglycerides as an independent risk factor and within diabetic populations their relationship to CHD risk appears stronger, it is unlikely that epidemiological studies will provide much further insight. More is likely to be gained from delineation of the pathological consequences of hypertriglyceridaemia on lipoprotein metabolism and atherosclerosis. Hypertriglyceridaemia is a major determinant of the distribution of LDL particles; it is associated with increased postprandial lipaemia and accumulation of atherogenic, cholesterol-rich remnant particles; it is associated with low HDL cholesterol concentrations and is associated with increased concentrations of important coagulation factors such as PAI-1. A current working hypothesis to explain the pathophysiology of diabetic dyslipidaemia is as follows. In the presence of insulin resistance and hyperinsulinaemia, hepatic VLDL output, particularly large VLDL, is increased. In the postprandial state, hepatic output continues and competes for the hydrolytic activity of lipoprotein lipase with exogenously derived lipid on chylomicrons. Postprandial lipaemia is prolonged with increased accumulation of remnants. Increased lipid exchange via cholesterol ester transfer protein leads to triglyceride enrichment of LDL and HDL. These particles are substrates for hepatic lipase, which leads to lipid depletion and small dense LDL and HDL. Small dense HDL is catabolized more rapidly to low HDL cholesterol concentrations.

As yet no clinical endpoint trials of lipid lowering performed specifically in diabetic populations have been reported. However, sufficient numbers of diabetic patients were included in the major statin secondary prevention trials to enable the reasonable conclusion that diabetic patients benefit to a similar extent to non-diabetics. Indeed, given the higher risk of diabetic patients, the absolute benefit is greater. Less consistent information is available for fibrate therapy. In the Veterans Administration HDL Intervention Trial (VA-HIT) there was a reduction in CHD events with gemfibrozil and this benefit was also seen in diabetic patients. However, in the Bezafibrate Infarction Prevention (BIP) study no overall benefit was observed with bezafibrate. For primary prevention there is little data available from clinical trials.

National and international guidelines on overall diabetic management and the prevention of cardiovascular disease include important targets for lipid management. The American Diabetes Association (ADA) and the recent Adult Treatment Panel III of the National Cholesterol Education Program in the USA make LDL cholesterol the primary target for lipid management with a goal of therapy <100 mg/dL (2.6 mmol/L). Statins are regarded as first-line therapy. In the presence of hypertriglyceridaemia (≥200 mg/dL), ATP-III provides an additional secondary goal of non-HDL cholesterol <130 mg/dL, recognizing the atherogenic potential of remnant lipoproteins. Low HDL cholesterol (<40 mg/dL) is recognized as a strong independent predictor of CHD although ATP-III does not specify a goal of therapy as evidence from clinical trials of the benefit of increasing HDL is considered insufficient. In patients with low HDL, the primary target for lipid management is LDL cholesterol. When LDL cholesterol is to goal the secondary target is non-HDL cholesterol when hypertriglyceridaemia is present. In Europe, the joint European guidelines have a somewhat less stringent goal of therapy for LDL cholesterol of <3.0 mmol/L.

For primary prevention, ATP-III has advocated that diabetes should be regarded as a CHD risk equivalent, i.e. diabetic patients should be treated as if they already had CHD (Expert Panel on Detection, Evaluation and Treatment of High Blood Cholesterol in Adults, 2001). This has major implications both in terms of compliance with multiple drug therapy and economic considerations. However, in the authors' opinion, this is likely to represent a major clinical advance in CHD prevention. In Europe, clinicians are likely to continue to use risk charts usually based on the Framingham model to calculate individual CHD risk (Wood et al., 1998). Many diabetic patients will fulfil the absolute risk requirements (20 per cent in 10 years) to justify statin therapy for primary prevention. A recent publication from the Sheffield group in the UK (not known for a cavalier approach to lipid lowering!) has advocated a lower CHD risk threshold for statin treatment of diabetes of 15 per cent over 10 years (Yeo and Yeo, 2001). It is likely that Europe will move towards the US position when ongoing primary prevention trials performed in type 2 diabetic populations without vascular disease are reported (Betteridge, 2001b), e.g. the Collaborative Atorvastatin Diabetes Study (CARDS) in the UK, the Atorvastatin as Prevention of Coronary Heart Disease in Patients with Type 2 Diabetes (ASPEN) in the USA. CARDS is a multicentre, randomized, placebo-controlled, double-blind, clinical trial of atorvastatin 10 mg daily in approximately 2800 patients with type 2 diabetes (aged 40–75 years) who have normal or only moderately raised serum lipid levels and no previous CHD or other macrovascular disease. The patients have one or more other risk factors (hypertension, smoking, retinopathy or microalbuminuria). The primary efficacy parameter is the time to the first occurrence of fatal or non-fatal MI (including silent infarction), acute CHD death, coronary revascularization procedure or stroke. The ASPEN trial involves approximately 2250 patients. It is a combined primary and secondary prevention trial comparing placebo to atorvastatin 10 mg/day. The primary endpoints are similar to those in CARDS, which should allow future combined subgroup analysis. The Fenofibrate Intervention and Event Lowering in Diabetes Trial (FIELD) is a randomized, controlled trial comparing micronized fenofibrate (200 mg/day) with placebo in approximately 8000 men and women with type 2 diabetes. It is a combined primary and secondary prevention trial. The primary endpoints are coronary mortality and coronary events.

The HPS contains a large subgroup of diabetic patients (Armitage and Collins, 2000); a total of 5963 (aged 40–80 years) with 2913 (49 per cent) with no evidence of cardiovascular disease. The preliminary results announced at the AHA (November,

2001) revealed a significant benefit for simvastatin therapy (40 mg/day) compared with placebo, with 279 events in the treated group compared to 427 in the untreated, placebo group. Clearly more detailed information will be available in the future from this study and the others mentioned above. The question will be should all type 2 diabetic patients receive statins or should they be targeted to those at higher risk calculated by new risk assessments based on UKPDS and perhaps HPS? Time will tell; in the meantime the authors adopt an aggressive approach to lipid management together with hypertension in their type 2 diabetic patients in addition to doing their best to optimize glycaemic control.

Clearly, type 1 diabetic patients are also at increased risk of vascular disease, particularly those with proteinuria and hypertension. A small number of type 1 patients (615) were included in the HPS, which will probably be too small to analyse. Otherwise there is no clinical trial evidence to guide the clinician. NCEP ATP-III makes no distinction in its recommendations between type 1 and type 2 patients. The physician caring for type 1 patients clearly needs to make a judgement as to when and if statin therapy should be instigated, taking into account age, microvascular complications, the lipid profile and other risk factors.

In conclusion, the management of the diabetic patient should not only encompass best endeavour at glycaemic control compatible with a good quality of life to reduce microvascular risk but also attention to major risk factors for macrovascular disease including dyslipidaemia. LDL cholesterol is the major therapeutic target with a secondary target of non-HDL cholesterol in some patients. Statins are the preferred lipid-lowering therapy for the majority of patients.

THE PATIENT WITH PERIPHERAL VASCULAR DISEASE

In national and international guidelines for the management of dyslipidaemia and statin treatment, patients with peripheral vascular disease (PVD) are included in the high-risk secondary prevention group, together with CHD patients. Despite this, it is the authors' impression that risk factor management and therapy are suboptimal in this group. It is clear that PVD patients, whether identified as claudicants or on the basis of reduced ankle-brachial pressure index, have high CHD risk (Winder, 2000). Why in some individuals atherosclerotic-related disease should present first as PVD is unknown. There is some evidence that the accumulation of cholesterol-rich remnant particles as seen in type III dyslipidaemia and type 2 diabetes have predilection for this vascular bed as well as the coronaries.

Early angiographic studies pointed to the potential benefits of lipid lowering in delaying progression of femoral atheromatous plaques, the Cholesterol Lowering Atherosclerosis Study (CLAS), for example (Blankenhorn et al., 1991). There are no clinical outcome studies of lipid lowering in specific PVD patients; however, some information can be gleaned from studies such as 4S. In this study examination of clinical assessment and adverse event data provided some data on the development of PVD. In the simvastatin group there were 52 recorded cases compared with 81 in the placebo group ($P = 0.008$). This observation has been confirmed by the preliminary results of the HPS, which contained a large number ($n = 2701$) of patients with PVD. In the PVD group, 332 vascular events were observed in the simvastatin group compared with 427 in the placebo group. After allowance for non-compliance, the authors concluded that simvastatin (40 mg daily) for 5 years would prevent 70 major vascular events in 70 out of every 1000 patients with PVD. On the basis of these data, physicians and primary care groups need to liaise with vascular surgeons to ensure that treatment protocols encompass PVD patients effectively.

THE PATIENT WITH CEREBROVASCULAR DISEASE

Patients with overt cerebrovascular disease (CVD) in the view of the authors should be carefully assessed for statin therapy. They are known to be at high risk not only for further CVD but also for CHD events. The realization that CVA patients might benefit from lipid lowering has been relatively recent, perhaps related to early epidemiology studies. Age is clearly an important risk factor for CVD; in those >80 years the annual risk is >2 per cent (Manolio et al., 1996). In addition, other important risk factors are hypertension, diabetes mellitus and impaired glucose tolerance, cigarette smoking, increased alcohol intake, high fibrinogen levels and heart disease, amongst others. With regard to plasma cholesterol concentrations, epidemiology studies did not point to a consistent and strong association between CVD risk overall and cholesterol (Prospective Studies Collaboration, 1995). In some studies, a positive correlation was observed with atherothrombotic stroke, but a possible negative association with haemorrhagic stroke (Neaton et al., 1992). Given the less than overwhelming epidemiological data, it is not surprising that CVD patients were not considered for cholesterol-lowering therapy despite the inclusion of other atherosclerotic disease being included with CHD as high risk in guidelines such as the NCEP.

It was data from the statin studies that pointed to the benefit of cholesterol lowering and stroke prevention. In the overview of randomized trials, Hebert and colleagues (Hebert et al., 1997) found a 29 per cent reduction in stroke. In the LIPID trial, not included in this meta-analysis, a 19 per cent ($P = 0.048$) reduction in stroke was observed (White et al., 2000). The recent preliminary results from the HPS have provided confirmatory evidence on stroke reduction based on more than 20 000 men and women (see page 277). Overall, there were 456 (4.4 per cent) strokes in the simvastatin-treated group compared with 613 (6.0 per cent) in the placebo group, a 27 per cent reduction ($P < 0.00001$). There was no excess of haemorrhagic stroke in the treated group. Importantly, this study recruited men and women at high risk of vascular disease including 3280 patients with established CVD. The authors estimated, after allowance for non-compliance, that statin treatment for 5 years would prevent major vascular events in approximately 70 of every 1000 with previous stroke, irrespective of cholesterol level, age, sex or other treatments.

The mechanism(s) by which cholesterol lowering with statins reduces stroke risk remain to be determined fully. It was suggested that the reduction in stroke observed in the statin trials was secondary to the reduction in CHD. Although CHD reduction is likely to contribute, it does not fully explain the findings. It is likely that reductions in atheromatous plaque regression and plaque stabilization play important roles. This is supported by studies using B-mode ultrasound, which have shown that cholesterol lowering retards progression of extracranial carotid atherosclerosis. However, perhaps more important than the degree of stenosis is plaque stabilization. It appears that echolucent or homogeneous carotid plaques (suggesting lipid-rich plaques) are associated with increased stroke risk.

It is the authors' opinion based on the above discussion that patients with CVD should receive therapy. Clearly, clinical judgement is important in targeting those who are likely to benefit most, taking into account quality of life issues. More information will become available from the Stroke Prevention by Aggressive Reduction in Cholesterol Levels (SPARCL) study, which compares atorvastatin to placebo in approximately 4200 patients with minor stroke or TIA; the primary outcome measure is the effect on total stroke.

THE PATIENT WITH CHRONIC RENAL DISEASE

Despite advances in renal support for patients with end-stage renal disease, cardiovascular mortality (myocardial infarction, cardiac arrest, cardiomyopathy, pulmonary oedema and arrhythmias) is markedly increased, the relative risk being higher in younger age groups. For example, in the USA, those dialysis patients aged below 45 years have a 100-fold excess cardiac mortality compared to the general population. Furthermore, patients with less severe degrees of renal impairment also have significantly increased vascular risk. It is likely that factors other than coronary atherosclerosis contribute to this increased risk, particularly left ventricular hypertrophy. Renal failure is associated with dyslipidaemia characterized by modest elevations in LDL cholesterol (much higher in nephrotic syndrome), low HDL cholesterol and moderate hypertriglyceridaemia. In addition to these quantitative changes, qualitative abnormalities include accumulation of cholesterol-rich lipoprotein remnants (partially hydrolysed chylomicrons and VLDL) and a shift in LDL density distribution to smaller, denser particles. This constellation of abnormalities has been termed the atherogenic lipoprotein profile and is found in the metabolic syndrome and type 2 diabetes mellitus. Indeed, insulin resistance is common in renal impairment. Lipoprotein(a) concentrations are also increased in renal impairment.

It is likely that dyslipidaemia contributes to the increased vascular risk in patients with renal impairment. There are as yet no outcome trials of lipid-lowering therapy in this condition but ongoing trials will provide much needed information on which to make clinical decisions. The Die Deutsche Diabetes Dialyse (4D) study in Germany compares atorvastatin 10 mg/day with placebo in patients within 6 months of dialysis. Baseline lipid entry criteria are LDL cholesterol ≤4.92 mmol/L (190 mg/dL) and total triglyceride ≤11 mmol/L (1000 mg/dL). The combined primary endpoint is cardiovascular mortality, fatal myocardial infarction, sudden death and non-fatal infarction. A further study aimed at patients at an earlier stage of disease is the Heart and Renal Protection (HARP) study coordinated in Oxford, UK. This study compares simvastatin or a combination of simvastatin with the cholesterol absorption inhibitor ezetimibe to placebo in 4000 patients with chronic renal failure.

Clearly, extra care is required when using lipid-lowering therapy in patients with chronic renal failure. The fibrates are generally contraindicated. The statins can be used safely but care needs to be taken in patients taking the immunosuppressant drug cyclosporin A. Concomitant use of this drug leads to increased plasma levels of statins and can increase the risk of rhabdomyolysis. However, if low doses of statin are used, this combination has proved safe. Furthermore, there is an increasing body of evidence that statins may reduce the risk of organ rejection in kidney recipients. The mechanism of this benefit remains to be fully elucidated but may involve reductions in T-cell cytotoxicity and interleukin production.

THE PATIENT WITH HIV ON HAART THERAPY

Increasing numbers of these patients are referred to lipid clinics. Combination and retroviral therapy (highly active antiretroviral therapy, HAART) often comprising a combination of HIV-1 protease inhibitors (e.g. amprenavir, indinavir, lopinavir, nelfinavir, ritonavir, saquinavir), nucleoside reverse transcriptase inhibitors (NRTIs) (abacavir, didanosine, lamivudine, stavudine, zalcitabine, zidovudine) and sometimes with non-NRTI compounds (efavirenz, nevirapine) has transformed the outcome of HIV patients. Many patients referred to the lipid clinic have undetectable viral load and normal CD4 counts. Excellent as this approach is to the management of the primary condition, it has become clear that it is at the expense of significant metabolic side-effects, which could have an important impact on future well-being and also acute severe complications. This has been the subject of an excellent review (Mooser and Carr, 2001).

Lipid changes (hypertriglyceridaemia, reduced total and HDL cholesterol and accumulation of small, dense LDL particles) have been described in individuals with asymptomatic HIV infection. These changes may be a response to chronic infection rather than a specific response to HIV. Correlations have been observed with various immune and inflammatory markers.

Once established on HAART, dyslipidaemia becomes a common problem and is more severe in those patients who develop the often distressing complication of lipodystrophy. Lipodystrophy typically results in lipoatrophy affecting the face, limbs and upper chest with fat accumulation around the abdomen and at the back of the neck. Insulin resistance with glucose intolerance and occasionally frank diabetes is an important accompanying feature. Lipid changes can occur early after initiation of therapy and was described first in patients receiving the protease inhibitor, ritonavir. Persistent increases in plasma triglycerides of 200 per cent and more, with plasma cholesterol increases of around 30–40 per cent, were observed as early as a week. Lipid abnormalities have also been observed in children with HIV and non-HIV volunteers. Some patients develop severe hypertriglyceridaemia (fasting triglyceride >11 mmol/L) such that the risk of pancreatitis is an important management consideration. Other protease inhibitors also lead to hypertriglyceridaemia but the effects appear to be less severe than with ritonavir. Therapy with protease inhibitors is also associated with elevations in total cholesterol, reductions in HDL cholesterol and increases in lipoprotein(a). Of the protease inhibitors, indinavir appears to have a less marked effect. The NRTIs do not appear to produce dyslipidaemia whilst there is heterogeneity amongst the non-NHRTs; efavirenz therapy is associated with hypercholesterolaemia whilst nevirapine is not.

Clearly, the mechanisms by which protease inhibitors produce these dramatic metabolic effects are likely to shed new light on the control of adipogenesis, lipid metabolism and insulin resistance. Currently these mechanisms are not fully understood. However, there have been significant recent advances. At a physiological level, the dyslipidaemia appears to be associated with hepatic overproduction of VLDL rather than impaired clearance. Triglyceride-rich lipoprotein production from Hep-G2 cells is stimulated by protease inhibitors. At a molecular level, important genes in hepatic lipogenesis controlled by the transcription factor, SREBP-1c (the concentration of which was increased in hepatic cell nuclei), are activated in ritonavir-treated animals. Retarded degradation of apoprotein B may also contribute to VLDL overproduction.

As mentioned previously, dyslipidaemia and insulin resistance are observed more frequently in those patients who also develop lipodystrophy; hypertriglyceridaemia correlates with the degree of lipodystrophy. Recent experimental work points to a possible role for SREBP-1c in the lipodystrophy. In tissue culture experiments, ritonavir-treated 3T3 preadipocyte cells showed an abundance of the cleaved active form of SREBP-1c. A mouse model of lipodystrophy, generated by over-expression of the active form of SREBP-1c, shows in addition to lipodystrophy, dyslipidaemia, diabetes and hypoleptinaemia. In this model leptin treatment corrects the dyslipidaemia and hyperlipidaemia but not the lipodystrophy, pointing to a direct role for leptin in the insulin resistance. In these mice, insulin receptor substrate 2 is reduced due to chronic hyperinsulinaemia. This leads to impairment of insulin-mediated inhibition of hepatic gluconeogenesis and continuous activation of SREBPs. These two processes further increase plasma concentrations of glucose and lipids and enhance the vicious circle. The lipodystrophy syndrome associated with HAART treatment clearly has features in common with this important new animal model. A further area of intense interest involves the possible cross-talk between SREBPs and the retinoid X receptors (see pages 215–16), which could have profound effects of insulin resistance and dyslipidaemia.

Given that HAART has rendered HIV a chronic condition, one is faced with a possible long-term exposure to a dyslipidaemia and the possibility of atherosclerosis. Alteration of the HAART regimen to more metabolically friendly drugs is often not an option. Severe hypertriglyceridaemia is a risk for pancreatitis. The authors' approach is to treat severe hypertriglyceridaemia (fasting triglyceride >11 mmol/L) by lifestyle measures (low-fat, low-refined carbohydrate diet, weight reduction, limitation of alcohol intake) together with high-dose omega-3 fatty acids (e.g. Maxepa capsules 10 capsules/day or Omacor 4 capsules/day). Fibrate therapy gives an additive effect.

The authors have managed many patients with random triglyceride concentrations in the 40–100 mmol/L range with these measures.

The more usual dyslipidaemia is characterized by more modest hypertriglycerid-aemia, hypercholesterolaemia, low HDL and small, dense LDL – which is similar to the dyslipidaemia of the metabolic syndrome, often called the atherogenic lipoprotein profile. Management involves lifestyle measures and, following an assessment of global vascular risk, attention to other risk factors. The authors' first-choice therapy is a statin if there are no contraindications. Protease inhibitors such as ritonavir inhibit cytochrome 3A4 which is important in the metabolism of simvastatin, atorvastatin and lovastatin. Pravastatin is not metabolized by 3A4. Drug area under the curve concentrations of statins are affected by co-administration of ritonavir and saquinavir. Minimal effects were observed with pravastatin, with a 4.5-fold increase for atorvastatin and a 32-fold increase for simvastatin. Fluvastatin is metabolized via cytochrome 2C9. There is thus a possibility of significant drug interaction of fluvastatin and nelfinavir. Theoretically, pravastatin or fluvastatin should have an advantage in avoiding drug interactions. However, in the authors' experience, lower doses of atorvastatin have proved effective and safe. All patients are warned to stop the statins if severe muscle pains and tenderness develop, suggesting myositis.

In HAART patients who develop type 2 diabetes, the authors use metformin as first-line treatment when dietary measures fail. Some patients with more severe disease have responded to night-time insulin (e.g. Insulatard) and daytime metformin. Some patients have required conventional insulin therapy.

Hopefully, in the future, new anti-HIV drugs will have fewer metabolic side-effects. In the meantime, the authors' view is that the metabolic abnormalities seen in these patients should be treated. There have been sporadic reports of unexplained premature CHD in treated HIV patients. Ongoing large cohort studies will provide further information on the vascular risk. Perhaps new information of benefit to, not only the HIV community, but also to the general population with insulin resistance/dyslipidaemia will emerge as the mechanisms of these adverse effects are understood in detail.

REFERENCES

Armitage, J. and Collins, R. (2000) Need for large scale randomised evidence about lowering LDL cholesterol in people with diabetes mellitus: MRC/BHF heart protection study and other major trials. *Heart* **84**, 357–60.

Berenson, G., Srinivasan, S.R., Bao, W. *et al.* (1998) Association between multiple cardiovascular risk factors and atherosclerosis in children and young adults. *N Engl J Med* **338**, 1650–6.

Betteridge, D.J. (2001a) Dyslipidaemia and diabetes. *Pract Diabetes Int* **18**, 201–7.

Betteridge, D.J. (2001b) Lipid-lowering trials in diabetes. *Curr Opin Lipidol* **12**, 619–23.

Blankenhorn, D.H., Azen, S.P., Crawford, D.W. *et al.* (1991) Effect of colestipol-niacin therapy on human femoral atherosclerosis. *Circulation* **83**, 438–47.

Collins, R., Peto, R., MacMahon, S. *et al.* (1990) Blood pressure, stroke, and coronary heart disease. Part 2. Short-term reductions in blood pressure: overview of randomised drug trials in the epidemiological context. *Lancet* **335**, 827–38.

EuroAspire I and II Group. (2001) Clinical reality of coronary prevention guidelines: a comparison of EuroAspire I and II in nine countries. *Lancet* **357**, 995–1001.

Expert Panel on Detection, Evaluation and Treatment of High Blood Cholesterol in Adults (2001) Executive summary of the third report of the National Cholesterol Education Program (NCEP) Expert Panel on Detection, Evaluation and Treatment of High Blood Cholesterol in Adults (Adult Treatment Panel III). *J Am Med Assoc* **285**, 2486–97.

Hebert, P.R., Gaziano, J.M., Chan, K.S., Hennekens, C.H. (1997) Cholesterol lowering with statin drugs, risk of stroke, and total mortality: an overview of randomized trials. *JAMA* **278**, 313–21.

Herrington, D.M., Reboussin, D.M., Broshihan, K.B. *et al.* (2000) Effects of estrogen replacement on the progression of coronary-artery atherosclerosis. *N Engl J Med* **343**, 522–9.

International Diabetes Federation (2001) *Diabetes and Cardiovascular Disease: Time to Act.* IDF, Executive Office, 1 rue Defacqz, B-1000 Brussels, Belgium.

Jick, H., Zornberg, G.L., Jick, S.S., Seshadri, S. and Drachman, D.A. (2000) Statins and the risk of dementia. *Lancet* **356**, 1627–31.

Jönsson, B. (2001) Economics of drug treatment: for which patients is it cost effective to lower cholesterol? *Lancet* **358**, 1251–6.

Kannel, W.B. (1983) High density lipoproteins: epidemiologic profile and risks of coronary artery disease. *Am J Cardiol* **52**, 9B–12B.

Krone, W. and Müller-Wieland, D. (1990) Hyperlipidaemia and hypertension. In *Baillière's Clinical Endocrinology and Metabolism*, Vol. 4, No. 4 (ed. D.J. Betteridge), Baillière Tindall, London.

MacMahon, S.W., Macdonald, G.J. and Blacket, R.B. (1985) Plasma lipoprotein levels in treated and untreated hypertensive men and women. The National Heart Foundation of Australia risk factor prevalence study. *Aerterioscler Thromb* **5**, 391–6.

Manolio, T.A., Pearson, T.A., Wenger, N.K. *et al.* (1992) Cholesterol and heart disease in older persons and women: review of an NHLBI workshop. *Ann Epidemiol* **2**, 161–76.

Mooser, V. and Carr, A. (2001) Antiretroviral therapy-associated hyperlipidaemia in HIV disease. *Curr Opin Lipidol* **12**, 313–19.

Neaton, J.D., Blackburn, H., Jacobs, D. *et al.* (1992) Serum cholesterol level and mortality findings for men screened in the Multiple Risk Factor Intervention Trial. *Arch Intern Med* **152**, 1490–500.

Neil, A., Rees, A. and Taylor, C. (eds) (1996a) *Hyperlipidaemia in Childhood*, Royal College of Physicians, London.

Neil, H.A., Silagy, C.A., Lancaster, T. *et al.* (1996b) Garlic in the treatment of modern hyperlipidaemia: a controlled trial and a meta-analysis. *J R Coll Phys* **30**, 329–34.

Pearson, T.A., Laurora, I., Chu, H. and Kafonek, S. (2000) The Lipid Treatment Assessment Project (L-TAP). A multicentre survey to evaluate the percentages of dyslipidaemic patients receiving lipid-lowering therapy and achieving low-density lipoprotein cholesterol goals. *Arch Intern Med* **160**, 459–67.

Prospective Studies Collaborative Group (1995) Cholesterol, diastolic blood pressure and stroke; 13000 strokes in 450 000 people in 45 prospective cohorts. *Lancet* **345**, 1647–53.

Schnyder, G., Roffi, M., Pin, R. *et al.* (2001) Decreased rate of coronary restenosis after lowering of plasma homocysteine levels. *N Engl J Med* **345**, 1593–600.

Shepherd, J., Blauw, G.J., Murphy, M.B. *et al.* (1999) The design of a Prospective Study of Pravastatin in the Elderly at Risk (PROSPER). *Am J Cardiol* **84**, 1192–7.

Shepherd, J., Blauw, G.J., Murphy, M.B., et al. (2002) Pravastatin in elderly individuals at risk of vascular disease (PROSPER): a randomized controlled trial. *Lancet* **360**, 1623–30.

Stamler, J., Vaccaro, O., Neaton, J.D. *et al.* (1993) Diabetes, other risk factors and 12 year cardiovascular mortality for men screened in the Multiple Risk Factor Intervention Trial. *Diabetes Care* **16**, 434–44.

Stampfer, M.J. and Colditz, G.A. (1991) Estrogen replacement therapy and coronary heart disease: a quantitative assessment of the epidemiologic evidence. *Prev Med* **20**, 47–63.

Stein, E.A., Illingworth, D.R., Kwitorovich, P.O. *et al.* (1999) Efficacy and safety of lovatastin in adolescent males with heterozygous familial hypercholesterolemia: a randomized controlled trial. *J Am Med Assoc* **281**, 137–44.

Tomlinson, B. (2000) Implications of high blood lipid levels in the hypertensive patient. In *Lipids and Vascular Disease: Current Issues* (ed. D.J. Betteridge), Martin Dunitz, London, pp. 133–50.

UK Prospective Diabetes Study (UKPDS) (1998) Effect of intensive blood-glucose control with metformin on complications in overweight patients with type 2 diabetes (UKPDS 34). *Lancet* **352**, 854–65.

White, H.D., Simes, R.J., Anderson, N.E. *et al.* (2000) Pravastatin therapy and the risk of stroke. *N Engl J Med* **343**, 317–26.

Williams, R.R., Hunt, S.C., Hopkins, P.H. *et al.* (1988) Familial dyslipidaemic hypertension. Evidence from 58 Utah families for a syndrome present in approximately 12 percent of patients with essential hypertertension. *J Am Med Assoc* **259**, 3579–86.

Winder, A.F. (2000) Lipids and non-coronary vascular disease. In *Lipids and Vascular Disease: Current Issues* (ed. D.J. Betteridge). Martin Dunitz, London, 121–32.

Wood, D.A., De Backer, G., Faergeman, O. *et al.* (1998) Prevention of coronary heart disease in clinical practice. Recommendations of the second joint task force of the European Society of Cardiology, European Atherosclerosis Society and European Society of Hypertension. *Eur Heart J* **19**, 1434–503.

Yeo, W. and Yeo, K.R. (2001) Predicting CHD risk in patients with diabetes mellitus. *Diabetic Med* **18**, 341–4.

ECONOMIC ASPECTS

The cost of CHD in industrialized countries is enormous. In 1996 in the UK, CHD cost the health-care system about £1.6 billion. The cost of hospital care accounted for 54 per cent of expenditure and drugs 32 per cent. Only 1 per cent of the total was spent on prevention. When production losses from death and disability and payments for social support are added, the total cost of CHD exceeds £10 billion. This represents a cost more than double that for any other single disease for which cost analysis has been carried out. UK figures are, however, dwarfed by US estimates for 2000, when total cardiovascular costs are projected to exceed $325 billion with CHD directly accounting for $118.2 billion.

In the UK, the National Health Service provides 90 per cent of health care with purchasers having an increasing influence on the provision of services by providers. In contrast to other countries, the UK, with centrally cash-limited funds, has been able to control health-care costs despite the pressures of an ageing population, expensive medical advances and increased demands from the population. The amount expended on health as a percentage of gross domestic product is considerably less than other westernized countries (Table 12.1), but it is debatable whether this represents efficiency or underprovision of care. In the USA, health-care providers dominate the purchaser/provider relationship but the system is undermined by 30 per cent of the population being either uninsured or inadequately covered.

Any initiatives to improve the health of individuals or a nation should be evidence based. This means that decisions should be based on the conclusions of randomized trial evidence and a consideration of the benefits and risks of the intervention against the pre-intervention prognosis. Unfortunately, as the number of health-gain initiatives is potentially large and as resources are finite, new initiatives must also satisfy economic considerations. In future, cost-effectiveness parameters should be built into the design of all randomized controlled trials.

The large-scale statin trials have revolutionized thinking about lipid lowering and have shown benefits to patients and health services across a spectrum of risk covering

TABLE **12.1** • Spending on health care in different countries as percentage of Gross Domestic Product

Country	% GDP
USA	13.9
Germany	10.7
Switzerland	10.0
France	9.6
Sweden	8.6
Netherlands	8.5
Australia	8.4
European Union average	8.0
Italy	7.6
New Zealand	7.6
Spain	7.4
UK	6.8
Ireland	6.3

TABLE **12.2** • Numbers needed to treat for the major statin trials

Trial	Events prevented	NNT	Follow-up (years)
WOSCOPS	NF MI/CHD death	45	4.9
AF/TexCAPS	NF/F MI UA CHD death	50	5.2
4S	NF MI/CHD death	12	5.4
CARE	NF MI/CHD death	33	5.0
LIPID	NF MI/CHD death	28	6.1

F, fatal; NF, non-fatal; UA, unstable angina.

both primary and secondary prevention. The numbers of patients, however, who could benefit are large and the costs high so clinicians and purchasers of health care are charged with developing policies for treatment to avoid poorly targeted and inefficient prescribing to maximize the cost-effectiveness of the intervention.

The 'number needed to treat' (NNT) concept is increasingly used by health professionals to gauge the impact of an intervention. This is calculated from the evidence of outcome event trials by the formula:

$$1 \div \text{treatment event rate} - \text{control event rate}$$

NNT data should be interpreted with some care as the original measurements of statistical uncertainty that applied in the original trials are usually omitted in their calculation.

The NNTs for the statin trials are shown in Table 12.2. From the table it can be seen that using 4S data only 12 patients need be treated over 5.4 years to prevent one CHD event.

The NNT reduces if the baseline absolute risk of the group under investigation increases. For example, in CARE, the NNT for the diabetic sub group reduces to 12 and

TABLE **12.3** • Comparison of the numbers needed to treat to prevent one event over 5 years with different cardiovascular interventions

Intervention or trial	Events prevented	NNT
Severe hypertension DBP 115–129 mmHg	Death, CVA, MI	3
CABG L main stem	Death	6
Aspirin for TIA	Death, CVA	6
4S	Death, NF MI, revascularization, CVA	6
Warfarin for AF	Stroke	7
Aspirin post-MI	CV death, CVA, MI	12
Beta-blocker post-MI	Death	20
ACE inhibitor for LV dysfunction	CV death or CHF hospitalization	21
WOSCOPS	Death, NF MI, revascularization, CVA	26
Mild hypertension DBP 90–109 mmHg	Death, CVA, MI	141

CHF, congestive heart failure.

in the 65–75 age range to 11. Similarly, if the 40 per cent of higher-risk WOSCOPS men, whose absolute risk is ≥ 2 per cent over 10 years, are isolated, the NNT becomes 22. Adding other events prevented and recalculating the figures to a standard 5-year period allows comparison with other important cardiovascular interventions (Table 12.3).

Statins are clearly clinically effective and with over 200 000 patient-years of experience, apparently safe, but are they cost-effective? There are four main methods of economic evaluation:

■ **Cost minimization analysis.** Here two interventions are compared only in terms of cost, the cheapest being the preferred option. No account is taken of differing effectiveness.

■ **Cost-effectiveness analysis.** Here costs are compared with units of outcome. For example, in a cholesterol management programme, the costs of screening, testing, professional time, monitoring and treatment can be related to a 1 mmol/L drop in cholesterol for a hypercholesterolaemic individual. A more common comparison is the cost per life year gained.

■ **Cost–benefit analysis.** This requires the benefits of an intervention to be valued in purely monetary terms. Consideration is given to the valuation of production gains or how much an individual would be willing to pay for the intervention. The analysis can be difficult to interpret.

■ **Cost–utility analysis.** This is an extension of cost-effectiveness and relates both the quantity and quality of life gained from a health-care intervention. For example, a year of full quality life is one QALY (quality-adjusted life year).

The 4S study revolutionized the attitudes of clinicians towards statins and well-designed economic evaluations support the clinical evidence. Johannesson *et al.* (1997) estimated the cost per life year gained with secondary prevention for men and women from 35 to 70 years old for the cholesterol range 5.5–8.0 mmol/L. The range was £2375–£17 125 from a hypercholesterolaemic 70-year-old man to a 35-year-old woman

TABLE **12.4** • Cost effectiveness of different health and safety interventions

Intervention	Cost per life year saved in GB£
Statin – secondary prevention	5000–6000
Statin – primary prevention	14 000–21 000
Beta-blocker for hypertension	12 000
Dialysis for chronic renal failure	28 000
Road works/building	62 000
Drivers' air bag	250 000
Airline smoke hood	750 000

with low cholesterol. When indirect costs (such as lost productivity) were added, treating younger patients actually saved money.

A second analysis, by Jönsson *et al.* (1996), incorporated the data from 4S on reduced hospitalization costs and calculated that each life year gained cost £5502. Several other studies have confirmed this figure for secondary prevention with minor variations. This is well within the limits normally considered as acceptable in sophisticated health-care systems (in the USA, interventions are considered highly cost-effective if each life year saved costs <$20 000, moderately cost-effective in the range $20 000–60 000 and expensive >$70 000). Recent economic evaluations of mammography in women aged 50–69 years are associated with a cost of £8561 per life year gained and numerous other studies confirm that statins are cost-effective compared with other interventions, both medical and non-medical (Table 12.4).

Estimates for cost-effectiveness in primary prevention have proved much more variable. The WOSCOPS investigators calculated the discounted costs per life year gained to be £20 375 across the study population and £13 995 in the higher risk 40 per cent. Other investigators, perhaps with political axes to grind, have inflated the figures significantly. The variations can be accounted for by the use of different methodologies and the failure to incorporate the effects of reductions in other long-term morbidity consequences such as heart failure, stroke and unstable angina. The cost savings involved in stroke reduction alone are significant and are rarely accounted in analyses.

In most studies of the cost-effectiveness of lipid lowering, the estimates are based on treatment targeted at threshold concentrations of cholesterol. As cholesterol levels by themselves are poor predictors of risk, it is more appropriate to target levels of absolute CHD risk and the paper by Pickin *et al.* (1999) estimates the cost per life year gained of four levels of CHD risk: 4.5 per cent per annum equates to the absolute risk of subjects with CHD in the placebo group of 4S, 3 per cent reflects the advice on statin prescribing issued by the Standing Medical Advisory Committee in the UK, 2 per cent the level endorsed by the Joint European Task Force and 1.5 per cent, the level of CHD risk in the primary prevention trial WOSCOPS.

The gross discounted costs per life year gained including drug costs and potential savings in health-care costs for the four levels of absolute risk are shown in Table 12.5.

TABLE **12.5** • Implications of targeting statin treatment at four CHD risk levels, showing the NNT, cost-effectiveness and implications for the UK population

	CHD events per year			
	4.5%	**3.0%**	**2.0%**	**1.5%**
NNT for 5 years	13	20	30	40
Cost per life year gained (£)	5100	8200	10 700	12 500
% UK adults above threshold	5.1	8.2	15.8	24.7
Annual cost (£millions)	549	885	1712	2673

In the UK, approximately 4.8 per cent of the adult population requires secondary prevention and subjects for primary prevention, at a 3 per cent CHD risk level, comprise a further 3.4 per cent. This means that, at least, 8.2 per cent of the UK population will require treatment at an annual cost equivalent to 25 per cent of the present expenditure on community prescribed medicines. It is difficult to envisage how more aggressive intervention at lower levels of risk will be affordable at current prices in a country with such high levels of CHD. Cost-effectiveness is of course country specific and different levels of intervention reflect the political and social pressures of each community on each nation's health-care system. In the USA current NCEP guidelines suggest cholesterol lowering would be applicable for 28 per cent of the population.

Sadly, the implementation of the evidence for the benefit of lipid lowering is inadequate. Few diabetic patients reach their LDL cholesterol targets and even in secondary prevention, Pearson reports from the USA that only 18 per cent reach the LDL cholesterol goal of <2.6 mmol/L. EUROASPIRE 2, recently announced, shows an improvement in lipid-lowering prescribing in secondary prevention but 59 per cent are not achieving the European LDL cholesterol goal of 3.0 mmol/L. The blame does not solely rest with physicians, as studies show up to 50 per cent discontinuation rates for lipid lowering medication 12 months from initiation. Issues surrounding compliance are discussed in Chapter 10.

Few medical treatments have received the intensity of cost speculation accorded to lipid-lowering therapy and this is appropriate, given the scale of the problem and the potential for benefit. Few classes of drugs, however, have been shown to extend life significantly and there are cost savings to be made in other areas of prescribing (for example, anti-ulcer and non-steroidal anti-inflammatory drugs). Inevitably, with patent expiries, statin costs will reduce and cost-effectiveness will increase.

Bonneux *et al.* (1998) calculated that eliminating CHD in the Netherlands would increase life expectancy by 1.9 years (2.5 per cent) but lifetime expected costs of health care would rise by 6 per cent, as survivors developed other costly conditions in their added years. Eliminating dementia instead would have no impact on life expectancy but, by contrast, would lower health-care costs by 6 per cent, a much more appealing proposition for government paymasters. The issue should become a humanitarian one of quality, not cost-effectiveness and physicians are reminded that the aim of prevention is to spare people from avoidable misery and death, not to save money on the health-care system.

COMMISSIONING SERVICES FOR THE PREVENTION AND TREATMENT OF CHD

The scale of the problem and the impact of the mortality and morbidity involved, make CHD prevention and treatment the major health priority in many countries. Local agreements for service provision must balance sophisticated medical interventions, such as revascularization procedures, against the health gains of other forms of prevention and care, some of which may be of less proven effectiveness. Commissioning of services should ideally be evidence based, aimed at local priorities and national targets and reflect the increased role of primary care. Only in primary care can the major burden of continuing primary and secondary prevention be addressed.

In some health-care systems, primary care teams are now able to influence the provision of services for their patients either directly through purchasing (budget holding or locally based purchasing) or indirectly through advisory roles to commissioning agencies. Primary care thus finds itself at the centre of a coordinated programme for CHD prevention and treatment (Figure 12.1).

Whilst the effectiveness of some forms of health promotion in primary prevention is unproven, much of the fall in CHD death rates since the 1970s is attributable to CHD risk-factor reductions. The evidence for secondary prevention is strong, particularly for cholesterol lowering, cessation of smoking, BP reduction and the use of other drugs such as aspirin, beta-blockers and ACE inhibitors in heart failure. Targeting secondary prevention first will produce short-term gains, primary prevention being a longer-term strategy. Unfortunately, 75 per cent of those with CHD under 65 years of age are first diagnosed when they have a heart attack. As 25 per cent of people with heart attacks

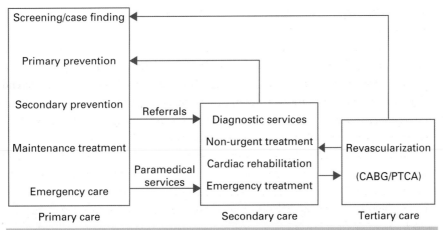

FIGURE **12.1** • Coordination of primary, secondary and tertiary care for CHD prevention and treatment.

SERVICES FOR THE PREVENTION & TREATMENT OF CHD

die before reaching hospital, secondary prevention is not always applicable.

The care of the patient with myocardial infarction can be improved in terms of prioritized ambulance dispatch, improved CPR education and availability and high technology facilities. The needs of the elderly, women and certain ethnic groups (such as South Asians) need to be addressed. Services for angina (improved access to exercise ECG, angiography and rapid assessment chest pain clinics) and for heart failure (improved access to echocardiography) should be reviewed. There is considerable variation in the provision of cardiac rehabilitation and revascularization services. For example, few districts in the UK achieve acceptable norms for revascularization (600 CABG and 400 PTCA per year per million population).

If primary care teams can work with secondary care authorities to produce a strategy responsive to individual needs with effective prevention programmes, major falls in CHD mortality and morbidity will result.

REFERENCES AND FURTHER READING

Bonneux, L., Barendregt, J.J., Nusselder, W.J. *et al.* (1998) Preventing fatal diseases increases healthcare costs: cause elimination life table approach. *Br Med J* **316**, 26–9.

Caro, J., Klittich, W., McGuire, A. *et al.* (1997) The West of Scotland coronary prevention study: economic benefit analysis of primary prevention with pravastatin. *Br Med J* **315**, 1577–82.

Johannesson, M. (2001) At what coronary risk level is it cost-effective to initiate cholesterol lowering drug treatment in primary prevention? *Eur Heart J* **22**, 919–25.

Johannesson, M., Jönsson, B., Kjekhus, J. *et al.* (1997) Cost effectiveness of simvastatin treatment to lower cholesterol levels in patients with coronary heart disease. *N Engl J Med* **336**, 332–6.

Jönsson, B., Johannesson, M., Kjekhus, J. *et al.* (1996) Cost-effectiveness of cholesterol lowering. Results from the Scandinavian Simvastatin Survival Study (4S). *Eur Heart J* **17**, 1001–7.

Pearson, T.A., Laurora, I., Chu, H. and Kafonek, S. (2000) The Lipid Treatment Assessment Project (L-TAP). A multicentre survey to evaluate the percentages of dyslipidaemic patients receiving lipid-lowering therapy and achieving low-density lipoprotein cholesterol goals. *Arch Intern Med* **160**, 459–67.

Pickin, D.M., McCabe, C.J., Ramsay, L.E. *et al.* (1999) Cost effectiveness of HMG-CoA reductase inhibitor (statin) treatment related to the risk of coronary heart disease and cost of drug treatment. *Heart* **82**, 325–32.

CHAPTER 13

CASE STUDIES

The following 20 case studies represent practical examples from our experience of managing the treatment of dyslipidaemia in patients with varying risk factor profiles. The lipid profiles are measured in mmol/L (Table 13.1) and can be assumed to represent fasting levels.

TABLE **13.1** • Lipid profiles

Total cholesterol – HDL – LDL							
20–95		**100–195**		**200–295**		**300–395**	
mg/dL	mmol/L	mg/dL	mmol/L	mg/dL	mmol/L	mg/dL	mmol/L
20	0.5	100	2.6	200	5.2	300	7.8
25	0.7	105	2.7	205	5.3	305	7.9
30	0.8	110	2.9	210	5.5	310	8.1
35	0.9	115	3.0	215	5.6	315	8.2
40	1.0	120	3.1	220	5.7	320	8.3
45	1.2	125	3.3	225	5.9	325	8.5
50	1.3	130	3.4	230	6.0	330	8.6
55	1.4	135	3.5	235	6.1	335	8.7
60	1.6	140	3.6	240	6.2	340	8.8
65	1.7	145	3.8	245	6.4	345	9.0
70	1.8	150	3.9	250	6.5	350	9.1
75	2.0	155	4.0	255	6.6	355	9.2
80	2.1	160	4.2	260	6.8	360	9.4
85	2.2	165	4.3	265	6.9	365	9.5
90	2.3	170	4.4	270	7.0	370	9.6
95	2.5	175	4.6	275	7.2	375	9.8
		180	4.7	280	7.3	380	9.9
		185	4.8	285	7.4	385	10.0
		190	4.9	290	7.5	390	10.1
		195	5.0	295	7.7	395	10.3

(continued)

TABLE **13.1** • *(continued)*

Triglyceride

100–195		200–295		300–395		400–495		500–600	
mg/dL	mmol/L	mg/dL	mmol/L	mg/dL	mmol/L	mg/dL	mmol/L	mg/dL	mmol/L
100	1.13	200	2.26	300	3.39	400	4.52	500	5.65
105	1.19	205	2.32	305	3.45	405	4.58	505	5.71
110	1.24	210	2.37	310	3.50	410	4.63	510	5.76
115	1.30	215	2.43	315	3.56	415	4.69	515	5.82
120	1.36	220	2.49	320	3.62	420	4.75	520	5.88
125	1.41	225	2.54	325	3.67	425	4.80	525	5.93
130	1.47	230	2.60	330	3.73	430	4.86	530	5.99
135	1.53	235	2.66	335	3.79	435	4.92	535	6.05
140	1.58	240	2.71	340	3.84	440	4.97	540	6.10
145	1.64	245	2.77	345	3.90	445	5.03	545	6.16
150	1.70	250	2.83	350	3.96	450	5.09	550	6.22
155	1.75	255	2.88	355	4.01	455	5.14	555	6.27
160	1.81	260	2.94	360	4.07	460	5.20	560	6.33
165	1.86	265	2.99	365	4.12	465	5.25	565	6.38
170	1.92	270	3.05	370	4.18	470	5.31	570	6.44
175	1.98	275	3.11	375	4.24	475	5.37	575	6.50
180	2.03	280	3.16	380	4.29	480	5.42	580	6.55
185	2.09	285	3.22	385	4.35	485	5.48	585	6.61
190	2.15	290	3.28	390	4.41	490	5.54	590	6.67
195	2.20	295	3.33	395	4.46	495	5.59	600	6.78

Glucose

50–250				260–500			
mg/dL	mmol/L	mg/dL	mmol/L	mg/dL	mmol/L	mg/dL	mmol/L
50	2.78	190	10.55	260	14.43	400	22.20
60	3.33	200	11.10	270	14.99	410	22.76
70	3.89	210	11.66	280	15.54	420	23.31
80	4.44	220	12.21	290	16.10	430	23.87
90	5.00	230	12.77	300	16.65	440	24.42
100	5.55	240	13.32	310	17.21	450	24.98
110	6.11	250	13.88	320	17.76	500	27.75
120	6.66			330	18.32		
130	7.22			340	18.87		
140	7.77			350	19.43		
150	8.33			360	19.98		
160	8.88			370	20.54		
170	9.44			380	21.09		
180	9.99			390	21.65		

The reader should evaluate each patient's global risk by multifactorial risk assessment and formulate a management plan, which should include not only a therapeutic strategy (e.g. change diet, stop smoking, add medication) but also an idea of the goals required to achieve a reduction in cardiovascular risk. Plans should be realistic and achievable and should reflect the evidence base of modern clinical practice.

A commentary from the authors is provided after the case studies. Where quoted, percentage CHD risk estimates are calculated using the Framingham risk function incorporated into the 'Cardiac Risk Assessor' software developed by Professor Paul Durrington at the University of Manchester, UK. LDL measurements are calculated using the Friedewald formula (all units in mmol/L; if using mg/dL, the factor is 5, not 2.19):

LDL cholesterol (mmol/L) = Total cholesterol − HDL cholesterol − (total triglyceride)/2.19

AUTHORS' COMMENTS

CASE 1

48-year-old company director

Unstable angina (troponin negative)	TC 4.3
6 weeks ago	HDL 1.2
PTCA and stent insertion	TG 1.3
Ex-smoker	
BP 146/88	
No relevant family history	
BMI 26	
Alcohol 26 units per week	
Aspirin, clopidogrel, beta-blocker, statin	

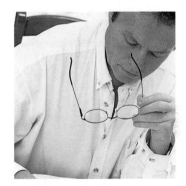

JMM

This patient was started on a statin during his admission and has already achieved target lipid levels, including a calculated LDL cholesterol of 2.5 mmol/L. Primary care has an important role to identify these patients, check their interventions and target achievement and foster compliance with medication, lifestyle change and rehabilitation programmes. I would encourage this man to eat healthily, lose weight, drink less and exercise more. There is certainly a case for adding an ACE inhibitor and this would improve his blood pressure control.

DJB

He has certainly reached the current goals of therapy of both NCEP ATP-III and the joint European guidelines. I agree that fostering compliance is a very important issue, particularly with multiple drug therapy. The aspirin/clopidogrel combination appears to have clear benefits in the CURE study. Following the HPS results it is likely that LDL targets will be reviewed in that high-risk individuals with baseline LDL cholesterol <2.6 mmol/L showed benefit with statin therapy. However, how low to lower LDL remains an open question and we await the results of TNT, IDEAL, SEARCH and other studies comparing standard to more aggressive LDL lowering. I personally would measure his homocysteine and advise folic acid supplementation if necessary. I do not know his pre-treatment lipid profile but certainly with any young CHD patient family screening for risk factors should always be considered.

CASE 2

60-year-old store manager

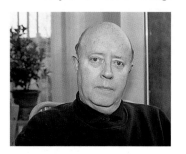

MI 4 years ago	TC 4.8
Ex-smoker	HDL 1.0
BP 134/80	TG 0.9
No relevant family history	
BMI 24	
Alcohol 14 units per week	
Aspirin, beta-blocker, statin	

JMM

This man is another secondary
prevention priority patient and needs an appropriate range of advice but at 3.4 mmol/L, his calculated LDL cholesterol level is too high. I would titrate his statin dose upwards, if possible, monitoring the changes at 6-weekly intervals. Plant stanol or sterol margarine might be helpful.

DJB

His LDL is clearly not to goal. In my experience the most common reason for this is failure to use an adequate statin dose. Market research studies confirm the generally low average statin dose, lower than used in the endpoint trials. The greatest LDL reduction is with the first dose of statin with an average of 6 per cent further LDL cholesterol reduction when the dose is doubled. I agree that functional foods such as the stanol ester and plant sterol products should be considered. Appropriate use of these products could be equivalent to two statin dose titrations. If he is on maximum statin dose a more potent statin in terms of LDL lowering could be considered. If he is on a maximal-tolerated dose, add-in therapy with a low dose of anion-exchange resin is a possibility. This would need to be well separated from his other medication to avoid absorption problems. I would suggest one Omacor fish-oil capsule/day, given the GISSI trial results.

CASE 3

53-year-old banker

Asymptomatic	TC 7.6
Smokes 15 a day	HDL 1.1
BP 170/102	TG 2.3
Maternal uncle has angina	
BMI 28	
Alcohol 20 units per week	

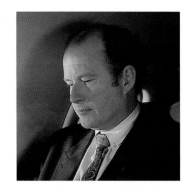

JMM

Multiple risk factors are active here, including the pattern of mixed hyperlipidaemia. Calculated CHD risk, using the Framingham risk function, exceeds 30 per cent over 10 years. There is plenty of scope for lifestyle change including the management of hypertension, cessation of smoking and dietary alteration. Losing weight may improve blood pressure and lipid levels and increasing exercise might facilitate this. If progressive improvement in global risk cannot be demonstrated in 6–9 months, I would start a statin.

DJB

It would be interesting to know the age of onset of CHD in the maternal uncle, together with any known risk factors. The possibility of familial combined hyperlipidaemia should be considered. The primary care physician or secondary care lipid clinics are both well placed to organize family screening, which may help with diagnosis. The risk charts underestimate risk in familial dyslipidemias. I would certainly want to know if there is family history of type 2 diabetes and would measure his fasting glucose. He does have several features of the metabolic syndrome. Lifestyle changes have been shown to decrease progress to diabetes in patients with impaired glucose tolerance. I would suggest a statin drug. In patients with a concomitant hypertriglyceridaemia a higher dose of statin is often required. If his LDL cholesterol is reduced to goal and his triglycerides remain raised then non-HDL cholesterol is a secondary goal of therapy. Clearly hypotensive medication should be considered.

CASE 4

58-year-old headmistress

Asymptomatic	TC 8.2
Smokes 20 a day	HDL 1.3
BP 144/86	TG 2.1
Mother angina, maternal aunt	
MI aged 65	
BMI 24	
No alcohol	

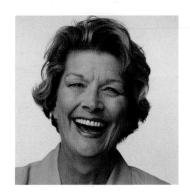

JMM

This menopausal lady's 10-year CHD risk is 20 per cent. She could improve her risk profile significantly by stopping smoking. Her LDL cholesterol is high and her blood pressure borderline at a time that rates of CHD for women begin to equate to those of men. I would concentrate on lifestyle change, but if she were unable to modify her risk profile, lipid modification with a statin would be indicated.

DJB

Her family history is very important. Her maternal aunt had an MI at 65 years and mother has angina. At what age did CHD symptoms begin? Are there any known risk factors? It is important to remember that the risk charts do not take into account family history. I would suggest a statin.

CASE 5

50-year-old insurance salesman

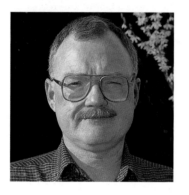

Asymptomatic	TC 5.2
Non-smoker	HDL 0.7
BP 132/84	TG 1.8
Paternal grandfather angina aged 82	
BMI 26	
Alcohol 14 units per week	

JMM

At first sight, this man's apparent lack of risk factors is reassuring. His HDL cholesterol, however, is low and, when calculated, his 10-year CHD risk is 15.1 per cent. This is roughly the population risk in the West of Scotland Coronary Prevention Study (WOSCOPS) where treatment with a statin was found to be beneficial. Losing weight, eating healthily and intensifying his exercise regimen would also help.

DJB

Low HDL cholesterol is an important risk factor as emphasized by ATP-III. Furthermore, when calculating risk using the joint European charts, risk is underestimated when HDL is low. He is not particularly overweight and he is not a smoker yet his HDL is very low. I agree that weight reduction and appropriate physical activity could help increase his HDL. Statin treatment is likely to be beneficial – his calculated LDL is 3.7 mmol/L. Clearly trials (AFCAPS/TexCAPS) indicate benefit at this risk level but health economic constraints may apply in some countries, as the number needed to treat is higher. This may prove a less important factor as statins lose patent and become available as generic. I nowadays always advise functional foods in addition to other lifestyle measures.

CASE 6

27-year-old actor

Asymptomatic	TC 9.5
Non-smoker	HDL 1.0
BP 124/62	TG 1.1
Father died MI aged 49; paternal uncle angina aged 52; paternal grandfather died suddenly aged 54	
Wife just had twins	
Early arcus and tendon xanthomata	

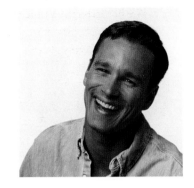

JMM

Familial hypercholesterolaemia (FH) is one of the commonest inherited conditions, in most populations, affecting up to 1 in 500 people. This is similar to the prevalence of type 1 diabetes and yet much under-diagnosed. Here there is a clear family history of early coronary death, there are obvious physical signs and high levels of LDL cholesterol. Diet and medication are appropriate but I would consider referral to a specialist centre for advice.

DJB

Despite his young age, this man merits aggressive cholesterol lowering with statins as first-line therapy. Sadly, some primary care physicians would mistakenly use the risk prediction charts in this situation; this is inappropriate. Analysis of the Simon Broome Register indicated a 100-fold excess mortality in young adults with FH. This man is best managed in a specialist lipid clinic. High-dose statin therapy is required given the starting LDL of $\cong 8\,mmol/L$. Combination therapy with the addition of an anion-exchange resin or, in the near future, specific cholesterol absorption inhibition may be required. The new 'super' statins would clearly have a role. It is the author's clinical practice to perform periodic non-invasive cardiac assessments in high-risk FH patients with a low threshold for cardiac referral. It is highly likely that he has an LDL receptor defect. In some centres, genotyping is available and if a mutation is identified, this aids family screening, which is an important responsibility of the clinic; given the autosomal dominant inheritance, this will have a 50 per cent positive pick-up rate. Although the diagnosis of FH can be made on cord blood, it is the author's practice to test children at around 10 years. Fortunately, it is highly likely that our patient's wife does not have FH. However, it would be reassuring to see the wife's lipid profile. Homozygous FH is, thankfully, extremely rare. However, if this were a possibility, genetic counselling and early screening would be mandatory given the need for intensive therapy. The question of family screening should be addressed sensitively, particularly in relation to the children. Strong reassurance is the rule and the potential excellent prognosis should be emphasized given the early detection and treatment. Very rarely, this clinical picture can be seen in FDB as discussed in Chapter 3.

Case studies

CASE 7

39-year-old secretary

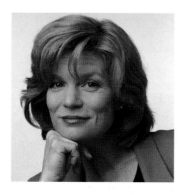

Asymptomatic	TC 11.0
Non-smoker	HDL 1.1
Father died MI aged 39	TG 12.6
BMI 26	
No alcohol	
Tubero-eruptive xanthomata	

JMM

From a family history of early coronary death, the suspicion that a genetic defect might be active is confirmed by the finding of tubero-eruptive xanthomata on this patient's elbows and the grossly abnormal lipid profile. Despite its rarity, remnant hyperlipidaemia is to be found in family practice and the metabolic and physical abnormalities respond well to treatment.

DJB

Remnant hyperlipidaemia (dysbetalipoproteinaemia; type III) is rare but important to recognize because of the high risk of vascular disease and sometimes pancreatitis. She should be referred to a specialist lipid clinic. She is highly likely to demonstrate E2 homozygosity; her VLDL isolated by ultracentrifugation will show an increased cholesterol/triglyceride ratio and her lipoprotein electrophoresis, a broad-beta pattern. She probably has familial combined hyperlipidaemia in addition to E2 homozygosity leading to type III phenotype. Hypothyroidism, diabetes and other secondary causes should be excluded. Family screening would be worthwhile. Fibrates can be effective in this condition but the author's first choice is a statin. Sometimes combination with a fibrate is necessary. Lifestyle and nutrition are important as always. Insulin resistance, which is common in this situation, will be helped by weight loss and exercise. The blood glucose should be monitored periodically. Effective treatment rapidly leads to disappearance of the xanthomata for which the patient is usually extremely grateful.

CASE 8

41-year-old programmer

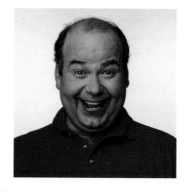

Recurrent abdominal pain and vomiting	TC 9.0
Smokes 20 per day	HDL 1.0
BP 116/74	TG 23.7
No relevant family history	
BMI 28	
Alcohol 7–20 units per week	

JMM

Plasma becomes milky in appearance when triglyceride content exceeds about 11 mmol/L. Triglyceride levels in excess of 10 mmol/L increase the likelihood of acute pancreatitis, which may be the explanation for this patient's abdominal pain. This patient needs specialist advice from a lipid clinic.

DJB

He has the type V phenotype with hyperchylomicronaemia and raised VLDL as indicated by the raised cholesterol. He should be referred to a specialist centre. Severe hypertriglyceridaemia is most commonly due to secondary causes, particularly alcohol and diabetes. He does not drink to excess but it is important to check his glucose. Occasionally this phenotype can run in families and is described as familial hypertriglyceridaemia. It is likely that lipoprotein lipase or apoprotein C-II deficiency would have presented at an earlier age. This can be confirmed by the rapid response to a very low-fat diet and the measurement of lipoprotein lipase enzyme activity. Familial hypertriglyceridaemia does not respond rapidly to diet and lipoprotein lipase activity is measurable.

Treatment is with a low-fat, low-refined carbohydrate diet together with fish oil (Maxepa, 10 capsules/day or Omacor, 4 capsules/day) plus a fibrate. The diet is crucial in this condition and often the necessity of a low *total* fat diet is not appreciated. Compliance can be difficult and a single 'binge' may produce severe lipaemia and pancreatitis. Strong anti-smoking advice is needed, not only for the obvious reasons, but also as it exacerbates the hypertriglyceridaemia. I would also advise abstinence from alcohol. High-dose fish-oil will reduce hepatic VLDL output and is very useful in this condition, together with a fibrate. There is some evidence that antioxidant vitamins may reduce the risk of pancreatitis in these patients.

CASE 9

37-year-old shop assistant

Asymptomatic	TC 12.2
Non-smoker	HDL 0.9
BP 124/80	TG 4.5
Mother MI aged 52	
Maternal uncle and grandfather MIs aged 49 and 56	
Xanthelasmata	

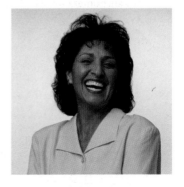

JMM

The revelation of an adverse family history in a patient with a severe mixed hyperlipidaemia suggests the possibility of familial combined hyperlipidaemia. More common than FH, presentation is in adult life and differentiation from 'common' hyperlipidaemia is sometimes difficult.

DJB

She should be referred to the lipid clinic. Given the family history and this lipid phenotype she could have FH or FCH. Tendon xanthomata on her or a family member would
point to FH, as these do not occur in FCH. Genetic studies of the LDL receptor might
help if a receptor mutation is found. Screening the surviving family might show the differing lipoprotein phenotypes typical of FCH. Unfortunately, there is as yet no definitive marker of this condition. Treatment is the same. She needs high-dose statin,
together with diet and lifestyle measures. Non-invasive cardiac monitoring is also
important given the early onset of CHD in her mother. Insulin resistance is often seen
in FCH and fasting glucose should be monitored periodically. She should be encouraged
to undertake regular appropriate exercise and lose weight if necessary. Occasionally
combined therapy of statin plus fibrate is required.

CASE 10

38-year-old chef

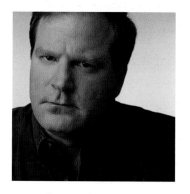

Asymptomatic	TC 9.4
Non-smoker	HDL 1.6
BP 156/94	TG 3.9
No relevant family history	
BMI 35	
Alcohol 15 units per week	
Xanthelasmata	

JMM

This patient's mixed hyperlipidaemia almost certainly relates to his obesity.
Xanthelasmata, whilst very non-specific, often correlate with elevated triglyceride levels,
which in turn are often markers of obesity or excessive alcohol consumption. His calculated 10-year CHD risk is low at 7.2 per cent so I would concentrate on weight reduction by realistic goal setting and supportive follow-up to benefit his blood pressure and
lipid profile.

DJB

He is markedly obese which contributes to the mixed hyperlipidaemia but he has a reasonable HDL – perhaps he is drinking more than he admits to. It is important to check
his glucose and thyroid function. Weight reduction is the first line of therapy, which
should not only improve his lipids but also his blood pressure. He needs follow-up and
possible therapeutic intervention if lifestyle measures fail. He may be a candidate for
anti-obesity drugs such as orlistat or sibutramine. The latter would require careful blood
pressure monitoring.

CASE 11

46-year-old dress designer

Type 2 diabetes mellitus diagnosed	TC 5.5
1 year ago	HDL 1.0
Ex-smoker	TG 3.4
BP 128/76	
Mother type 2 diabetes mellitus and	
peripheral arterial disease	
BMI 25 (was 28)	
Alcohol 7 units per week	
Gliclazide (glycosylated Hb 5.8 per cent)	

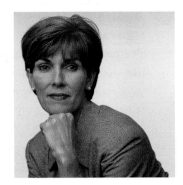

JMM

This lady has made considerable efforts since diagnosis but still shows a typical diabetic dyslipidaemia. She is at high lifetime risk of atherosclerotic disease and the presence of diabetes eliminates any premenopausal cardioprotection. Calculated LDL cholesterol is 3.9 mmol/L, which is well above target. I would start treatment with a statin as the evidence base for benefit is stronger but a fibrate would also be acceptable.

DJB

She has done well to reduce weight. Many physicians would have prescribed metformin as first-line oral agent; perhaps she was intolerant of it. I wonder whether she still needs the sulphonylurea now. The recent ATP-III report of the NCEP regards diabetes as a CHD risk equivalent with an LDL goal of <100 mg/dL (2.6 mmol/L). If this is achieved and the hypertriglyceridaemia persists, a secondary goal is non-HDL cholesterol of <130 mg/dL (3.37 mmol/L). My first choice drug would be a statin. The HPS has provided considerably more data on the benefits of simvastatin in the prevention of CHD and stroke in people with diabetes. I am surprised her BP is so good. This needs monitoring and it is my routine practice to look for microalbuminuria. I have a low threshold for prescribing ACEs.

CASE 12

48-year-old postal worker

Second-generation Pakistani	TC 7.3
Impaired glucose tolerance	HDL 0.7
Non-smoker	TG 3.8
BP 170/102	
Paternal uncles with MI aged 46 and 53	
BMI 25, waist circumference 98 cm	
Xanthelasmata and arcus	

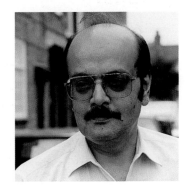

JMM

The clustering of hypertension, impaired glucose tolerance, central obesity, low HDL cholesterol and elevated triglycerides suggests the presence of the insulin resistance syndrome. Besides the specific management of his lipids, blood glucose and blood pressure, attention to diet and exercise are important. His 10-year CHD risk is 26.4 per cent but Framingham calculations seriously underestimate risk in such individuals.

DJB

The metabolic syndrome is highlighted as a target for CHD prevention in the ATP-III report of the NCEP (see Chapter 5). This clustering of risk factors associated with insulin resistance is associated with high vascular risk. Optimal management represents a major challenge to physician and patients given the importance of lifestyle measures and the need for multiple drug therapy. His LDL is 4.9 mmol/L (189 mg/dL). This is the first major lipid target with a goal <2.6 mmol/L (100 mg/dL). I would use a statin. If the hypertriglyceridaemia persists (>200 mg/dL; 2.3 mmol/L), a non-HDL cholesterol <130 mg/dL (3.33 mmol/L) becomes a secondary target. Generally, a higher dose of statin is required in the presence of hypertriglyceridaemia. The low HDL is an important risk factor and attention should be given to lifestyle measures. Additional drug therapy may be required. Nicotinic acid increases HDL but is relatively contraindicated in insulin resistance. Statin/fibrate combination is occasionally warranted with increased safety monitoring (gemfibrozil should not be used in combination therapy). I would also consider metformin therapy. Both lifestyle measures and metformin have been shown to reduce the rate of progression of IGT to frank type 2 diabetes. Clearly, blood pressure control is important and combination therapy may be needed to achieve treatment goal (<130/85 mmHg). ACE inhibition should be part of the antihypertensive therapy. A current focus of attention is to identify patients at an earlier stage than diabetes so that preventive measures can be instigated, both for CHD and for diabetes. It would thus be sensible to screen his family if possible.

CASE 13

42-year-old construction worker

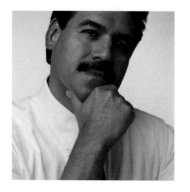

Asymptomatic	TC 7.6
Smokes 20 per day	HDL 1.7
BP 154/90	TG 4.4
Maternal grandfather CVA aged 64	
BMI 28	
Alcohol 56 units per week	
Xanthelasmata	

JMM

This is the typical mixed hyperlipidaemia often associated with alcohol abuse. Whilst potentially 'cardioprotective' at lower amounts, higher alcohol consumption is associated with increased CHD. Lifestyle change might improve this patient's BP and BMI as well as his lipid profile.

DJB

Clearly, the focus of this man's management is the reduction of alcohol intake – this may be easier said than done. This is the likely cause of his hypertriglyceridaemia, increased HDL and his blood pressure. The family history of stroke could be highlighted to him. It is important to check his glucose. As in other cases of hypertriglyceridaemia plus the high alcohol intake, his liver function tests are likely to be abnormal, most often due to fatty liver. In my experience, changing lifestyle in this type of patient is difficult, with advice on alcohol reduction and smoking cessation falling on stony ground. This degree of alcohol intake is a relative contraindication to hypolipidaemic drug therapy.

CASE 14

44-year-old housewife

Asymptomatic	TC 7.6
Non-smoker	HDL 1.7
BP 130/82	TG 4.4
No relevant family history	
BMI 24	
Alcohol 10 units per week	

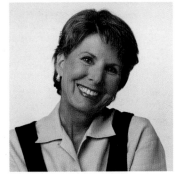

JMM

Occasionally families are encountered where levels of HDL cholesterol are very high. High HDL cholesterol is associated with longevity and although the total cholesterol is raised, the patient can be safely reassured.

DJB

This patient illustrates the importance of obtaining a full lipid profile. She has a substantial HDL, even for a woman, such that her total/HDL cholesterol ratio is below 3. She has no other risk factors and no family history of CHD. It would be interesting to look further into the family history – longevity has been described in families with high HDL. Although total cholesterol/HDL cholesterol ratio is an excellent predictor of risk in epidemiological studies, in the individual patient, anomalies can be seen. In the future, better measures of HDL and reverse cholesterol transport system may be available as more is learned about this process. If this patient had CHD I would lower her LDL with a statin.

CASE 15

60-year-old businesswoman

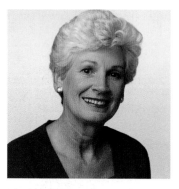

Stable angina	TC 6.2
Ex-smoker	HDL 1.4
BP 140/82	TG 1.3
Both parents died CHD in their 70s	
BMI 27 (was 25)	
Aspirin, beta-blocker, ACE inhibitor	
Original TC 6.6, best ever (on full dose statin) 5.6	

JMM

This lady never really showed a good response to her statin, despite apparently good compliance. Weight gain was always a problem and eventually she was found to have an elevated TSH. Hypothyroidism is common and often difficult to diagnose without an index of suspicion. Her lipid profile improved dramatically when treatment with thyroxine was started.

DJB

In my lipid clinic I discover unsuspected hypothyroidism in about six patients per year. Hypothyroidism is usually associated with hypercholesterolaemia but may be associated with any lipid abnormality. Anecdotally, hypothyroid patients given statins are more likely to have muscle aches and pains. In patients with muscle side-effects check the TSH. Hypothyroidism is, of course, a cause of increased concentration of the muscle enzyme CPK.

CASE 16

55-year-old butcher

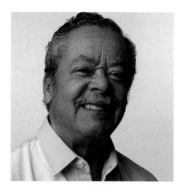

Claudication	TC 6.1
Ex-smoker 1 year	HDL 1.1
BP 124/80	TG 1.8
Brother angina aged 62	
BMI 27	
Alcohol 21 units per week	
4.5 cm abdominal aortic aneurysm	

JMM

Cholesterol lowering in patients with non-coronary arterial disease has been much neglected by health professionals but is now clearly established by the findings of the Heart Protection Study. This man is more likely to die of CHD than his peripheral atherosclerosis and merits aggressive intervention with a statin as well as aspirin and lifestyle advice. His aneurysm needs continuing monitoring as elective surgery may be indicated in due course.

DJB

This man should have effective statin treatment.

CASE 17

76-year-old ex-social worker

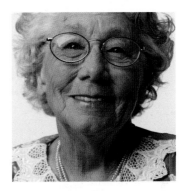

Asymptomatic	TC 7.9
Non-smoker	HDL 1.4
BP 142/66	TG 1.8
Bother died MI aged 58	
BMI 26	
No alcohol	

JMM

Although the relative benefits of cholesterol lowering in older people at high risk of a vascular event are now established, there is still debate about treating older people at lower levels of risk. Despite this, the absolute benefits of treatment may be greater (because the elderly have more CHD events). In this elderly lady, I would check thyroid function but would not proceed beyond lifestyle advice.

DJB

I certainly treat elderly people with established CHD as the benefits are seen relatively early. For primary prevention it is a matter of judgement. The HPS provides good evidence for treating the elderly high-risk population. The PROSPER study will provide further information on the elderly at lower risk. In my opinion, in the next few years, lipid-lowering therapy will be offered more extensively to the elderly just as antihypertensive therapy is. The absolute benefit may be considerable.

CASE 18

70-year-old ex-electrician

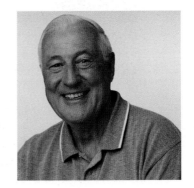

Branch occlusion left middle	TC 5.9
cerebral artery	HDL 1.2
Smokes 2 per day	TG 1.5
BP 168/78	
No relevant family history	
BMI 27	
Alcohol 7 units per week	

Case studies

JMM

Together with stopping smoking and post-stoke rehabilitation, aspirin is clearly indicated. The PROGRESS trial has recently informed us of the benefits of treating hypertensive stroke survivors with a 28 per cent reduction in stroke recurrence. Stroke victims are at high risk of other major vascular events and the HPS now also mandates statin therapy.

DJB

Ongoing studies such as SPARCL will contribute further information on the benefits of statin therapy in patients with stroke. The physician clearly needs to take on board quality of life issues when assessing these patients.

CASE 19

50-year-old bus driver

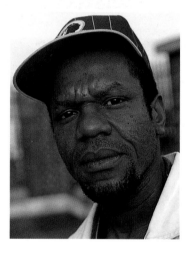

Hypertension on treatment	TC 7.6
Smokes 20 per day	HDL 0.9
BP 156/96 (pre-treatment 166/102)	TG 2.9
Paternal uncle CVA aged 50	
BMI 28	
No alcohol	
Thiazide diuretic and beta-blocker	

JMM

The blood pressure of Afro-Caribbeans is notoriously difficult to control with beta-blockers and ACE inhibitors. As both thiazides (in standard dose) and beta-blockers have adverse effects on lipid metabolism, I would use a long-acting calcium antagonist or an alpha-blocker. Formulations of very low dose thiazides are still awaited. His CHD risk, based on pre-treatment blood pressure, exceeds 30 per cent over 10 years and lipid-lowering treatment is indicated.

DJB

His HDL is below the tenth centile and the combination of hypertriglyceridaemia and an LDL/HDL of >5 puts him at high risk – he has the so-called atherogenic profile. The beta-blocker (if it does not have vasodilator properties) is likely to exacerbate his hypertriglyceridaemia and low HDL. The thiazide at high dose (5 mg or greater) may exacerbate his lipid problems. It is important to exclude glucose intolerance as he has several features of the metabolic syndrome. It is important to check compliance issues with the antihypertensive therapy. Weight reduction, if possible, would help. In the presence of hypertriglyceridaemia, a higher dose of statin is generally needed to achieve LDL goal.

CASE 20

58-year-old waiter

MI 2 years ago on a statin, aspirin and a beta-blocker	TC 4.4
Non-smoker	HDL 1.4
BP 126/78	TG 1.1
Brother has angina aged 64	
BMI 25	
Alcohol 14 units per week	
Complaining of muscle aches	

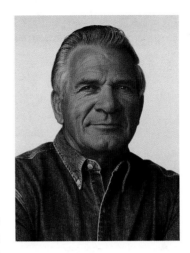

JMM

Muscular aches and pains are common symptoms in the general population but in a patient taking a statin should alert the clinician to the rare possibility of drug-induced myositis and I would check this patient's CPK. The results can be hard to interpret as there is significant intra-individual variation but when levels exceed 10 times the normal upper limit, the statin should be stopped.

DJB

In the large placebo-controlled clinical trials there is little difference between statin therapy and placebo in terms of muscle symptoms. However, it is not unusual to encounter patients in the clinic with complaints of muscle pain and normal CPK. Clearly, it is important to emphasize the importance of the therapy and exclude other causes. Reduction in statin dosage may help in persistent problems and I usually advise the use of cholesterol-lowering functional foods. If the patient is completely intolerant, then second-line agents such as resins and fibrates are an option.

INDEX

Full names of clinical studies and their abbreviations are shown in the list of abbreviations in pages xi–xvi

abbreviations xi–xvi
ABCA1 gene 15–16
abetalipoproteinaemia 88
accidents/cholesterol association 238–9,
    240
ACE inhibitors 168, 290
acipimox 214, 301
adolescents 311–13
AFCAPS/TexCAPS (study) 225, 227,
    251–3
    hypertensive patients 325
    women 317
Africa 33
age considerations 103
    cholesterol screening 96–7, 297,
        303–4
    see also adolescents; children; elderly
        patients
alcohol
    alcohol consumption 47, 48, 137–40
        primary care guidelines 300
        sensible drinking 165
        wine 48, 140, 188
    effects on lipids 139
    types of 140
    units of measurement 138–9
alpha-blockers 326
angiographic trials 254–64
    clinical events in 264
    combination drug therapy 257–9
    diet and lifestyle 255–7
    single drug trials 260–2
    summary table 256
animal studies 16, 133
anion-exchange resins 313
anticoagulant therapy 310
antihypertensives 70, 325–6
antioxidants 140, 186–90
    clinical trials 187, 260, 263–4, 276

antiretroviral drugs/therapy 70, 333–5
apical sodium-dependent bile acid
        transporter (ASBT) inhibitors 231
apoproteins 5–6
    apoprotein A-1 5–6, 70
    apoprotein B 68, 77–8, 109
        effect of drugs on 70
        familial ligand defective 76–8
    apoprotein C 6
        C-II deficiency 68, 85
    apoprotein E 6, 9, 82–3
    apoprotein(a) 20–1
    remnant particle disease 82–3
arcus senilis (corneal arcus) 72, 73, 81
arterial endothelial dysfunction 279–80
ASAP study 187, 263–4
ASPEN study 329
ASPIRE study 289
aspirin 290, 309
ATBC study 188
atenolol 168
atherogenesis 16–21
atherosclerosis
    coronary 103
    in familial hypercholesterolaemia 75
    historical aspects 23, 24
    personal history of 104–5
atherosclerotic plaque 19, 23–4, 108–9
atorvastatin 221, 224, 300, 335
    clinical trials 263, 270–2, 329, 332
ATP III 65–8, 310, 328–9, 330
    recommendations for CHD
        prevention 152–4
AVERT study 270–1
AY-9944 221
azithromycin 137

BECAIT study 260
bendrofluazide 325

beta-agonists 70
beta-blockers 168–9, 290, 309, 325, 326
beta-carotene 188
bezafibrate 217–20, 301
    clinical trials 132, 219, 260, 261,
        274–5
    diabetic patients 328
bile acid sequestrants 208–10, 301
BIP trial 132, 219, 261, 274–5
    diabetic patients 328
birth weight, low 57
blood pressure 110–11, 167, 190–1
blood tests, primary care guidelines
        297–8, 304
body mass index (BMI) 124–5, 172
British Doctors Study 103, 114
British Family Heart Study (BFHS)
        161, 293
British Hyperlipidaemia Association
        312–13
British Regional Heart Study 36, 40–4,
        117
broad beta disease *see* remnant particle
        disease
bupropion 162–3

C-reactive protein (CRP) 136–7
Caerphilly Collaborative Heart Disease
        study 116
Cambridge Heart Antioxidant Study
        (CHAOS) 187
Canada, CCAIT (trial) 260
cancer/cholesterol association 240
captopril 168
carbamazepine 70
carbohydrates 29, 184–6
CARDS (study) 329
CARE study 224, 267–8
    elderly patients 322

hypertensive patients 325
stroke reduction 55
women 317
CARET 188
carotenes 186, 188
case studies 345–61
CCAIT (trial) 260
cerebrotendinous xanthomatosis 90
cerebrovascular disease 331–2
cerivastatin 221, 227
change, stages of change model
150–1
CHAOS study 187
children 311–13
primary care guidelines 302
smoking 113–14
China 33, 46
Chlamydia pneumoniae 137
cholesterol
CHD and 105–7
chemistry 3–4
Cholesterol Papers (Law et al.) 52–6,
239–41, 243
conclusion 240–1
classification of levels 153
dietary 180
effect of drugs on 70
hepatic synthesis 10, 11
historical aspects 23
homeostasis 13
lipid profiles 345
low levels 50–2
normal levels/variations 49, 97–8
plasma transport 12
primary care target levels 302, 305
screening kits 99–100
and stroke 54–6
cholesterol efflux regulatory protein
(CERP) 15–16
cholesterol esters 4, 5
cholesterol-lowering drugs 208–30
clinical trials 236–86
Cholesterol Treatment Trialists'
Collaboration 280
cholestyramine 208–10, 301
clinical trials 209–10, 245–7, 260
chylomicron remnants 8–9
chylomicrons 7–8
familial chylomicronaemia syndrome
85–7
cigarette smoking 161–3
consequences of 114–15
damage mechanism 116
primary care guidelines 300

as risk factor 38
risk reduction 116–17
see also smoking
cigarettes
tar content 116–17
taxation 114
ciprofibrate 217–20, 301
CLAS (studies) 213, 256, 257–8,
330
classification of lipid disorders 63
clinical trials
angiographic trials see angiographic
trials
lipid-lowering see lipid-lowering
clinical trials
ongoing 169, 280–1, 326
see also specific trials and individual drugs
and drug groups
clofibrate 214–15, 216, 219–20
clinical trials 213, 218, 243
cocoa 189
coffee 191–2
colesevelam 301
colestipol 208–10, 301
clinical trials 258
common polygenic hypercholesterolaemia 72, 80–1
communication skills 159
community-based prevention of CHD
292
compactin 221
compliance 291–2
contraceptives, oral 318
corneal arcus 72, 73, 81
Coronary Drug Project 213, 214, 218,
245, 253
corticosteroids 70
creatine phosphokinase (CPK) 226
cut-points, in children 312
cyclosporin 70, 333

DART (trial) 182, 184
dementia 323, 343–4
diabetes 117–23, 326–30
control of 170
hyperglycaemia and CHD 119–20
insulin-resistance 120–1
insulin-resistance syndrome 45
mortality 118–19
prevalence 117–18
prevention 123
primary care guidelines 300
WHO classification 118
in women 317

Diabetes Atherosclerosis Intervention
Studies (DAIS) 261
diabetic dyslipidaemia 121–2
diabetic neuropathy 122–3
diagnosis 63–91
primary dyslipidaemias 71–87
rare disorders 87–90
secondary dyslipidaemias 69–71
diet 28–9, 172–207
antioxidants 186–90
calorie-controlled 174
carbohydrates 29, 184–6
dietary fibre 184–5
effects on lipids 201
fat in 176–84
food choices 197–9
fruit and vegetables 32–3, 47, 189
guidelines 199–200, 203, 300
historical aspects 24
lifestyle studies 255–7
Mediterranean diet 47, 182, 197
migration studies 27, 45–6, 182
miscellaneous factors 191–6
Oslo Study 243–4
potassium/sodium 190–1
strategies 196–201
vegetarian/vegan 196
weight loss 172–5
Western diet 102
wine-drinking 48, 140, 188
diuretics 168, 326
docosahexaenoic acid (DHA) 210
dolichols 225
doxazosin 169
drinking see alcohol
drug-induced dyslipidaemia 70, 325
drugs (lipid-lowering) 208–32
the future 230–1
primary care guidelines 300–2, 305
see also clinical trials
dysbetalipoproteinaemia see remnant
particle disease
dyslipidaemia
classification 63
diabetic 121–2, 327–8
drug-induced 70, 325
hypertension and 324–5
primary 71–87
as risk factor 327–8
secondary 69–71

economic aspects 338–44
economic development 28–34
4S study 267, 340–1

economic aspects *cont.*
  industrialization 28
  socio-economic status 40–4
  statins 340–1
  urbanization 29
eggs 180
eicosapentaenoic acid (EPA) 178, 181,
    210
elderly patients 322–3
  hypertension 169
  primary care guidelines 297, 302, 303
epidemiology 23–59
  studies between populations 34–5
  studies within populations 36–52
ethnicity 44–6, 105
etofibrate 217
EUROASPIRE studies 289, 290, 342
Europe, smoking in 113
European Atherosclerosis Society,
    guidelines 65, 66
European Coronary Risk Chart 142,
    144–6
exercise 163–5
  benefits of 130–1, 164
  dangers of 164–5
  guidelines 164, 300
  lack of 38, 129–30, 131
  physical fitness 128–9
ezetimibe 231

Factor VII 20
familial chylomicronaemia syndrome *see*
    lipoprotein lipase deficiency
familial combined hyperlipidaemia
    (FCH) 72, 78–80
familial hypercholesterolaemia (FH)
    12, 16, 17, 71–6, 77
  SCOR trial 256, 258–9
  screening 76, 100
familial hypertriglyceridaemia 72
familial hypobetalipoproteinaemia 52, 88
familial LCAT deficiency 87–8
familial ligand defective apoprotein B
    (FDB) 72, 76–8
familial phytosterolaemia 195–6
family history 38, 104
fat in diet 176–84
  modifying 196–201
FATS (study) 213, 256, 258
fatty acids
  biochemistry 177–9
  isomers 178, 179
  omega-3 181, 210–11, 301, 311

fenofibrate 217–20, 301
  clinical trials 260, 261, 329
fetal nutrition 57–8
fibrates 214–21, 301
  clinical trials 273–5
  see also individual drugs
fibre in diet 184–5
fibric acid derivatives *see* fibrates
fibrinogen 69, 131–2, 217–18
FIELD trial 329
Finland
  Finnish Mental Hospitals Study
      243–4
  Helsinki Heart Study 109, 218–19,
      238, 247–8
  North Karelia project 292
  Seven Countries Study 34–5
fish eye disease 88
fish oil 181–2, 210–12, 311
flavonoids 140, 186, 188–9
fluvastatin 221–30, 300, 335
  clinical trials 273
folic acid 311
food industry 204–6
4D study 332
4S study 224, 227, 264–7, 309
  economic aspects 267, 340–1
  hypertensive patients 325
  stroke reduction 55
  women 317
Framingham Point Score 142–4, 149
Framingham Study 36–8, 103
France 47–8
  Lyon Diet Heart Study 47, 182–3
Friedewald formula 65
fruit and vegetables 32–3, 47, 189

garlic 192
gemfibrozil 56, 216–17, 218, 220, 301
  clinical trials 261–2, 273–4
    Helsinki Heart Study 109, 218,
        238, 247–8
  diabetic patients 328
gene therapy 233
genetic factors 104
geographical differences 24
Germany, PROCAM Study 46
GISSI-Prevenzione trial 187, 311
Global Burden of Disease study 25–7
glucose 38
  impaired tolerance 117–19
  lipid profile 346
glycaemic index 185–6

GREACE study 272
Greece, Seven Countries Study 34–5

HARP study 333
HDL (high density lipoprotein) 7–8,
    14–15
  abnormalities 72, 89
  CHD protection and 18–19, 106–7
  classification of levels 153
  effect of drugs on 70
  guideline levels 67
  lipid profile 345
  measuring 63–4, 99
  trends in levels 37
  in women 315–16
HDL Atherosclerosis Treatment Study
    (HATS) 259–60
health care costs 338–9
health professionals, time-constraints
    290–1
Heart and Estrogen/Progestin
    Replacement Study (HERS)
    319–20
Heart Outcomes Prevention (HOPE)
    study 187
Heart Protection Study (HPS) 187,
    189–90, 275–8, 331
  diabetes 329–30
  elderly patients 322
  hypertensive patients 325–6
  stroke reduction 331
Heidelberg study 255, 256
Helsinki Heart Study 109, 218, 238,
    247–8
heparin 70
Heparin Extracorporeal LDL
    Precipitation (HELP) system 233
hepatic cholesterol synthesis 10, 11
hepatic lipase 8, 11
hepatic triglyceride synthesis 10
hepatosplenomegaly 72, 86
high-risk patients, primary care
    guidelines 303
highly active antiretroviral therapy
    (HAART) 70, 333–5
HIV infection 333–5
HMG CoA reductase inhibitors *see*
    statins
homocysteine 134–5, 311
homocystinuria 134
hormone replacement therapy (HRT)
    318–22
Hungary 32, 33

hydroxymethylglutaryl coenzyme A reductase inhibitors *see* statins
hyperalphalipoproteinaemia 89–90
hypercholesterolaemia
  common polygenic 72, 80–1
  familial *see* familial hypercholesterolaemia
  polygenic 72, 80–1
  primary care, drugs for 300–1
  primary care guidelines 298
  radical therapy 232–3
  statins in 224
hyperglycaemia, as risk factor 119–20
hyperhomocysteinaemia 135
hyperinsulinaemia 121
hyperlipidaemias
  classification 63, 64
  primary care, drugs for 301–2
  refractory 232–3
  type II 63
  type III *see* remnant particle disease
hyperlipoproteinaemia, classification 64
hypertension 324–6
  antihypertensives 70, 325–6
  consequences of 110
  control of 165–70
  definition 111
  dietary salt and 190
  elderly patients 169
  primary care guidelines 299–300
  as risk factor 38, 109–12
  in women 317
Hypertension Optimal Treatment (HOT) trial 167–8
hypertriglyceridaemia 20, 328
  atherogenic changes accompanying 108
  familial 72
  primary care, drugs for 301–2
  primary isolated 81–2
hyperuricaemia 120
hypoalphalipoproteinaemia 89
hypothyroidism 69–70

ileal bypass 232
  POSCH study 232, 256, 262
illness and serum lipids 98
immigration studies 27, 44–6
industrialization 28
inflammatory markers 135–7
insulin resistance 120–1

insulin resistance syndrome 45
intention to treat 241
isotretinoin compounds 70
Italy, Seven Countries Study 34–5

Japan 32–3
  Seven Countries Study 34–5
Joint British recommendations for CHD prevention 151–2
Joint British Societies Coronary Risk Prediction Chart 142, 143
Joint European Societies recommendations for CHD prevention 152

LCAT *see* lecithin cholesterol acyltransferase
LDL (low density lipoprotein) 9, 12–14
  atherogenesis and 16–18
    modified LDL 17–18
  CHD protection and 105–6
  classification of levels 153
  effect of drugs on 70
  extracorporeal removal 233
  Friedewald formula 65
  guideline levels 66, 67
  LDL receptor pathway 13–14
  LDL receptor structure 12
  lipid profile 345
  measuring 64–5
  plasma LDL levels 14
  primary care target levels 302, 305
  subfractions 18
  trends in levels 37
  in women 315–16
LDL-related protein (LRP) 9
lecithin cholesterol acyltransferase (LCAT) 6
  see also familial LCAT deficiency
left ventricular hypertrophy (LVH) 111
Leiden Intervention Trial 255
Lifestyle Heart Trial 255–7
lifestyle studies 255–7
  changing people's habits 159–71
  dietary change 196–201
  exercise 163–5
  see also diet; exercise; smoking
linoleic acid 179, 181
lipaemia retinalis 72, 86
lipase 4
lipid clinics 305–6

lipid-lowering clinical trials 236–86
  primary prevention 242–8
    combined primary/secondary prevention 275–80
    statins 248–53
  secondary prevention 253–75
    angiographic trials 254–64
    combined primary/secondary prevention 275–80
    with fibrates 273–5
lipid-lowering drugs/therapy 48, 208–35
  in children 313
  cost effectiveness 341
  the future 230–1
  gene therapy 233
  high risk patients 303
  in hypertensives 325–6
  ileal bypass 232
  lipoprotein removal 233
  liver transplantation 232
  mechanisms of benefit 278–80
  portacaval shunt 232
Lipid Research Clinics (LRC) studies 209–10, 238, 245–7, 253–4
LIPID study 224, 268–70
  hypertensive patients 325
  stroke reduction 55, 331
  women 317
Lipid Treatment Assessment Project (LTAP) 289
lipoprotein lipase deficiency 72, 85–7
lipoprotein removal 233
lipoproteins 5–21
  atherogenesis and 16–21
  classification 6
  high density *see* HDL
  intermediate density 11
  lipoprotein(a) 20–1, 68, 109
  low density *see* LDL
  metabolism 5–16
  structure 5–6
  very high density 9–10, 65
  very low density 9–10, 65
LIPS study 273
liver
  cholesterol disposal 9
  disorders 70–1
  transplantation 232
  see also hepatic *entries*
Lopid Coronary Angiographic Trial (LOCAT) 261–2

Los Angeles Veterans Study 243–4
lovastatin 221–30, 300
    in adolescent boys 313
    clinical trials 224, 251–3, 258, 260
low birth weight 57
Lyon Diet Heart Study 47, 182–3

macroalbuminuria 122, 123
margarine 193
Maxepa 211, 301
measurement of lipids 63–9
Mediterranean diet 47, 182, 197
menopause 315
    HRT and 318–22
meta-analysis techniques 237–8, 239
metabolic syndrome 67
metformin, HAART patients 335
microalbuminuria 122, 123
migration studies 27, 44–6, 182
MIRACL study 271–2, 310
mixed hyperlipidaemia, primary care,
    drugs for 301
MONICA programme 29–30
Monitored Atherosclerosis Regression
    Study (MARS) 260
monounsaturated fatty acids 179,
    180–1
mortality
    rates 25–34
    world-wide causes 26
MRFIT Study 36, 39–40
Multicentre Anti-Atheroma Study
    (MAAS) 260
myocardial infarction 24
myopathy 226
myositis 221, 227

National Cholesterol Education
    Program (NCEP) 65–8, 94,
    311–12
National Health Service 338
National Heart Lung Blood Institute II
    study 256, 260
National Service Framework for
    Coronary Heart Disease 295–6
nephrotic syndrome 122, 123
Netherlands, Seven Countries Study
    34–5
neuropathy, diabetic 122–3
New Zealand Cardiovascular Risk
    Prediction Charts 142, 147
NHANES 2 (survey) 187
Ni Hon San Study 27

niacin see nicotinic acid
nicofuranose 301
nicotine replacement therapy 161–2
nicotinic acid (niacin) 212–14, 301
    clinical trials 258, 259–60
North Karelia project 292
number needed to treat 339–40
nurse-led clinics in primary care 294–5
Nurses' Health Study 180, 192–3
nuts 192–3

oat bran 184–5
obesity 43–4, 124–8
    abdominal 67
    central obesity 125
    consequences of 127
    diabetes and 125
    drug therapy 175–6
    measurement 124–6
    prevalence 127–8
    as risk factor 126–7
    WHO classification 124
    in women 317
oestrogen 70, 103, 186, 315
oestrogen replacement therapy
    318–22
omega-3 fatty acids/fish oils 181,
    210–11, 301, 311
oral contraceptives 318
orlistat 175–6
Oslo Study 117, 243–4
osteoporosis, statins and 321–2
OXCHECK project 161, 292–3
Oxford Vegetarian Study 196

P/S ratio 179
PAIP trial, stroke reduction 55
pancreatitis 86
Pansuola 191
paraoxonase 19
passive smoking 116
patients, as barriers to implementation
    of CHD prevention 291
peripheral vascular disease 330–1
personality types 133
phenobarbitone 70
phenytoin 70
physical activity see exercise
phytoestrogens 321
phytosterols 193–6
pitavastatin 230, 231
PLAC-I clinical trial 260
plant sterols 193–6

plasminogen activator inhibitor 1
    (PAI-1) 120, 132, 218
polysaccharides, non-starch 184
polyunsaturated fatty acids 181–4
population strategy 92, 93, 204–6
portacaval shunt 232
POSCH study 232, 256, 262
Post Coronary Artery Bypass Graft trial
    262–3
potassium in diet 190–1
pravastatin 221–30, 300, 335
    clinical trials 55, 224, 248–51, 260,
        267–8, 268–70
    PROSPER study 56, 323
pregnancy 302, 318
prevention of CHD
    in the community 292
    guidelines 150–4
    obstacles to 290–2
    in primary care 292–4
    services for 343–4
primary care
    lipid management guidelines
        296–305
    nurse-led clinics 294–5
    prevention of CHD 292–4
    screening in 96
primary dyslipidaemias 71–87
primary isolated hypertriglyceridaemia
    81–2
primary prevention, in the elderly 323
Primary Prevention Project (PPP) 187
primary prevention trials 242–8
    combined primary/secondary
        prevention 275–80
    lipid-lowering clinical trials 242–53
    statins 248–53
PROCAM study 46, 106
progestogens 70
PROSPER study 56, 323
protection from CHD, HDL and
    18–19
psychosocial risk factors 133–4
pyridoxine 311

Quetelet's index see body mass index

raloxifene 321
referral, from primary care, guidelines
    302, 305
remnant particle disease 9, 20, 72, 82–6
renal disease, chronic 332–3
renal failure 122, 123

retinoids 70
reverse cholesterol transport 15–16
rhabdomyolysis 227
risk
　global risk 102
　plasma triglycerides and 20
　relative/absolute 141
risk assessment 140–50
　tools 142–50
risk factors 24–5, 56–7, 101–55
　British Regional Heart Study 40–4
　Framingham Study 36–8
　immigrants in the UK 44–6
　modifiable 102, 105–9, 299
　　non-lipid 109–50, 159–71
　MRFIT Study 39
　non-modifiable 102, 103–5, 299
　phases of acquisition in developing
　　economies 29
　physical inactivity 129–31
　primary care guidelines 299, 303,
　　304
　psychosocial 133–4
　stroke 54–6
　thrombogenic 131–3
　in women 315–18
　see also individual risk factors
ritonavir 335
rosuvastatin 230–1, 300
roxithromycin 137
Russia 31

St Thomas Atherosclerosis Regression
　Study (STARS) 255, 256, 257,
　260
salt 190, 191
saquinavir 335
saturated fatty acids 178, 179
Scandinavian Simvastatin study see 4S
　study
SCOR trial 256, 258–9
scoring systems 142–50
screening 92–100
　age considerations 96–7, 297, 303–4
　children/adolescents 311–13
　equipment 99–100
　familial hypercholesterolaemia 76,
　　100
　individual (high risk) strategy 92–3,
　　93–100
　laboratory variation and sampling
　　errors 98–9
　methods 95–6

near site testing 99–100
　population strategy 92, 93
　in primary care 96, 297–8, 303–4
　screening tests, criteria 94
　secondary prevention 93
　selective/non-selective 94–5
　United States 31
SCRIP 256
secondary dyslipidaemias 69–71
secondary prevention, in the elderly
　322–3
secondary prevention trials 253–75
　combined primary/secondary
　　prevention 275–80
　with fibrates 273–5
selective oestrogen receptor modulators
　(SERMs) 321
selenium 186
serotonin 51–2
Seven Countries Study 34–5, 36
sex differences 103–4, 313–14
　LDL 18
　mortality rates 26, 27
　see also women
Sheffield Risk Table 142, 148
simvastatin 196, 221–30, 300, 309, 335
　clinical trials 55, 224, 259–60, 263,
　　264–7, 275–8
　see also 4S study
sitostanol 194–5
sitosterol 196
sitosterolaemia 89
smoking 43–4, 112–17, 163–5
　cessation of 161–3, 309
　fibrinogen levels 132
　harm reduction 163
　life expectancy 115
　mortality 115
　passive 116
　prevalence 31
　risk to women 317–18
　young people 113–14
　see also cigarette smoking
socio-economic factors 40–4
sodium in diet 190–1
Southampton Heart Integrated Care
　Project (SHIP) 294–5
soya 193
SPACE trial 187
specialist care 305
statins 221–30, 300
　in adolescents 313
　adverse effects 225–6, 300

clinical efficacy 222–5
clinical trials 224–5, 248–53,
　264–70, 275–80
　elderly patients 323
cost-effectiveness 309, 340
cost per life year gained 340–1
drug interactions 226, 310
economic evaluation methods 340
indications 228
mechanism of action 221–3
osteoporosis and 321–2
pharmacology 222–5
pleiotropic effects of 228–30
and stroke 56, 280
sterol regulatory element binding
　proteins (SREBPs) 13–14, 334
Stockholm Ischaemic Heart Disease
　Study 213
stress 38, 133–4
stroke
　risk factors 54–6, 111
　statins reducing risk 56
Stroke Prevention by Aggressive
　Reduction in Cholesterol levels
　(SPARCL) study 332
sugars 185
suicide/cholesterol association 238–9,
　240
Syndrome X 120

tamoxifen 321
Tangier disease 19, 87
tendon xanthomata 72, 73–5
thiazides 169, 325
thrombogenic risk factors 131–3
thyroid disorders 69–70
tibolone 321
time constraints 290–1
tobacco advertising 163
trans fatty acids 180
treatment
　priorities, primary care guidelines
　　299, 304
　services for 343–4
　see also lipid-lowering drugs/therapy
triglyceride-lowering drugs 212–32
triglycerides
　atherogenesis and 19–20
　chemistry 4
　classification of levels 153
　cut-points, NCEP 67
　effect of drugs on 70
　hepatic synthesis 10

triglycerides *cont.*
  lipid profile 346
  post-prandial concentrations 108
  as risk factor 107–9, 316
  serum testing 97, 99
  in women 316
triparanol 221

ubiquinolone-10 186
ubiquinones 225–6
under-treatment 289–90
United Kingdom
  CHD statistics 28
  immigrant populations in 44–6
  Prospective Diabetes Study
    (UKPDS) 168, 327
  smoking in 113
  see also entries beginning with British
United States 30–1
  Framingham Study 36–8, 103
  lipid guidelines 311–12
  MRFIT Study 36, 39–40
  National Cholesterol Education
    Project (NCEP) 65–8, 94,
    311–12
  Seven Countries Study 34–5
  smoking in 113
unsaturated fatty acids 178
urbanization 29

VA-HIT (trial) 56, 109, 218–19,
    273–4, 274–5
  diabetic patients 328
valproate 70
vastatins *see* statins
vegetables 32–3, 47, 189
vegetarian/vegan diet 196
vitamin B12 311
Vitamin C 186, 187
Vitamin E 186, 187
vitamin supplementation 187, 189
VLDL (very low density lipoprotein)
    9–10, 65

waist-hip ratio (WHR) 125–6
weight 38
  low birth weight 57
  see also obesity
weight loss 172–5
wine 48, 140, 188
women
  CHD and 313–22
  cholesterol-lowering trials 241,
    252
  diabetes in 317
  HDL cholesterol 106
  hormonal effects 315
  menopause and HRT 318–22
  parity 314–15

pregnancy 302, 318
primary care guidelines 302
risk factors 315–18
SCOR study 258–9
serum lipid variations 98
sex roles 313
World Health Organization
  Cooperative primary prevention trial
    132, 218, 243, 244–5
  hyperlipidaemias/hyperlipopro-
    teinaemias classification
    63, 64
  MONICA programme 29–30
WOSCOPS (study) 55, 225,
    248–51
  economic aspects 341

xanthelasma 73, 74, 81
xanthomata
  eruptive 72, 86
  in familial hypercholesterolaemia
    73–5
  lipoprotein lipase deficiency 86
  palmar 84
  remnant disease 84
  tubero-eruptive 72, 84

Yugoslavia, Seven Countries Study
    34–5